The Price of Passion

The Price of Passion

Carla van Raay

EBURY
PRESS

1 3 5 7 9 10 8 6 4 2

Published in 2008 by Ebury Press, an imprint of Ebury Publishing
A Random House Group Company
First Published in Australia as *Desire: Awakening God's Woman*
by HarperCollins*Publishers* Pty Limited in 2008

The Random House Group Limited Reg. No. 954009

Addresses for companies within the Random House Group can be found at
www.randomhouse.co.uk

A CIP catalogue record for this book is available from the British Library

The Random House Group Limited supports The Forest Stewardship
Council (FSC), the leading international forest certification organisation. All
our titles that are printed on Greenpeace approved FSC certified paper carry
the FSC logo. Our paper procurement policy can be found at
www.rbooks.co.uk/environment

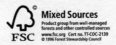

Mixed Sources
Product group from well-managed
forests and other controlled sources
www.fsc.org   Cert no. TT-COC-2139
FSC   © 1996 Forest Stewardship Council

Printed in the UK by CPI Cox & Wyman, Reading, RG1 8EX

ISBN 9780091923204

To buy books by your favourite authors and register for offers visit
www.rbooks.co.uk

For Aaron

Love is an inescapable reality
that knocks you
senseless
takes your breath away
and leaves no heart beating
but its own

Nirmala, *untitled poem*

CONTENTS

FOREWORD BY AARON

My name is Aaron and I am Carla's partner in this story. I am proud of Carla for writing about our journey for you to read.

We are all human beings who struggle to live separately and together within our relationships. We can have lives of indifference and aloneness. Or we can challenge ourselves to overcome our fears of being open and expose our rich and sensitive lives — a complex waterfall of endless moments.

I prefer to take a shower in the waterfall of my life. I spent too long worrying about what I thought of myself, and made myself depressed and defeated and tired in many ways. I don't want that to be my whole life.

I am looking for light. I am looking for kindred spirits to be my friends. Carla was a spark of life and light in my early manhood. The cogs and wheels of life brought her back to me after thirty years as a bright torch to help me look into my dark places. I am looking for closure in those dark places.

This is Carla's story, from her point of view. She is a brave woman. I am challenged by her openness, her innocence, her fearlessness at revealing herself so nakedly.

This story is also about my nakedness.

Nakedness isn't really so bad after the fear has evaporated. What may be left is the very fine and noble soul. We all, in our own way, tap into the same kind of inner life that Carla has. We all fall down and we all try to get up again. I hope you enjoy realising this — I truly have.

Love can come, love can go. Only the love you give can remain.

May you all enjoy sharing Carla's story as much as I have.

God's love to all.

Aaron

PREFACE

 My first book, *God's Callgirl*, was the frank story of my journey from sexual guilt to radiant innocence. What has happened since the publication of that book is even more extraordinary: it is a love story of the kind that wrings awe from my heart. The divine intelligence that I surrender to every day showed itself to be more compassionate, more creative and more astonishingly loving than I could dare imagine. This book is the story of one woman's blossoming into true love. I am sixty-five as I write. May this be an inspiration to all who know that to love is the only way to live, and that it is never, ever too late.

When I was growing up, sex was everywhere — lustful, hurting. Its yellow, dirty light darted from the eyes of my grandfather, my father's brothers, my father himself, and some of the men in my neighbourhood. I felt it warily. I had to be on my guard always, so as not to be taken by surprise as I was so often as a child.

At eighteen, I chose to become a nun and made a vow of chastity: that would take care of sex, wouldn't it? No, it did not! It refused to go away. I even experienced spontaneous orgasms, and in such awkward places as the convent's chapel.

I left the convent and married, still without knowing what sex was all about. Then I experienced irresistible chemistry and all-engrossing sex with a much younger man — not my husband. This was the catalyst for me wanting to explore my sexuality through prostitution, and God's Callgirl was born.

The Price of Passion is about sex in a relationship such as God's Callgirl never experienced. Life arranged for me to meet up again with the man who introduced me to real sex: Aaron. He was nineteen and I was thirty-four when we first met. Thirty years later, we found that the energy between us was still the same, and we continued where we'd left off — only this time we were so much older, we'd experienced different pasts, had built up different habits of thinking and doing. The relationship became a powerful healing for both of us. We discovered that wholesome sex can heal the deeply ingrained attitudes that develop from hurtful experiences and less-than-enlightened choices.

Passion has a price. It may be paid gratefully or not, but it has to be paid. This fact is one of the many lessons within this story.

May you, the reader, share in my journey. I hope my story will inspire you to immerse yourself in any healing your soul longs for.

Carla

DIONYSUS HERE, CARLA

Easy is right. Begin right
And you are easy.
Chuang Tzu

 Ever since the publication of my first book, *God's Callgirl*, the story of how I became a nun, then a prostitute and healed from both those choices, I'd sensed a sea change coming on. What it would look like, or what area of my life it would touch most, I had no idea.

I left my safe haven in Denmark (Western Australia) — my secure one-bedroom unit with a glorious garden built up over ten years, my cosy lifestyle with friends I love, my spa in the backyard — to answer a strong pull towards the city of Perth. First I was offered a friend's house to look after for three months; then came an invitation from two good friends to share their newly built home. I lived there for a year until the house was sold. My next move was to a mansion on the river at Applecross, as a live-in housekeeper. I had my private living space at street level and worked three mornings a week upstairs. I had been there for about a year and a half when my quietly regulated life suddenly changed.

A couple of weeks after an article about *God's Callgirl*, with my photo, appears in the local Sunday newspaper I get a message on my answering machine. A male voice: 'If you're the Carla I think you are, and you have a daughter called Caroline, then I'd like to talk to you.' He says his name is Aaron, and he leaves his phone number.

You know that strange feeling you get when you see a phone number and you're sure you've rung it sometime in the past, but have no idea when or who it belongs to? My eyes gain focus — the way eyes do when they travel back through time — and connect the phone number with an address I knew thirty years ago. A rush of memories comes.

Aaron, the nineteen-year-old with long blond hair whom I had an affair with as a married woman. He was like an angel or a lesser god, straight from the Pantheon, a young Dionysus lent to me for two weeks, no longer. An affair that spanned our drive from Perth to Panawonica in the north-west of Western Australia, and ended so suddenly when he went back to work there and I continued on to Wickham, where my work and my husband waited for me. The affair was the end of my marriage and the beginning of my sexual flowering. As for Aaron, he was one person I never expected to hear from again. At nineteen, Aaron had his whole life in front of him. At thirty-four, I was married, had a baby daughter, a complex past, and some serious growing up to do.

I phone the number. His mother picks up. 'Wait a sec; I'll get him for you.' She doesn't bother to find out who's calling. A whirlwind has been set in motion without me knowing it. The simple action of picking up a phone has begun to move deep waters waiting behind dammed walls.

Aaron comes to the phone and we exchange the fewest of words to confirm who we are. Then my unbelieving ears hear, 'Can I come over to see you *now*?' It sounds more like, *Don't dream of saying no;*

that's not possible. I surprise myself by saying yes; this getting together is happening as fast as the way we parted.

It is already getting dark. I live and work as housekeeper in a house by the river. Hardly anyone knows how to find the little metal gate that leads onto my verandah, set among a row of pencil pines near the end of a steep driveway, almost at the edge of the water.

I grab a torch and stand at the top of the driveway so I can signal Aaron. I'll be able to tell from the hesitant way the driver approaches that it's him.

The car swings in and stops beside me. The window is open. 'Bend down!' says a voice, and a face appears. I do as I'm told and get a kiss planted firmly on my lips. This is Aaron's way of breaching thirty years.

I am totally unprepared for what happens next. He steps inside my house, pushing his big energy before him. It envelops me before his body reaches me for our first hug and my knees are already buckling, because that energy — the feeling of him — is exactly the same. And now I know that I have never forgotten him. Now I remember how special our connection was, and realise that in thirty years I have never come across this quality again. It's shocking, overwhelming. How could my conscious mind have forgotten this? How can it take me by such surprise now? I have known all my life that I wanted what we had during those amazing two weeks. Some part of me had convinced myself that I would never have it again, I guess. So I stopped looking. And now here it is. Unmistakably. Unbelievably.

I'm in his big arms. I rest my head against his shoulder and feel his belly against mine, pumping out his excitement. The energy between us ignites old, dusty light bulbs one after the other, filaments still intact, until we stand in a veritable pool of light. I immerse myself in the feeling, captivated, and he catches me as I lose my balance. He finally pushes me away and I instinctively head for the kitchen bench —the nearest solid object to hold me up. I turn to have a good look at him.

Aaron, my Dionysus, whom I met thirty years ago.

Dionysus, who was made the scapegoat for all things licentious after he fell from grace with Roman society. Dionysus, the energy of sexual and sensual exuberance and spontaneity, unfortunately replaced by Bacchus, god of drunkenness, debauchery and crudeness, and then by Apollo, the sun god, representing order, industriousness and reason.

Dionysus, whose energy is what women long for, what too-rational souls are afraid of, and what religions suppress with all their power. It was Christianity that put horns on Dionysus and called him the devil. It is religion of all kinds that engenders the great malaise and guilt around sex and sensuality.

Aaron's full-bodied, unimpaired, innocent sexuality, his unashamed erotic sensuality, takes my breath away. It oozes out of the pores of his skin; it is concentrated in the touch of his hands, in the look of his eyes, and, as I will discover, in the strength of his penis. The penis that responds so readily, that is so patient, so deeply respectful of the female energy, knowing how to arouse it and keep it aroused. Aaron's sexuality is all-male without the macho, and elicits the all-female, free of the need to control. Dionysus would be proud to be compared to Aaron.

Aaron has found a chair to sit on and smiles with mild amusement. 'You've been lonely a long time then?' he asks, and spontaneously opens his arms to me. I'm bent over, feeling pale and hot in turns. I decide to sit down as well. Not on his lap, Carla; not yet. Don't be that foolishly eager; get a hold on yourself.

My blond god has turned fifty. His hair is no longer what it was; it's very short and grey all over. His face has broadened out; his forehead has some deep wrinkles just above the nose and his chin has developed the flesh of middle age. His foot —

'What's wrong with your foot?' I ask.

'Someone hit my Achilles heel with a hockey stick a few weeks ago and now it hurts like hell all the time.'

'Oh.' It explains his hobble as we walked to my gate in the dark.

I keep looking. The honey skin is lined, but still has a youthfulness about it. The shape of his head is the same as I remember it; the silhouette of his head and shoulders used to drive me wild when I was thirty-four going on sixteen. That mouth, so well delineated it makes me think of a rosebud. And his eyes ... his eyes have exactly the same hypnotic attraction. They are still carelessly beautiful, still so steady, deep-set and mysterious under those dark eyebrows that set them off perfectly.

His hands. They are a part of him that hasn't aged. Aaron's strong hands are unscathed; still have that manly innocence. His arms? I can't see them; they're covered with a black windcheater. His legs are enveloped in unflattering grey tracksuit pants, thick socks sticking out from the end and fleecy-lined ugh boots. My Dionysus is not wealthy and doesn't know how to impress with dress. He drives an old Colt and has been out of work for the last couple of years. I will hear his stories, but not tonight. He asks if he can put his foot up on a chair, and I suggest he sits on my couch and stretches his leg out on it.

My place is small; it takes only a few steps from kitchen to lounge room. Once at the couch, he lies down on it and catches my arm as I pass. I find myself pulled down beside him. It's a fairly narrow space for two bodies; before I know it, I have one leg over his torso to make it easier to lie together.

All the while, Aaron watches me intently. He seems to sense what's going on inside me, and waits patiently for my feelings to settle down and for me to come to grips with his sudden presence. I feel at a disadvantage. Aaron appears cool and collected; he smiles indulgently, highly pleased with himself, while I'm behaving like a foolish maiden. We lie still, looking at each other, becoming used to the gentle rhythm that is building up between us: breathing in, breathing out. Our eyes gradually meet our souls, long before our lips touch and feel the edge of thirty years of hunger.

I can't remember exactly what happens after that, except that we make love that first evening. It is as natural as rain touching the leaves of a tree; as inevitable as waves crashing on the shore; as incredible as salmon mating upstream after a perilous journey. We haven't seen one another in thirty years. I've been celibate for twelve years, and Aaron has been alone for six. Now we are entering a whirlwind. For both of us, long-held assumptions will shift under our feet; ideas will change; some concepts, very familiar, will disappear forever. But we don't know all this in our first love-making. We are simply babes in the wood.

UNWRAPPING THE PRESENT

And my soul,
I have come to see,
is both spirit and flesh.
St Teresa of Avila

 'You're so CLEAN!' he raves. 'Clean! Clean! I love your smell, and how you taste. It's still the same as it was back then. You're clean like an angel-woman.' And he gathers me up in his arms like a man gathers a treasure. His own clean energy is like a benediction.

'I can still see that innocent child–woman in you,' he says. 'Your face and personality are still the same.'

It's a few days after our reunion and we talk about those two weeks we spent together thirty years ago.

'You were my first girlfriend, you know.'

'What?'

I was his first girlfriend? I think back to his manner then: it was considerate, hesitant, because he hadn't wanted to intrude on a marriage. But I'd never guessed that it was his very first time.

He has an important question to ask me. 'Carla, why did you, a married woman, decide to make love to me?'

I look at Aaron, and my mind travels back.

I remember that it was me who made the first tentative move towards him. We were lying in the back of my station wagon while one of Aaron's friends drove us some of the way from our respective mining communities to Perth. Aaron was taking a break from work, and I was going to meet my parents, who had flown from Melbourne to Perth to visit my sister and catch up with me as well.

Aaron was politely reserved, keeping his lanky body quite still in the back of the car, one arm under his head, looking at me and smiling now and again. Untold thoughts were going through both our heads, but it was me who wriggled my body closer to his. Aaron's eyes grew wide; he still didn't move, but watched me intently. It was those eyes that drew me closer; nothing in them said, 'Don't do this, Carla.' Our magnetised bodies did the rest. We lay in each other's arms, and knew the world to be a very good place.

He smelled good; his breath was so sweet, his hands like none I had ever known. I was completely captivated, and no conscience in the world could have drawn me from this newfound heaven. I had married a good man for whom I had been trying to crank up loving feelings. The sex we had was nice. I hadn't known what to expect other than nice. I didn't know what to expect from Aaron either, but it wasn't until many years later that I realised the sexual energy between us had been of the best: the best match physically, the best respect, the best appreciation, the best feeling of *Oh wow, I'm home!* The best except for one thing: we didn't have a deep friendship as a basis for our liaison. We were just rawly enjoying each other. We didn't have the time to mature the connection we felt into something that was based on a real knowledge of each other as people. As it turned out, that was what we'd both longed for ever since, when life taught us that what we'd had back then was rare. But it was too late by then; we'd been out of contact for many years.

I never thought I'd see Aaron again. We were both exhausted when we finally reached Panawonica. The sudden pang of parting went deep, but it was expected. Aaron didn't even kiss me before he left, and he didn't look back as he strode into the men's quarters. I was a married woman again, and had to return to Wickham and my husband.

Only ... I couldn't be James's wife any more. I couldn't do unfulfilling sex any more; it wasn't fair to him or to me. Something had awoken in me that was unstoppable. I needed to explore this thing called sex!

Thinking that it was sexual experiences I craved, I started my long career as a callgirl, and enjoyed those years while I flowered as a woman. Then, for five years, I had an exclusive relationship with Hal, a man I fell in love with, before going back to prostitution and the experience of many different kinds of touch. And I *still* didn't encounter what I'd had with Aaron.

I look at him now, all these years later, and try to answer his question.

'I'd worked in the men's mess at the Wickham mine, where I was surrounded by single men. None of them affected me sexually at all. I was married and wasn't interested in any of them.' I stare at the floor, concentrating. 'With you, I experienced an intense chemistry for the first time in my life.'

Aaron listens with bated breath. I am doing him an honour, telling him how he was the one guy who could make me quite insane.

'You were a chemistry virgin,' he concludes.

A chemistry virgin? Never heard that before, but it sounds good.

'Remember the electricity we felt when I was showing you how the gears in the car worked and our hands touched?' I say.

Yes, he does remember. I had seen his astonished face then, and he mine, but it was me who was more affected. This sensation was a first for me, and it confused me. That touch created a wave of desire to know more. What would happen if I touched him again?

It's so strange making love with Aaron again. My eyes are perpetually trying to adjust: he seems nineteen, but he is fifty; he seems fifty, but he is nineteen. To compound the confusion, he brings along photos;

among them, one taken of him at Panawonica. It's not a good photo, rather blurry, but it shows those magnificent long, strong arms and those capable, but gentle hands that are still the same. He takes on a careless pose in the picture, one hip jutting out, legs in a pair of jeans, feet in regulation work boots. His curly, blond, shoulder-length hair gives him away as a mine worker far from home; a fish out of water.

Aaron lasted six months as a machine operator, then went back to university to continue his studies.

Aaron has a sense of the numinous, the unseen forces that shape our lives. 'Everything you've experienced has brought you to now,' he says. 'Everything you did, including going into a convent, was part of what you had to go through so we could be like this now.'

We lie back and let that statement run its rills of energy through us. Gratitude wells up from my abdomen to my heart and spreads in delicious waves through my body, bringing tears to my eyes.

'We met, we found out we liked each other, and we never forgot each other's essence. We did all our growing away from one another. We went through all that shit and came to ourselves, and then we found each other again.'

'We could have missed each other! We could have gone through life and never crossed paths again!' That's me, creating horror; shallow breaths in rigid chests.

'Not possible,' says Aaron. 'It's only *us* who do all this. *We* arranged our lives, and we did it on purpose.'

'We did that?'

'We trusted the future to some part of ourselves. We knew exactly what we were doing. This is how we wanted it — to come together when we were able to see who we were without any garbage getting in the way. Just imagine: would we have survived our own paranoia? Our neuroses would have made us eat each other alive. We would have destroyed that incandescent beauty waiting in a chrysalis state. To find our naked essence, and to find that it's the same essence in both of us — that's the treasure we waited for.'

Alone, I confide my thoughts to my journal, compelled to write. I've abandoned the book I was working on; I need to get down what is overwhelming me now, hoping that the writing process will help clarify my thoughts and feelings. I write as if talking directly to Aaron.

Aaron, we've known each other again for two weeks now.

Last night, you brought photos with you, ones you secretly took of me on our journey back to the north-west.

I know what you see in them; it's what I saw in you the moment you walked in my front door — the pictures in our minds that have haunted us both for thirty years. So now we are each in love with who we were back then — transformed into older bodies, but essentially the same person. To me it is an agony to have grown so much older, to know the limitations of this relationship. It is breaking my heart, even as I understand that I am overwhelmed with gratitude for what I have — this love that seems to be bigger than me.

You can see me, Aaron; you call me gentle. No one, no one at all, has seen this in me to tell me. The gentleness you feel comes from the deepest respect I have for what I am touching. I'm not just touching your body. I'm touching your soul, and myself, in a way that's hard to explain, even to myself.

I recognise myself in you. You say that I'm vulnerable — yes, you are too. Innocent — yes, very — and sweet beyond belief.

I showed you another photo, one taken by a friend in Wickham after my return, and it sent you into a spin. I was sitting on the verandah in my bikini, right fist under my chin, elbow resting on right knee, eyes softly smiling, face wistful, and hair long, straight and carelessly tied. Silver blond, you called it, and you remembered my skin, like satin, you said. You couldn't stop saying 'Wow!' and walked around the room with the picture and kept telling me what you saw in it. Hopefully this mesmerisation is only a trigger for something deeper. You said that you felt strangely unsettled, disturbed, distracted. Now you're beginning to know how I've been feeling these last two weeks! I think of you and gulp with the sudden remembrance of having you inside me. My pelvis goes up involuntarily. My hands go all over my body, enjoying how I recall the feel of your energy. I've been alone for such a long time.

I take a break from writing and sit back to dream. During those years of isolation in Denmark, a small town on the south coast of Western Australia, I learnt to be with myself in an intimate, spiritual way. Life became my Beloved as I turned loneliness into intimacy with my deepest Self. There was so much in Denmark that was a beautiful reflection of my Beloved: the ocean, the trees, my garden, the gathering of friends ...

I rest in the arms of my Beloved whenever I am still. I look for my Beloved in all of life's shapes and events, every day.

It can be a strange thing, this love affair with myself. I go for a walk, or sit up in bed reading or listening to music, and my mouth lifts for a kiss. My lips are open; blood fills them to a feeling of ripe tenderness, and the faintest of brushes, like a zephyr wind, touches them. These moments are so spontaneous, and the kisses so much like a meeting of spirits, that it seems impossible for them not to take shape eventually in some physical form. This lover that is me, but also another, is somewhere out there. So far it is angels who have kissed me, but some day those lips will be of flesh and blood.

Year after year it was like that. I learnt that most amazing of all relationships: the spiritual relationship to God as my Beloved. This Beloved is in everybody and everything, and especially in my inner space. For years, I was embarrassed to talk about it to anyone; now I know it's normal for quite a few of my friends, and there's plenty of corroboration from the poetry of the ancient sages and saints.

My Beloved, you are closer to me than a lover;
You are with me in my waking and my dreams;
You are within the food I eat,
The air I breathe . . .

So goes a poem called 'Beloved II' by Barbara Barton, a lady of eighty-plus I met at a meditation group, who wrote a booklet full of similar songs of love.

I remember the day I went walking with my deeply spiritual friend Penny. It was a blustery day and it threatened to rain, but Penny and I braved it to the beach at Green's Pool, an hour or so before the sun was due to set. We walked briskly with the wind behind us — to beat the clouds, perhaps — but there was no mercy: the rain caught us and, after some gentle warning, huge drops pelted us. We were soon soaked to the skin, but kept walking north, towards the fading light and the purple–blue clouds that shifted as if under a painter's wet brush. After we reached the rocks, glistening with browns and ochres, we turned into the wind again. As we approached the wooden steps leading up to the car park above us, I turned to take a last look at the sky. An invisible artist was painting it in wild strokes with colours I'd never seen before or since — greys and blues, melting and streaking with purples, in breathtaking beauty, rolling around the fading light as if playing a private game that we witnessed only because we were in what most people would call the wrong place at the wrong time. No human artist ever painted such beauty.

Penny and I hurried home to warmth and a cup of tea, both of us awed by this exhibition of our Beloved's artistry.

I come out of my reverie and continue my journal entry.

And along you come, Aaron, and suddenly I have my Beloved in
a manly physical form — yours. This takes me so deep, it pulls
tears from my core; tears of joy and gratitude and bliss. No wonder
I want to kiss you very, very gently, savour the fullness of your lips,
touch your soul through your lips. You don't know this, so you often

kiss in passion instead of tenderness, or simply try to copy me, to please me. You know how I enjoy kissing you, but I mostly feel alone when I kiss you — you don't meet me there yet. You don't know that I don't kiss easily. I don't even hug people much. I tell them I'm the shake-hands-and-walk-fast type.

But I love the depth that is slowly growing in you. I love to be close to you, to feel your energy, our legs entwined, to be at peace like that, breathing deeply, drinking in love and presence, even leaving sex to another time.

Your gift to me is to bring me alive to what has been hidden in myself, in a way I shall never lose again.

I realise with a shock that, sexually, I've been winding down, imagining myself slipping under the ground to merge blissfully with nature in a peaceful death. I have spent much of the past twelve years in celibate silence, loving the miracle of the flowers and plants that grew in my garden, all the while allowing myself to grow old, to imperceptibly lose my life force in favour of ultimate peace.

And now I've met my Beloved in Aaron.

THIS LOVE KNOWS ITS AGE

Love knows no age
Leo Buscaglia, chapter title from his book *Love*

 I walk outside and am kissed by the air. I lift up my face and the sun comes and strokes it, so beautifully it makes my feet lift from the ground. Oh! The sensuousness of just walking! One moment, *this* moment, and the bliss of being here, in a body, taking this one step.

I do my housework, turn on a tap. How can the act of turning a tap be sensual? Anything can be when I am in a relationship with my Beloved, meeting in the present moment.

Aaron, you are a catalyst for awareness of what is right in front of me. So beautiful.

And then, incredibly, my mind takes over with the temptation to immerse myself in the pleasure of being admired and wanted. I hurt so much from being older, from the age of my body. How I want to be younger and more voluptuous! How I regret the thinness of my ribcage, the wrinkles in my neck and on my face and body, the lack of shape in my breasts, the presence of hard lumps there.

How can you stand it? When will you say, *Well, that's enough. Sorry,*

Carla, but my libido has carried me away from you because I met so and so, who is twenty years younger, not fifteen years older?

I write in my journal again:

> I can feel the mental and emotional tension like a cloak,
> like a piece of clothing I'm putting on for size;
> it's that obvious.
> If I keep this on for comfort, something else will die,
> something that I can't put my finger on as yet.
> I feel the need to stay in the moment and not make a security
> out of anything.
> I want to live for whatever the moment brings,
> for whatever comes out of infinite, unknown possibilities.
> Right now, it is giving me the magic of a relationship evolving.
> My intuition tells me this:
> The best chance of the magic staying
> is by not making any demands on it.
> Keep your primary relationship with your Beloved intact.

I'm so free to love when I remember this, free to lie back in the arms of my Beloved in the sea of Life. I know that the metaphors are getting a bit mixed up here. I also know that in spite of everything I know right now, I will forget.

I look in the mirror and see myself and can't believe what I see.

You must be blind, Aaron. The past, probably, blinding you to the present. I don't want you to suddenly wake up to having an ageing woman in your arms.

You never say anything about my body that you appreciate — except my hips. You do seem to like my hips a lot, and appreciate me wanting you, yes.

I'm crying deep tears inside. I'm letting myself come to terms with reality, and it hurts. I've never seen myself so old before. It makes me weep to have missed out on such a big chunk of life. It's a bit like dying. This is what it feels like to weep for the dying of the light. I thought I had already done that, back in Denmark, where I was ready to slowly meditate myself into the grave. But this fresh taste of sexual love has made me want to grasp life anew; it shows me what I've missed. In all my past relationships, all my previous love-making, there was never such a touching of souls as now. Ironically, it is my maturity that makes me feel as intensely as I do. In my young days, the body had its intensities. Now it is the soul, in a body that is no longer young, that can feel exquisitely. The paradox is torture. My body can no longer adequately reflect my feelings or match their depth. It's cruel, devastating.

How am I going to get over this? I should appreciate what is here, however fragile. This love is like a flower, so delicate as it blazes in its beauty. Yet it seems destined to last for only the shortest of time. A white light, a concentration of energy in a moment, an explosion. I think I want to die, I said once. But I don't feel ready to face the ashes of the aftermath. The price of passion is deepest doubt.

'Put some of that lubricant on you,' he says. 'I understand about older women getting drier down there. It's alright!'

The tube of Eros lubricant has a permanent place now on the top ledge of my well-made wooden bed. Is there anything this man doesn't understand; anything he can't take in his stride? He seems determined not to judge anything about me. His priority seems to be to make me feel comfortable, to get over my hesitation about being older.

'You're a bit wrinkly,' he said when we were naked for the first time and I had to leave the bed for something, exposing my body — my buttocks, to be precise. He doesn't say that kind of thing any more. In a way, he has gone beyond what my body looks like to feel the person inside it.

What really gives me discomfort is the state of my breasts. Only a few weeks ago, my GP was convinced that the big, hard, angular lump he could feel in my right breast was cancerous. He booked me in for tests straightaway. It turned out the lumps were cysts — a big one that broke into two smaller, rounder ones. Due to the lack of tissue in my breasts, they were very easily detected by touch.

I still think of my breasts as mutilated by the scar from an operation I had ten years ago to remove several small lumps. The doctor must have known that so many lumps were unlikely to be carcinogenic, but I didn't know any better at the time and allowed his surgeon mate to operate on me the day after my consultation. The hard, irregular lumps kept on coming.

Aaron just isn't into touching my breasts. He ignores them altogether. Perhaps their small size doesn't impress him. I don't want to ask him; it's a turn-off for me just thinking about my breasts. What will he think when he eventually discovers the lumps? I don't dare imagine. But I do want him to touch my nipples. They are super-sensitive and even more responsive than my clitoris.

Aaron's first touch on my nipples is desultory — an unenthusiastic response to the news that they are sensitive. He twiddles them.

'That hurts,' I say.

He gives up.

It's a week later when he says the obvious, 'You've got a lump there,' and points to it. It's detectible even without touch.

'Yes,' I sigh, not looking at him. 'It's just a lump, though,' meaning, *I know all about it, and it's not cancerous if that's what you're hinting at.*

Aaron drops the subject and takes his attention to other parts of my body, but the next time we're together he ever so gently rests the tip of one finger on each nipple and caresses them with hardly a movement, watching my face. The sudden kindness takes my breath away and my back arches in pleasure. He smiles and takes me in his arms, pressing me tightly to his chest, flattening what little there is of my breasts against himself.

'It would be good if you filled out a bit,' he says in passing some time later.

I have every intention of doing just that. Six months ago, I stopped eating wheat and dairy because of a digestive reaction to both and became the thinnest I've ever been. I plan to take body-building food supplements to build up some form.

'Massage of the breasts will increase the blood flow,' says my naturopath when I tell him my problem. 'The extra attention will help as well.' He recommends that I go to the gym and stop hormone-replacement therapy. 'The lumps will dissolve,' he says.

What? The lumps are due to the years of HRT? I'd always thought that my shapeliness depended on hormone replacements. What will happen to my shape when I stop taking them?

I learn about phyto-oestrogens, black cohosh, don quai and licorice tea — all contributors to feelings of female wellbeing and all available over the counter. And I phone the Menopause Institute of Australia, which recommends (based on a phone consultation) a program of natural progesterone and a tiny amount of natural oestrogen. I can now look forward to correct hormonal balance, extra energy and a more consistently good mood.

'I regret not being older,' Aaron says.

When I hear this, something tugs at my heart. It's the regret that I'm not younger. Why would he want to be older, I ask him.

'So you can feel more at ease with being the age you are,' he says.

Well, I don't want him any older. I love the way he's full on with his sexual energy, the way he still appeals to young girls because of his pheromones. Does he know how sexy he is without doing anything overtly sexual, in spite of his daggy appearance?

I don't want him any older. But being older myself gets to me sometimes, and maybe he can feel that. Maybe that's why he said what he did.

I dance, as I often do, in the open space between my dining table and the lounge room. It's my favourite way of exercising, stretching. I put on a CD and move to an invisible hand guiding my steps and gestures. Tonight, I decide to dance naked and to watch myself in the large mirror I've propped up on my camphor box against the wall of the dining area.

For the first time, I see what Aaron sees: a person so thin that her ribs are sticking out. The waist is also very thin, and the torso flat and sinuous, but oh, those ribs! I gulp. Have I lost so much weight? Apparently so. My breasts are tiny protuberances in this skinny whole; only the nipples stand out. The sight is depressing and my sexual energy droops. My dancing becomes a physical exercise instead of an ecstatic celebration.

There's more: a large purple bruise on the back of my right thigh. I've not noticed it before, and I can't recall bumping myself there. The bruise is about eight centimetres across. I know from past experience that it will stay for quite some time, then turn yellow before it finally disappears.

I've gone back to wanting to be desired by a man, wanting to make a good impression. What I see here is suddenly not good enough.

I notice how this kind of thinking brings down my energy. How easy it is to fall into this trap. With it comes the thought that I'd better hang on to Aaron because it would be impossible to find another good man who'd be interested in me. From this perspective, it seems so difficult to be in my other space, where everything is alright the way it is. In this space, thoughts of the Beloved seem alien.

I sit still, and slowly recapture myself.

There's only one sane thing to do: to accept the body I have once again, warts and all.

That bruise, yes; and the scrawniness in my neck, yes; and the spider-veins inside my right thigh, and my broken nails, wrinkly hands, and thin arms with sinews and bumps on them.

My bottom used to be tantalisingly pert; recently, it's acquired an extra lump beneath each cheek. I accept them; I accept all the flaws, leaving out nothing.

Those small breasts, in particular.

As I do this, I feel my sexual energy return, as if it had been banished and is now allowed back in. I decide to put on some clothes.

Skimpy clothes — my new black miniskirt and a slinky pink top that sets off my large nipples. I dance, and the dance takes me. I try different tops, and dance again. Skirt, no skirt; red knickers, no knickers. I feel free, as I used to before a man came into my life to complicate things.

And then it's time to go to bed and sleep in deep peace.

MY FLESH-AND-BLOOD BELOVED

I look at your body, dear . . .
an altar is every pore and hair on every body —
confess that, dear God,
confess.

St John of the Cross, *A Vital Truth*

 He wants to take a look down there.

'It's quite petite,' he says.

I'm intrigued by his observations. My experiences have been almost exclusively with men and men's varying penises, but Aaron, of course, has seen a few vulvas in his life.

'Your labia are very neatly put together,' he says smiling, 'not flapping about like the petals of some big blooming flower.'

I look at him with my arms around the back of my head, amused.

'I just want to know where to put my dick exactly right,' he explains to my interested face. 'You're much like a young girl, you know — I like the little sparse hairs [how he brushes off the fact that at my age I've lost quite a bit of my bush!] and the fact that they're blond, just like the hair on your head. In fact, you're just what I want: you're thin, you're tall and blond, and sexually you respond like a young woman. You really do.'

22

He looks at me with wonder in his eyes, as if to say, *How is this possible?* Then he lies down beside me and takes me into his arms, and I can feel his gratitude for coming home to what his soul has longed for: a woman friend who takes him into her heart, just as he is, because, at her age, the bitterness of life has been burnt out.

Having sex is quite a work-out for Aaron; in fact, it's his favourite sort of work-out — I think he'd prefer to limit exercise to sex! It's a good way to lose weight, he says. He works up a sweat. Sitting on top of me, taking a breather, he wipes his short hair with his hand and sends a shower of droplets onto my face.

For weeks at the beginning, when Aaron and I make love he refuses to have an orgasm. He never explains it, and I make the assumption that he wants the sex to last. Finally, I ask him about it.

'I was too afraid to come in you,' he says.

'Too afraid of what?'

'I'm used to getting spat out after sex. Sex has caused a lot of problems for me. It took a while for me to trust you enough to come in you.'

This is an inkling of a problem I shall hear more about in the future. Aaron's been hurt.

'I want you to have it all,' he says, hunched on his elbows, looking earnestly into my eyes. 'Whatever I can give you, I want to give, but you must ask for it. Right now, what do you want?'

'I want to kiss you.'

'Then *move* to kiss me,' he orders, gently, firmly. Even so, he advances his face towards me as he speaks, and meets my mouth before my head is half-raised from the pillow.

The pleasure centre for Aaron seems to be in his penis. For me, there's no centre; my whole body becomes a field of pleasure. His gentle, careful, gradual penetration sends ripples of ecstasy through every vein, to the hairs of my scalp, the nails of my hands and toes. I have few words or metaphors to describe this when it happens.

Aaron is utterly in awe of it. 'What's it like for you, Carla? Tell me! Wow, can my penis do this?'

'I don't know if it's your penis or not,' I say. 'I'm having sex with *you*, not with your penis!'

'I want to know how to touch!' he moans, letting his face sink into the pillow. 'I want to know how to touch so your *soul* knows it, not just your body.'

He surprises me with his words. I *do* feel touched; not just by his hands, his lips or his penis, but by the deep innocence of his soul. Can't he see that?

'You already know how to touch, Aaron.'

He's pleased to hear me say this. The insecurity that lurks in him needs reassurance; he needs to know how he's received.

Aaron tells me to hold on tight, arms behind his head, legs behind his back, so he can move me down the bed, locked to him more tightly at the pelvis. 'Hang on, babe — we're going for a ride.'

My instant pleasure overflows, down my legs and arms and into my face. Aaron watches, fascinated by the response his action is having on me.

'My pleasure is to see you having pleasure,' he says. In case I think he's implying that he's doing it for me and not for himself, he adds, 'This is what I've wanted for so long. Now this is SEX!' he yells enthusiastically. 'This is having sex, babe!'

Sometimes, stating the obvious is such a turn-on. Especially when the words come out of Aaron's mouth.

'You give sex a good name, Carla,' he adds.

Aaron is slowly healing from the memory of the sting that too often came with sex in his past. He's still wary, like the black widow spider's mate, but he's learning to trust and that's allowing him to lose control in sex.

'Isn't that what everyone wants, babe?'

Aaron's not like some lovers I've known, who roll over and away after they come and are asleep in a jiffy. He stays close to me, his arms strongly around my shoulders that have been pulled around to face him, intent on being together in the aftermath of our intensity. It's a deep sharing of this experience, breathing in the new fragrances released in our love-making — his sweat, my skin, his semen, my vaginal juices, the sweetness in our rapid breaths.

And then, at last, come love words from Aaron.

'I love your body because it's yours.'

'I've never had sex like this before.'

'You're totally with me, no mind, no thoughts.'

'I can feel your kindness.'

'I feel safe with you.'

'Do you know how difficult it was for me to say those things?'

'I like the shape of your face,' he says. 'And your triangular eyes, so kind. Your profile reminds me of David Bowie!' He catches his breath. 'Is that why I liked him — because he reminded me of you?'

'You're the most complete woman I've ever met.'

'I've had great moments of passion, but not this wholeheartedness.'

'Our longing to be together is equal in both of us. You want me as much as I want you.'

THE FABRIC OF OUR LIVES

I did not know life was a fabric woven by my soul.
St Catherine of Siena, 'Until your own dawn'

 Lynda, my very best friend, wants to meet the man who has put such a spark in my eyes. She's offered to come to my place and cook Sunday brunch for us, and her husband, Don, from whom she is separated — and who is also a good friend of mine — is invited as well. Aaron isn't the socially outgoing sort and hesitates about the prospect of being put in close contact with strangers, even if they're my friends. Might it be that he doesn't want to put himself in a position of being sized up? Not that Lynda and Don are the critical kind; far from it. Their spiritual life is focused on the practice of accepting God (as they conceive of God) in all others. These two love genuinely and generously.

Aaron crosses my doorstep more decently dressed than at any time I've seen him. He's wearing a new green pullover knitted by his mother, and underneath is a shirt with a collar — a notch above the thin grey T-shirts I've seen him in so far. His legs, however, are still encased in the old grey tracksuit pants that are too short to cover his bum at the back, and too short in the legs to reach his sneakers. He only has a few winter clothes with him, he explained to me some time ago; the rest of his wardrobe is in Darkan, a town east of Collie in the south-west, where he has a house. He's temporarily living at his parents' home in Perth for the duration of his primary school teacher training here. I strongly doubt that those other clothes would be more flash than the ones he's brought with him. Aaron's not a dresser. He relies on personality.

Lynda, an apron covering her neat top and slacks, moves away from the stove to greet him with a big, warm welcome. After all, this is her best friend's lover, and she is so utterly delighted that this new animation has entered my life that liking Aaron is a given. Aaron shakes her hand politely. Don arrives a little later, almost dancing through the front door, showing his delight at being here for this occasion. His usual rather reserved, dignified manner is replaced by a boyish anticipation of good company.

Once we're seated, the conversation is spearheaded by Aaron. He starts by firing questions at Don in a manner that sounds more like an interrogation. No inflection at the end of the sentence to indicate a question mark; rather, a statement that sounds like an order: *Answer me, tell me, convince me with your answer that you mean what you say.*

Don is taken aback — but not offended. His answers are simple, non-defensive, spoken with as few words as possible. I can see his amusement. *Where's this guy heading?*

Aaron is pleased. 'Good,' he says, 'now we're friends. Let's shake hands.' And they do.

My mouth almost drops open. It's the first time that I've been with Aaron in company and I get to see a different side of him: the Aaron that has to be in control of the dynamics of a conversation, and has to impress others with his special brand of difference. *I'm different, I'm not run-of-the-mill, and I'm likely to be your superior.* I can see how this would work for a lot of people: they would be fascinated; and that's probably what he wants — their open-mouthed fascination. He won't get it from Don; nor from Lynda, who has returned to the stove while I mix a fruit-juice cocktail. All of us are aware of what Aaron is up to, and none of us is offended. This is a soul who has suffered much, that is plain, and who wants to make friends, that is also plain. The conversation continues in a good-humoured style.

Aaron says to Don, 'I want to ask you a meaningful question.'

'Go ahead,' Don replies.

Aaron wants to know what has been the most important thing Don has done in his life.

Lynda laughs at Aaron's audacity as she turns sweet-potato pancakes in the pan. The question is unexpected, but it doesn't take long for Don to answer.

'To start to meditate,' he says, simply and truthfully. He eyes Aaron gently, a soft smile around his lips. *How is Aaron going to take this?*

Well, Aaron takes it as a thing Don did in the past; that it *had* meaning, but surely he's not doing it any more.

'On the contrary, it's the single most important thing I do in my life,' Don assures him.

'So *why* do you meditate?' Aaron asks, with the attitude of: *Hey, dude, don't you know all the disciples left the commune more than a decade ago?*

Don's answer is even more surprising. 'To find the Truth.'

Aaron's next question is predictable. 'And what is the truth then?'

But Don doesn't take the bait. He doesn't side-step the question either. He simply says, 'I don't know.'

In the surprise-me-if-you-can stakes, Don is definitely ahead, but although he's one of the most intelligent people I know, he isn't pedantic. I guess he's simply stating something that is ultimately true. 'I honestly wish I knew what Truth is, but I don't,' he says again. He's quite willing to appear dumb rather than wise.

Aaron wants to shake hands with him again — his sign of approval. Why does he think Don needs approval? That a sign of his approval has some significance?

It's Don's turn to ask questions. He wants to know what kind of work Aaron has done in his life. Uh-oh! A leading question of the delicate kind, since it touches on the elaborate set of values Aaron has developed; values that fly in the face of society's norms. Aaron starts off by saying that he qualified as an architect. It took him ten years in three different universities to get his degree, but he finally did it. He doesn't add that after taking a first-hand look at what kind of work the run-of-the-mill architect has to do — the lack of creativity in all of it — and not daring to hope to be one of the rare few who are successful in selling their own unique designs, this put him off for life. He doesn't mention that he worked for mining companies as one of their most efficient dishwashers, or that he was also employed in a mine as a controller of machinery. Or that for ten years he drove a taxi, and won the Best Driver of the Year award while in the very same month being wrongly indicted for the sexual harassment of a passenger, which almost caused him to suffer a nervous breakdown. He could have added that his knowledge of geology, astronomy, the history of the world's wars and all things extraterrestrial would undoubtedly match that of a university academic on any of those subjects, but it just wouldn't occur to him.

'Did you practise as an architect?' Don asks.

'No,' admits Aaron. 'I trained as a computer programmer after that.'

'I wanted to know what you *did*,' Don reminds him. 'Did you work as a computer programmer then?'

'No, I didn't,' Aaron says, and, as if proud of the fact and to head similar questions, adds, 'I've been unemployed for most of my life.'

This isn't a shameful statement for Aaron, who has rebelled against society's demands for discipline, controlled behaviour and the need for productivity. Don isn't impressed, but he doesn't back off from this handsome man with obvious talents. He casually gets Aaron talking about how he earned his land and house — by building another house for a friend in the same town. No one asks about Aaron's building skills, but I know that although it's not something he'd trained for his skills are phenomenal. He puts things together solidly, with the greatest care and attention, and doesn't realise how unusual that is.

During this conversation I am cringing inside; and when I become aware of my cringing I cringe some more. But I can't help loving this man. I can see his shortcomings, and I can see where his self-confidence crosses over into a need to be in control or to be the top dog in the room. He often complains about others wanting to control him. How true that our complaints are most commonly about things we deny in ourselves! So what? I've decided to love Aaron unconditionally. In moments like this, I can feel the power in that.

Lynda joins us at the table. She loves to love with food and today she has excelled herself: our brunch is a feast.

Much of the conversation is about a movie Lynda and I watched last night, *Antonia*, made in my native language, Dutch. It brings up many topics for discussion: tribal loyalties, the power of tolerance, the power in the friendships of women, whether a group has the right to take the life of one of its own when this person becomes a destructive force; the response of killing that person versus a lifelong condemnation and forced control of that person.

Throughout the brunch, the affection between Lynda and Don is evident.

'These two people really love each other,' I explain in response to Aaron's wondering expression. 'It's just not appropriate for them to live together right now.'

When Lynda and Don have said their goodbyes, we sit opposite each other, Aaron's naked right foot on my lap so I can massage it.

'All my illnesses and physical symptoms are symbolic,' he ventures, giving me the opportunity to ask him what the hurt to his Achilles heel might mean. He knows it's his father, but what are the issues with his father?

'To get him out of my system,' Aaron answers, slightly annoyed, evasive.

I press the question. 'What is it you always wanted most from him but never got?'

Aaron doesn't have to think hard for the answer. 'His respect, of course.'

It's a complicated story, Aaron's psyche. I decide to leave it in peace and see what evolves. Life is busy finding ways of teaching both of us. Why push the river?

VERSES OF LOVE

 'Hi, babe,' he says when I answer the phone. 'I've just finished an assignment and want a break. Can I come over for half an hour?'

It takes him half an hour just to get here. It's nine when he opens the door and walks into my room. My music is in full throttle: Emma Shapplin giving her heart away fearlessly while her voice tries to match her passion. So nice to feel his arms around me: a perfect fit, he being just that much taller. He's in no hurry to let me go this time. His mouth softly touches mine. It doesn't open with eager, searching tongue. His lips just come back for more gentle contact.

I melt to feel his tenderness and my knees buckle. Does he notice? Yes, he grasps me more closely, keeps his eyes closed and keeps kissing. What can be written about kisses? *Sweeter than wine*, someone once wrote in a song.

More sensitive than a vagina, I think, is the mouth. This time, it is me who sticks out my tongue and starts to circle his lips with it, electrifying both of us, fainting with the pure pleasure of it. His lips are so tender, so soft, so undemanding, so responsive and full. He lets me take the lead — he enjoys this — until he surprises me with his sudden initiative. Kissing becomes an exploration of our very souls: *How are you, how have you always been, how is it possible that we can be together like this?*

'Let me get you off your feet,' I hear myself say, remembering his sore foot, and he opens his eyes in surprise, as if to say, *Are you inviting me to your bed?*

I can read his eyes and I say, 'You came here to rest and that's best done on a bed.'

He nods in agreement, sits on the side of my bed and takes off his sneakers and socks, laughing off the possibility that they might smell after their day of imprisonment. But they're not so bad today. He's a little overweight; his foot has impaired exercise for several months and the calories have been piling up.

He lies on the bed, legs spread-eagled in comfortable at-homeness, hands across his chest, eyes closed; he already seems on the way to a deep sleep. It's nine in the evening and he's had a hard day doing assignments.

I lie down beside him, fully dressed, and put my arm around him. My CD player has switched to a disc called *Verses of Love*. It was a gift from a girlfriend and I haven't heard it myself yet. 'Do you want silence?' I ask, but he says, 'No, I enjoy your music,' and we both listen. It's dramatic, strong — music with poems thrown in. Male voice, female voice, varied, lovely; classical, not croony. We don't hear a word of the poems. No doubt they're all advice about relationships and how love can break your heart.

I stroke his chest, put my hand under his thin T-shirt to touch his skin. We've already established that touching him like this is my way of showing affection; it doesn't mean I'm seducing him.

'I'm not used to that,' he says. 'In my family, there was no touching, and the females I've known always indicated they wanted me by touching me.'

'Well,' I answer, looking into grey eyes the same colour as mine, 'I just love to turn myself on by touching your body. It makes me feel sensual, and it makes me feel *you*, the *you* in there,' and I poke his chest.

He knows what I mean and smiles contentedly.

'Have your way with me,' he says. 'The real me loves it,' and he closes his eyes and smiles. 'But we're here to have a rest together, you know.' And he rolls onto his side, his head touching mine.

I can just make out his profile when I open my eyes. He's so peaceful. Our breathing is naturally synchronised, deep and content. His presence, the feel of him, is so much like a blessing that tears run down my face. He doesn't notice — they run down in a way that doesn't touch his cheek — but he opens up his eyes to share a look of wonder at what we're both experiencing.

'This is heaven,' he says, and shuts his eyes again, breathing gently. He lies on his back now, right arm under my shoulders, legs spread-eagled again.

We rest, until he rolls over and clasps me firmly in an embrace of sudden, shocking appreciation. The strength in his arms! He almost crushes me, but no, we can breathe like this, until he flips me over onto himself. I'm now lying on top of him.

'Lie still,' he orders.

I put my head on his chest, my legs wide open around his, pelvis on top of his.

Resting this way is not possible for long. Without thinking, without any plan for anything at all to happen, our breath seems to travel to our genitals. *They* move up and down instead of our lungs. Hmmm . . . nice . . . a new experience. Relax, enjoy. It is me who sits up and moves my pelvis over his in a more deliberate way. I'm still fully dressed in knitted skirt and long-sleeved top, while he wears his student's 'uniform' — grey tracksuit pants topped with a grey cotton T-shirt with slogan.

Might as well take down his tracksuit a bit and let skin touch skin. His penis is not totally flaccid but not stirring. I sit on top of it and move up and down, ever so gently, almost imperceptibly, leisurely. I watch his peaceful face; the lines on it have disappeared, especially the ones around his eyes. He's handsome like this; I can't always say that in broad daylight. His manly innocence is so easy to see with him lying still, lips apart as he breathes. His hair is very short — cropped almost to the skull. It suits him. He wears an earring in his right ear; I must ask him one day what that means. It gives him the air of a hippie — something he wouldn't like me to say, I feel, since I know from one of our earlier conversations that he definitely doesn't espouse their ideals. When did he have it put in? It doesn't add to his dignity. I bet it has to do with his individual, independent nature.

One hand comes up and feels my fanny, looks for my clitoris, strokes around it for a little while, withdraws again. I continue with my pleasure, in no hurry to do anything else, but the inevitable happens: his penis engorges to the point where it wants to rise. I lift myself up and, holding his penis in my hand, very gently let the tip of it touch the top of my vulva, rubbing it slowly. His penis rises another notch and I feel my wetness drip down. I slip the top of his penis a little way into my entrance, just a very little way. In answer, he moves his pelvis up and down with ease, gently, absolutely without any hurry. His penis doesn't need the support of my hands now, so I place my hands on his broad chest, caressing him. His eyes are still closed. He looks more and more like an angel, younger and younger, tantalisingly like the Aaron I used to know three decades ago. His arms and hands are most like they were back then: he was already muscular and beautiful at age nineteen, with fingers not long like an aristocrat's, but more like those of a practical man, or a man who can be practical when he wants to be, which describes Aaron exactly.

His penis enters more deeply now. He can't do much with his pants on, so I slip them from his legs. He cooperates silently, then suddenly flips himself over onto me, eyes full of mischief. He takes over, his rhythm gentle, his thrusting measured and gradual. He concentrates so hard that his tongue comes out and lodges in a corner of his mouth, giving his face a humorous mien. He pushes his penis all the way in and watches my face as the ecstasy of his touch floods me. I feel so deeply touched. Not just by his penis, but by his utter consideration, his total attention, his whole intuitive self — alive, gauging my acceptance and pleasure. (I would say 'to the point of feeling exactly like I feel', but he denies that. 'Lord knows what it is you feel about me,' he said once. 'All I know is, it must be good, and it's you doing this to yourself. I'm just a catalyst for your own pleasure.' I don't remind him that on another occasion he told me that he knew what women felt, because in good sex he'd felt their feelings.)

After a short while, I choose to respect the initial intention we both had of just resting, and I withdraw to lie beside him once more, draping his T-shirt over his still-erect penis, which begins to shrink again.

'I wake up in the morning with a happy dick,' he tells me out of the blue, as if this is what people talk about every day. 'It's full of blood, engorged but not erect. It isn't as if it's aching to jump on your bones. It just knows it's content, treated with respect. It isn't told it's bad, it isn't shrivelled up in fear and neglect, it isn't longing to be anywhere except with me. It's grown bigger since we met again, I'm certain of it.'

Aaron takes his dick in his hands and eyes it quizzically for size, to see how correct he is. I'm looking too, and want to gobble it up. I tell him so.

'No need,' he says, 'it's not on the top of my agenda. Rest.'

The subject of fellatio came up some days before. It was all part of his desire for me to take the lead 'at least half the time'. I told him that because of my past as a prostitute, where I took the lead most of the time since I needed to be in control of the situation, I was tired of taking the lead. He told me he was too: tired of pandering to women who left every move up to him. But there was more I had to tell him, since he hasn't read *God's Callgirl* and didn't know what lay behind my hesitation to take his penis into my mouth — however clean and beautiful it is — and let it come in me.

In the middle of the night, my daddy would come and surprise me with his horrible breath, like stinking fire. His hands were rough and the hairs of his chin hurt as he rubbed them against my cheek while trying to kiss my mouth. He did something worse — something so bad, I tried to go back to sleep again before it happened. He'd put a smelly thing in my mouth; it was hard and big and tasted terrible. He'd take it out after a while and my mouth could relax, but something awful was still there, something warm and sticky that made me want to cough. I longed for a drink of water that never came.

My daddy was my hero; I loved him unbearably, but I became terrified when his eyes started to glint. Especially after the age of six, when he hurt me badly. He wanted to scare me into never telling anybody, not even the priest in the confessional, about what he was doing with me. He'd nearly killed me then: his large, strong hands around my neck, shaking me, his bulging eyes burning into me; his feet kicking me low in the spine when I dropped to the floor and couldn't get my breath to answer him.

Yes, I understood! I wasn't to go to confession. I wasn't to talk to anyone. I was the baddest girl alive, who couldn't talk to my mother or the priest. I was so bad that God couldn't forgive me. My guardian angel abandoned me. My only hope was Lucifer, the devil, who surely had the power to keep me alive so I wouldn't go to hell. Every time my daddy came to me in the night, I was sure I would die, but if I prayed to Lucifer, he would perhaps keep me alive. He did, and I knew even then in my little heart that he would exact a price. What that was I only found out much later, when everything I tried to do to improve my life and get out of prostitution failed.

I was nine when I found myself wanting to hurt a naked toddler. I wanted to hurl that child to the ground, stomp on it, maul it with my hands, stab it with a stick, especially that tender part between her legs. I suddenly became aware of what I was thinking and hurried away, slinking along the street like a fox in the night; my eyes burning not with brightness but with shame.

What would make a child of nine want to maim and kill a toddler? I know the answer today: it is the envy of innocence. That little child represented what I had lost. I'd lost my innocence, and the loss had created a peculiar kind of anger that tried to find an outlet through the violation of someone else's treasure. I had no understanding of this as a child: only raw reaction. I now know more about the cycle of sexual abuse: that the violated feel compelled to violate others. Not only that; they want to get back what they've lost. They become like the pagans of old, believing that by killing something, the spirit of what they've killed will somehow be theirs. It's the excruciating longing for wholeness that drives those who abuse children.

'The abuse I suffered as a child was oral abuse,' I began to tell Aaron, tentatively. He eyed me from where he was lying on the bed, not sure he'd heard correctly. I was sitting on the edge of the bed with my back to him, turned just far enough to speak to his face. 'My father put his penis into my mouth to relieve himself into it.' I spoke the words quickly. 'It was a dirty and smelly thing.' Silence. This was too much for Aaron to take in all at once. He elbowed himself up, but I went on. 'I swallowed that stuff, and couldn't clean up afterwards. Developed whooping cough instead.'

Aaron sank back onto the bed. He couldn't comfort a woman who has experienced trauma of that kind.

'It's alright, Aaron. I can talk about it, and not feel overwhelmed or anything, but fellatio doesn't appeal just now.'

He took my hand silently, without squeezing it, eyes closed. I could feel his compassion, and also the fact that he didn't feel sorry for me. It was mostly a thing of the past. I survived it well. Now is now. And he's happy just to be with me.

Only hours later, I spontaneously caressed his penis with my tongue and lips. I did this often in my career as a prostitute: my tongue was swift and knew where to go and edge away to excite pleasure without exciting too much. I can do it with pleasure when

I feel safe. Aaron's so much in control of his body that I can be certain that he won't ever come in my mouth without being invited.

Now the topic of sharing taking the lead in love-making has come up again. Both the feminine in him and the masculine that worked so hard in the past to please a difficult partner want his woman to be assertive. With him on top of me now, the issue resolves itself naturally: I can't do much in this position! Aaron puts the fingers of his strong hands through mine and pins them to the pillows, making me more helpless, opening my chest wide. It's his version of bondage, where he enjoys the feeling of being in control. His masculinity asserts itself as soon as he knows the woman he's with is an active partner, not just passive. Holding me strongly like this gives him the chance to balance himself in a way that enables him to penetrate me in a different and potent way. Orgasms of the non-clitoral kind ride through me like waves on an ocean and I cry out.

'Are you hurting?' He stops suddenly, anxious.

I shake my head, smiling weakly. He gently recommences his rhythmic drive, sending me crazy. I beg him to stop, and he grins and lets me go. So much for not wanting to take the lead!

REALITIES

The mind tries to feel safe enough
to allow love
out into the open
Nirmala, untitled poem

 We're lying on the bed, him on his back, me with an arm over his chest, my right leg over his, and we have a conversation.

'God has blessed you with an extraordinary number of nerves in your vagina and clitoris.' This is Aaron being lovingly scientific. 'He made you into an extraordinary woman. Did you know you had this in you? Surely you must have enjoyed sex when you were a prostitute?'

'Yes, I did, very much sometimes, but not like this.'

Everything's new and different with Aaron — he should know this. The trouble with voicing such things is that words so easily bring the sacred down to the corny. I hesitate, but I owe it to him. 'You've taken me where I've never been before.' Pause. 'And then further still. And even further.'

He turns his face to see me. I move my head back a little because I know his eyes can't focus well close up.

'So *that's* what was happening,' he says. 'All I saw was ...' And he imitates the noises I made and the way my head moved.

'Stop it!' I yell.

He smiles, turns his head back again.

'Whenever I say something that makes me feel vulnerable, you say something silly!' I complain, but I don't feel blame. Instead, something inside me bursts into laughter.

Farting. It's one of the devastating things that can happen during sexual intercourse. A woman is particularly prone to it because her innards get squashed when her legs are up and around her man's torso, and even more so when her legs are under her man's armpits.

My farts are not nice ones. They're the bomb-out kind that make people faint. Control over these methane emissions isn't easy. Not only that; a woman's vagina can make trumpet sounds as the air gets released during some kinds of intercourse. You always hope that it won't spoil your man's romantic mood. The price of passion can be severe embarrassment.

Aaron lets himself sink down on his side of the bed after a fart quietly fills the space and hits him. 'You have wonderful social skills,' he says. 'You leave me for dead!'

After a moment, he has a comment: a typically Aaron one.

'I think it's the anger coming out of you from the time you had sex and didn't really want to do it. That part of you is healing now ... I don't think a woman should have sex unless she wants to be a lover. She shouldn't do it for money; then she can't be a lover. Sure, some women manage to do both. I think you did, for a time. Some women do it out of need. My old girlfriend Samantha, for instance. She needed so much to be wanted that she'd go with anybody. She was getting fucked for all the wrong reasons.'

Samantha. Samantha who still wants Aaron. She won't let go and phones his home in Darkan every night just in case he's there. He says he dreads her calls, yet can't bring himself to say, 'Sorry, I don't want to listen to you,' and hang up. Samantha seems to be an unshakeable part of his past. What would she represent in his own symbolic language?

It's coming to light more and more just how much Aaron's confidence in healthy relationships has been damaged by memories and interpretations of his experiences with previous girlfriends. His lack of guile with partners makes him vulnerable to rejection, and this has happened time and time again. Every one of his women started to doubt either his affection for them, his loyalty or his sanity. They'd ridicule him bitterly; they'd become paranoid about not being the centre of his universe and would turn into emotional wrecks he felt obliged to try to pacify. Eventually, this had worn him out.

Samantha — who had exhausted their relationship by going from one emotional drama to another for three years — trashed his house. This was after she'd told him she was ready to start living on her own and left. Three nights later, she returned and knocked on his window. He wouldn't let her in to start another drama; insisted that she keep to her word and go home. She became hysterical, accusing him of hiding a woman in the house.

'I've only been gone three days and you've got another girlfriend!'

Aaron couldn't persuade her that this wasn't true. When she started to smash his windows, he fled the house and hid among some bushes in the dark until long after she'd left.

You'd think this would be the end, but not for Aaron, whose loyalty goes beyond the ordinary.

'Did you take her back?' I ask.

'Yes, eventually. We were together for another three years, because she was my friend and I loved her. It took that long for me to realise that you can't make decisions for anyone else and you can't make anyone grow. With Samantha, I burnt out as far as rescuing women is concerned. I used to think that love could fix anything. But the best way to handle that kind of insecurity, where you can't talk it out, is to take them by the scruff of the neck, hang them over a cliff and let them go. It's *their* fear. I can't fix it; *they* have to face it sometime. You can only model something to a person, and then leave them to make a decision.'

Aaron swings himself around on the office chair as he talks.

'Samantha was a little girl emotionally. She enjoyed herself sexually, but wasn't prepared to let go of attachment. Her parents always cuddled her to make her feel better and less lonely, even when she was an adult. They tried to protect her from life. So she continued to solve her loneliness by always being with someone. She'd agree to anything to stay with me. She had no sense of individuality. She couldn't let go of the "us" thing. She wasn't strong enough to be on her own. If she wasn't in a relationship, she'd go with anyone who made a pass at her. That's how she got raped. After that experience, her anger would come up at every imagined sign of betrayal. When I wanted to visit a friend I'd met through Samantha — he was crippled and loved talking with me — she was angry. "No! You can't go and see my friend!"' Aaron sighs. 'Relationship is a bonus. To Samantha, it was an addictive pill.'

I'm interested in the incident he's glossed over: Samantha's rape.

'How did it happen, Aaron?'

'She rented a room from a couple who had two children. She was so innocent — and the guy raped her. He locked her up but she managed to escape. She was in hospital right after the rape when I had a dream about her. I was out in the bush at the time. I phoned, and raced back to be with her when I found out what had happened. She came running down the hospital corridor into my arms. She needed me.'

After splitting up with Samantha another three years later, Aaron made an unbreakable resolve: he'd no longer spend his time wondering who or how to be in order to avoid conflict. He'd just be himself and women could like it or leave him alone. Aaron regained his self-respect, but was left with a horrible wound: the wound of having lost trust in women and in the possibility of a good relationship. His radar for trouble became so honed that for six years he avoided having sex; not because he didn't find several women interesting, but because he could predict the run of events and it just wasn't worth it.

In me, he had something new: a woman who would make demands on him to come up to her standards, since he was living in her space. Was he going to measure up or leave? Was he going to handle the occasional conflict without throwing in the towel or feeling that he'd compromised himself?

Aaron has many bad memories, from childhood to as recently as his last relationship, and they have left their scars. It will take more insight than he's had to date to resolve them, since he's still full of justification for the anger and fear and the idea that he's a victim.

I've known the way out of many of my own delusions and illusions on my journey from extreme guilt and discomfort about who I was to the recovery of innocence. I just forgave and accepted who and what I was, one moment at a time. It was a truly humbling and a truly freeing time for me, since a new self-esteem arose spontaneously out of the ashes, one that wasn't so dependent on anyone's opinion. It rested on the feeling of myself as an eternal being, magnificent, powerful, loving, peaceful, both at rest and vitally alive.

Aaron has made many positive decisions in his life — miraculously, considering what he's gone through. When he was hauled before the courts on a false charge of sexual harassment as a taxi driver, he found that not a single person who knew the truth was willing to stand up for him. He's been much betrayed, if I am to believe his stories. The glitches in Aaron's world-view seem to come from the basement of his subconscious; not easy to gain access to all at once, nor safely as far as he's concerned.

'I killed three children,' Aaron says mournfully. He never wanted children, and made this plain to his then partner, Anika, again and again. The first pregnancy was a mistake on both their parts. He insisted on an abortion.

'I think the first was a mistake, but the second was just carelessness. She knew all along that I didn't want kids.'

'Did you use condoms?'

Aaron looks at me as if I am suggesting something irrational and unthinkable. 'No.' A sombre tone of voice. 'Then she betrayed me by ripping out her IUD. I made her have her third abortion.'

'Why would she rip out her IUD?' I asked.

'I don't know. Maybe she felt guilty about the other two foetuses she'd lost and wanted to replace them.'

'So why was this third abortion a reason for your breaking up?' I want to know it all.

'It wrecked her body, my trust in her, and our relationship.' He pauses. 'I left because the trust between us had been destroyed.' He looks bitter. 'You can't trust women; they all want to tie you down.'

I imagine the desperation that must have hung between them as the weight of what separated them became stronger than the love they'd shared for seven years. No more sex. No more relationship.

'I'm a very bad boy in her books,' he says quietly, flicking a pencil onto the desktop, swaying back in his chair.

He was thirty when he left her, and in the next fourteen years he experienced more sorrow via a series of relationships that all started happily but ended in disaster. Six years of being on his own and he meets up with me. He's become very practical about relationships in the meantime. 'People underestimate my ability to let go,' is a remark that sends an icicle into my heart. He's unattainable. He can't love, as I do, with pain. He will not have any more pain. Will not.

SIMPLE THINGS

And the greatest gift
God can give is His own experience.
Meister Eckhart 'To See As God Sees'

'Sometimes, to be is all that's necessary,' says Aaron, looking like a cherub after making love this Sunday morning. He voices his contentedness from his pillow, eyes closed, one hand under his head. Aaron loves to talk 'wise stuff' when he feels like this. 'All I know is that I exist,' he says. 'All I know is what I feel. Life is a sensation. The mind doesn't know a thing. It's a hanger-on. It's like the software in a computer, always doing calculations, always trying to figure out data about reality, to find out the truth as best it can. But *I* just exist.'

I sip my tea. I've made a pot for both of us and brought a tray back to bed, as well as a book, which I don't get to read now that Aaron's in one of his communicative moods.

'You are the *carer* of your mind,' he says. 'You care for your mind, and you just watch it do things. But you're *not* this mind. All you are is what you are, nothing more. I am. The rest is craziness really.'

'They mean a lot to me, those words, Aaron.'

I mull over them as I think of the way I've been pulled recently by the high-voltage meetings I've been attending at the National Speakers Association and others. Most of my friends and acquaintances there are highly successful and highly motivated people for whom I have great respect. I've been asking myself if I should be doing more to make myself like them — work harder, be more on the ball, make more money. But there's just not enough motivation. I'm content to do what I already do: write, keep up my website, respond to my emails, give talks when I'm invited, spend time with Aaron, my daughters and grandchildren, now and again invite friends over for dinner and attend the occasional spiritual gathering. This may change, of course, but at the moment, the river is flowing nicely: not too fast, not too slowly.

Perhaps I should do more to wake up further in the spiritual sense. I've read of such wonderful awakenings. The powerfully aware individuals I have had the good fortune to meet are a joy to be with and so stimulating. But again, I lack motivation. I'm content to be happy with myself, at whatever level I'm at or not. I'm so happy just to be, living one moment as it is, then the next, day in and day out, that I wonder if I'm fooling myself. But if I am, it's a risk I feel okay to take. I figure that if my deepest, truest self wants me to do something else, it will make that obvious.

In a lot of ways, I've wised up to this mind of mine. But not quite all of it, yet.

Aaron comes in with another pot of tea, to give me a surprise. There's a further surprise when I find out it's green tea, after pouring it into cups prepared with milk. It tastes good all the same. That's how he likes it, Aaron says. He wants me to get into my pink terry-towelling dressing gown so I'll stay warm as I sip. He perches his cup on the ledge above our bed, where it will cool down until it's lukewarm. In the meantime, he lies down and puts his arms around the sitting me, snuggling his head close to my chest, slipping a hand under my dressing gown to hold a breast.

'I love you, babe.' The words always come out with such tenderness. 'Relationship is about an exchange of energies. When you give me your love, it's easy for me to give you all I have. I love the way you melt into me; you give yourself to me and you trust me. I've always wanted to love like this.'

I smile and keep sipping milky green tea.

Aaron confides more of his soul to me.

'I used to think that because I survived on welfare for a lot of my life, I was a failure. Then I looked at the people who had everything — good job, big house, car, wife, kids, etc — and I saw that they yelled at each other. They weren't connected the way we are. I'm not successful the way they are, but I'm in the part of life I really value: I know how to connect and love. I feel successful in what matters in life.'

'I agree, Aaron. That's why I'm with you.'

I put the tray on the bedside table. He runs his hands over my body as I slide down the bed and then bend my back into his body. Our hands move over each other's available limbs; such a friendly thing to do, like petting a cat: it likes you petting her, but in return you get her magnetism. An exchange of energies.

'This curve, this shape — it's so familiar to me and such a turn-on,' he says, hands massaging up and down my body. 'You let me slip inside you,' he says, 'that's so nice.'

His words are ordinary, but the tone in his voice so appreciative. He isn't trying to turn me on or flatter me with his talk. That's what I like so much about Aaron: he doesn't seem to manipulate with words.

It's so easy and effortless, lying down on my side, keeping warm under the covers while making love in the cool of the early morning. I love it when he grips my shoulders so he can thrust in a more controlled way. I put my hands on his and feel the energy of love and desire. His left hand travels down to the curve of my hip and he holds it with his hand as he thrusts, then massages my entire back and pulls my head towards his for a kiss. At last

I hear him sigh a few times with deep contentment; it's over, and we lie still.

'Your tea's still waiting for you,' I say, as we break and exchange a kiss.

'That's alright; it can wait until next summer, when it's all warmed up again. Let's try it,' and he gulps it down. He likes it best when it's no warmer than this.

He asked me once whether I'd ever enjoyed doing sex doggy-style. 'Yes,' I say, 'quite a lot, but it was just having sex, not making love. I couldn't look at you if we did it doggy-style. It's much nicer face to face and being connected to you.' So he dropped it.

Today, he brings it up again. This time I say, 'OK, let's try it,' and stand at the edge of the bed, legs apart, and present my bottom. The height isn't quite right, so I climb onto the bed, resting on my knees and hands. Yes, perfect.

He enters me, and I gasp. He thrusts gently, and I gasp again. Every movement of this is a peak experience, more physically intense this way than any other. I can't see Aaron's face, feel lost in paradise. Then his left hand thrusts a bunch of sheet towards my moaning mouth; I'm making so much noise that he's sure it will travel upstairs to where my employers live. I laugh and cry and moan into the sheets until I can't take any more. He pulls out and rolls me over and my hand goes straight to my clitoris. He bends over and takes my nipples in his mouth. It's the first time he has given my nipples his undivided, enthusiastic attention. I feel shocking pleasure at this change in him; the pleasure rises and rises ... in a wave that arches my body up to his, my head off the back of the bed. This time it's his hand that stops my scream from travelling upstairs. Or, rather, his fingers. Instinctively, he knows that I'll take them into my mouth and make them part of my pleasure.

My body comes down ever so slowly, and now it's Aaron's turn. He wants to come inside me. 'This is for you,' he says.

'Are you sure?' I ask, because I don't want him to get tired.

'I'm sure,' he says, as if to say, *When I say something, I always mean it, girl*, and he lets his passion have its way inside me. It's a mingling of psychic juices that must generate some very special children somewhere in the world of spirit or earth.

Later, neither of us is tired. It's a lesson to me: there are moments when indulgence saps energy and there are moments when energy simply balances out. Here it was mostly done doggy-style.

'You're a virgin,' he says, 'because every time we make love, you're new. We go to ever new spaces. I'm a veteran; you're a child–woman. The wiser you get, the more you'll enjoy the quality of being a child–woman.'

I asked Aaron a question: 'Why did you come back into my life?' He wrote a poem shortly after, in response.

> *To show you who you are, he says.*
> *God's girlfriend — rather special.*
> *You smell nice, he says; I remember your smell:*
> *It's still the same.*
> *We are still the same people, though thirty years have gone between.*
> *Still exactly the same energy.*
> *You opened to me like a flower when I was nineteen*
> *You are still like this flower*
> *You still have the same innocence (still a convent girl)*
> *Yet so strong in your vulnerability.*
> *You left something of yourself in me, thirty years ago*
> *And I just had to find it again,*
> *So here I am, to tell you*
> *How much you have meant to me all these years.*
> *You set me up for life to feel good about sex.*
> *You showed me how a woman could appreciate what I had to give.*

> *Isn't it great that I'm a man, and I have a dick,*
> *And you're a woman, and you want me?*

'Can you feel this pull between us?' he asks, as he holds me very close against him. Our kisses have been endless; we can't get enough of each other's sweetness.

'Yes, of course.'

I've been aware of it as a living energy that pulls our entire bodies together from head to toe, but is strongest at our chests. Our hearts are wide open to each other. What we're feeling are the combined female and male energies coming together in our hearts, creating perfect balance. It's this balance that seems to create bliss. Neither of us wants to take any advantage of the other. We simply love each other with as much openness as we can give, and we want the pleasure to go on endlessly.

'We're friends forever,' says Aaron. With these words he defines our connection as a desire to be a force for good for each other, throughout eternity. 'We've made this bond elsewhere already; this is simply a reunion. We're like angel-spirits revelling in having a physical body, so happy that we're man and woman.'

I think of what he was like in the beginning: this rough diamond has become an exquisitely sensitive and present man with huge, soft hands and the most tender of willing lips.

TELL ME WHO YOU ARE

What part of heaven did he come from?
Adapted from a poem by Tukaram, 'That Angel
Talked Like a Sailor'

Aaron has a peculiar way of expressing what I call his Dionysian quality; he constantly thinks in pictures. Life isn't meant to be about chasing after money, he maintains; life is for living and loving. In the twenty-first century, Aaron/Dionysus has to go on unemployment benefits provided by the Apollos of the suburbs, who are willing to do disciplined study, think and work hard enough to pay taxes. This is a fact of life that Dionysus is learning to accept, and he's become willing to toe the line and eat humble pie to be a useful person in society and earn that money. But not just money for its own sake. He'll build a house with it, and then quit working to live in the house. With the money leftover, he'll grow a garden. Then he'll live on the smell of an oily rag and be happy, or so he tells himself. After all, he's done so already for many years; he knows how.

But is there the possibility that in a couple of years he may be transmogrified? Every chance, and perhaps no chance.

* * *

I confide my Dionysus theory to my friend Don, who is a mentor of sorts for me. He can give me a spiritual perspective on the inner workings of my soul.

'Carla, beware of concepts,' he warns, like a good instructor. His voice is always soft, his eyes earnest but never far away from a smile. 'You talk about Aaron as Dionysus and this might get in the way of being with who he really is in the moment. If you want to live in the innocence of love ...'

I get what he means. Concepts are at least one step removed from the real thing.

'No concept can define a person,' Don continues, 'and even when it seems to fit the model exactly, the fit is only on part of the model, never the whole, and even then only for that particular time, not always.'

Oh. Oh well, thanks, Don. I should have known that already, shouldn't I?

I go away feeling chastened. Privately, I believe that Aaron's a big improvement on any Dionysus.

He tells me about his place at Darkan as he lies on his back, one arm tucked under my neck and around my shoulder. 'My house and shed are full of recycled material,' he says. 'None of it's really junk. It's all got a purpose in the building plan.'

He goes on to describe some of it, trying to make it sound more attractive so I will visit him there, then suddenly pulls my face to his to kiss me on my mouth, and goes on talking. Does he know how he stops my heart when he does this? No, it's just how he is: he loves to love. But I can't see myself living in Darkan, ever.

The vision of his future home seems to me like a mixture of old cottage charm and space technology: a house built almost entirely of recycled material, but with white panels to hide things like light switches and gadgets that have all sorts of wondrous purposes, plus a round window in the meditation room, which will have carpets going up the walls, and lots of stainless steel in the kitchen. 'It'll mostly just be a large, open space,' he says. But for now it's a wooden house full of things he's picked up from the roadside. Lots of stainless steel pans, broken-down heaters and other things that will work when he gets around to repairing them with bits from other similarly broken-down items. He wants me to come and see it all.

'Will you come over and rough it with me for a weekend?'

'No way!' My answer is so unequivocal that it shocks him. I'm sure I wouldn't enjoy the experience, having roughed it years ago when establishing a community in rural Queensland with my two partners at the time, Hal and James.

'Darkan sounds like a cold and god-forsaken place; you won't see me there!' I continue. 'Has it got plumbing, this house of yours?'

'You mean piped water? Sure!'

'A flushing toilet?'

He doesn't answer straightaway, thinks up a funny response to make me believe it's not too bad, but I suspect the toilet is probably a hole in the ground, some way from the house, and it would be a bonus if it had a roof.

'You won't see me in Darkan!' I repeat.

He grins. 'Maybe you'll come over just to have a look when you've got time.' He hasn't given up.

It's just past six o'clock in the evening, Aaron's favourite time for coming around to my place. It seems that what usually happens when he comes around is one of three things: we sit and talk while we eat or sip tea; he improves my computer set up while I do house chores; or we go to bed. Tonight, we've done all three, and we're in bed, lying facing each other with our heads on the same pillow.

'Lie still. Look at me,' he orders. It's one of his favourite things, to lie at a certain distance so his eyes can focus and we can just gaze at each other. At first, it's quite uncomfortable: what's he thinking as he looks at me? I'm more comfortable lying closer to him, feeling his skin and energy. As I stare back, I feel an inclination to smile, and realise that it's an expression of my discomfort. Soon, though, a strange feeling takes hold of me as I realise this isn't about forming thoughts or opinions of each other. It is a beholding, a wondrous seeing. My tears well up and drop down. Aaron's face doesn't change. At last he sighs, and takes me into his arms. He feels the wetness of my face against his cheek, and holds me tighter.

'You choose your partner because it gives you the opportunity to be the man or woman you want to be,' Aaron says. 'You've had to do without love for a long time and I want to make it up to you.' He's aching to give me all he can.

'It's so easy with you,' he keeps saying, 'so simple. I can't get over how much you want me, and how it's not a trade-off with you. It's all just a giving of yourself.'

'You just love being loved!' I quip. And with that comes the idea that he doesn't really love me. What a sabotaging thought!

He loves what he sees because he sees himself reflected in me — that's fair enough. It's what he keeps saying: we're exchanging parts of ourselves. He's aware of me in him, and I've watched with astonishment the changes in his love-making, little things that add up to tenderness. He lies with his head towards the bed's end so he can take the sole of my foot and press it to his cheek. He dozes and wakes up to stroke my leg, reaches down and puts his hand over my vulva, parts the outer lips of my vagina and inserts part of his thumb, and we lie there like that, with one of my arms around his leg, a hand resting over his scrotum, until we both get too chilly and jump back under the covers.

We know each other so well now that our movements have become thoughtlessly coordinated, flowing effortlessly and unself-consciously. Our kisses stop for a moment, with both our mouths touching, open, breathing each other's breath, taking in each other's essence. He presses me against himself, and we lie there so close, so still, my cheek against the softness of his neck. He has entirely taken on the exquisite sensitivity that so astonished both of us when we first started to make love, so long ago.

And what is there of him in me? I feel I've become more assertive. I feel freer to say what I do and don't like. For example, when he comes in the afternoon and his stubble is like sandpaper, I ask him to shave before it starts chafing me. It's up to me to send him home when it gets late. I have the will to leave the bed so that he will follow suit, rather than wait for him to take forever and leave me asleep, romantic as that may sound. Late nights are ruinous for me. I always wake up early, so I need to get a good enough rest to face the next day energetically. At times, I've allowed us to spin it out to midnight and past: seven hours of making love. Now I tell him when I feel I've had the equivalent of a five-course meal and am totally satisfied, even though he might want to start dinner all over again.

It's 10 a.m. I've just come back from a long walk, during which I lost my scarf. I go out again in my car, tracing my steps all the way back, but can't find it. I feel how attached I was to that scarf: it was a sleek thing in vibrant purple and black that set off anything black I wore. My friend Laurian exclaimed 'Magnificent!' last time she saw it, and maybe 'magnificent' is similar to 'superior'. It was vaguely reminiscent of the splendour of cardinals, although they wear red as well as purple and black. Anyway, the scarf is gone, no longer belongs to me. Last Thursday I secretly criticised Aaron for being attached to *his* image, but now I get to see how attached I can be to the things I use to define *my* ego. Oh, the subtle, superior un-love of the thought that others would be better off if they listened to me! Aaron's just Aaron, my lover. Aaron doesn't need to change, not one little bit.

I think about my reaction to some of the things he does, like leaving urine on the rim of the toilet. Part of me thinks it's disgusting, and I can't help that reaction. But he can do this every day now and it won't matter. The freedom of that thought is exhilarating. His sinuses can stay blocked up and his foot sore, forever, until he wants to do something about it, and then it will be what *he* wants to do, not what *I* want.

I never thought this attitude would be possible. I've always believed that to be honest in a relationship, you have to tell your partner what you don't like about them, even if they don't want to hear. Honesty means something else to me now. It means honestly admitting that I love this man for who he is, not for what he does or doesn't do to flatter my ego. It means being honest when something about him might annoy me, because then it's time to accept both myself and him in spite of this annoyance. It means realising that it's such an enormous privilege to love, and for that love to mean something to someone else. It's such an immense privilege to be loved in return. What could possibly matter more than to preserve harmony so this love can flourish?

I'm not silly enough to think that a relationship will last just because two people decide to love each other. What do they do when differences of opinion arise? Aaron and I don't live together, so we're not as exposed to conflict as are other couples, who live in the same space day in, day out.

Would I enjoy living with Aaron? We're used to doing our own thing, and we both like having our own space. Even so, it's nice to just have him around when I'm busy. He comes around spontaneously sometimes and discovers that I have to prepare for a talk or for some other work and need to concentrate in silence. He takes out a book to study for college and it's really pleasant to have him there. One Sunday we spent the whole day like this: he studied and I wrote. The time was punctuated with kisses and fondles and occasional banter, until it was time to take a serious break and go to bed. I can't imagine a better sort of Sunday.

THE MOON IS FULL

Black holes are real.
So is the sun.
Carla van Raay on a clear day

 When I bought my bed, I decided on a sturdy structure with strong, flat railings on either end. I should've gripped the bed-end to steady myself as Aaron flips me over from a lying position on the pillows to get me on top of him. I'm getting used to the easy flow of this balletic movement, but this time I scream as I lose my balance for a second or two and see myself falling off the edge of the bed onto the floor. Aaron grabs me and pulls me back. Just as well he's so totally present and that his arms are so strong.

My nervous laughter of relief turns to the moaning of pleasure. He coordinates the lift of his buttocks with movements that bring his penis right against my pelvis, creating a sensation so intense that it's impossible not to scream softly. My employers have gone away for the weekend, so making a noise isn't really a concern.

He can see that the intensity of what we're doing isn't something I can sustain, so he says 'Hold on!' and turns me onto my back, struggling a little to get his legs back under himself. This way he's more in control and can stop when the intensity builds close to orgasm for both of us. He straightens himself, puts his hands on his hips, head back, and concentrates. Aaron has learnt to hold back indefinitely. We go on like this until I call a halt.

'Are you sore?'

'No, but my fanny's getting tired.'

He doesn't want to hear this at first. 'Tired fanny? You're not tired, but your fanny is?'

I close my eyes and lie still.

'Just let it come down gently,' I ask him, and he agrees. He holds his kneeling position while his penis slowly becomes more flaccid. He doesn't compromise by adding any movement to arouse it again and string out the process. At last he disconnects and lies down beside me. I immediately put my arm around his chest. He touches his head to mine as we rest. It's the end of our love-making for the evening, as far as I'm aware.

Half an hour later, Aaron lets me know he's still keen. He doesn't press me; just makes sure I understand that he would love it if we could connect again. I've recovered quite a bit and agree: let's do it. Aaron's delighted. When he enters me this time, my vagina is in a state of feeling I've never known. It hasn't come down from its previous aliveness.

The feeling electrifies him and his penis unexpectedly enlarges to the point of orgasm. He tries to pull back, but the end must be close. He asks breathlessly, 'Do you want me to come into you!'

When I blurt out, 'I want you, Aaron!' he still waits for me to come to a climax with him. 'Yes! Yes! Dammit, Aaron' is a clear clue and an explosion of light like an atom bomb envelops our loins when he lets go, and we travel into space.

Aaron's face is wet. I reach my hand up to touch it. 'It's not tears,' he assures me. 'It's not tears! It's just that I'm coming down now.'

He draws his hand through his hair and a fine shower of sweat droplets falls onto my face. I can taste their saltiness. His sniffles that have been absent these last three or so hours come back. His sinuses are blocked again.

He stays sitting up. I watch his straight shoulders — just like a Buddha's, I've often thought. In a few moments, he pulls himself away, suddenly aware that his knees are sore and that his limbs ache. 'That's why I don't like to orgasm,' he says.

'It's a shrivelled little nothing now,' he says almost ruefully, looking down at his crumpled penis.

His energy might have been on the low side when he asked if I wanted him to come into me before committing himself to orgasm. I didn't realise that he was asking to do me a favour. I don't want that: either he's dead keen or I don't need favours like this. A few moments ago, I was full of romance. Now, all romance has left my body.

He lies down, folds himself into my arms as I ask, 'Do you still enjoy being with me — right now?'

I'm wondering *how* far this romance has disappeared.

'My feelings haven't changed!' he hastens to explain. 'It's just that I have no desire left. I can't want your body just now.' He looks older, pale. 'All I want to do now is fade away and sleep.'

I feel his body relax as if on its way to sleep, but he won't let himself. I know what it is: he might snore when he sleeps and he hates that.

'Take a rest and sleep a bit,' I say. 'And it's alright to snore.'

'Really? Like this?' and he makes a loud snoring sound, and gives an embarrassed laugh.

I shrug my shoulders. 'Any way you like.'

A couple of weeks ago, I was appalled by his snoring. Right now, I don't mind it at all. I hold him while he falls asleep and starts to snore every bit as loudly as his pretend example. It disturbs me so little that I could fall asleep as well, but I'm not as tired as he is, so I just close my eyes.

He wakes up after a few minutes, turns his head to kiss me, and promptly falls asleep again. This happens three times before he wakes up to the fact that he must go. He turns around to face me so we can exchange some goodbye kisses. He can't go while I'm hanging on with one arm around him.

'Make it easy for us,' he says. 'Roll away from me.'

I release my arm and roll away to the cold side of the bed. I lie there on my back, feeling the wrench of being away from him. He notices and comes over to give me a kiss, smiling. He knows what's going on here: Carla's getting attached; Carla hurts when she's apart from him.

Aaron has a shower, and I make us both a cup of chamomile tea. It's past midnight. We sit across from one another at the table, but Aaron has to clear something up before he leaves.

'Don't get attached to me, Carla,' he says. 'I've been there, and it isn't worth the pain.'

I check inside myself. It's a timely look. I'm close to losing myself in him, but I don't think I will. I try to explain to Aaron why I won't get too attached. My words feel clumsy; I hope they don't sound strange.

'For the last ten years or so, my primary relationship has been with *life*,' I begin, 'and that's the same as with myself.'

Aaron seems to understand immediately; his face breaks out in a beaming smile and he extends his hand across the table.

'Let's shake on that,' he says, and I take his broad hand in mine.

We make our way to the front door. He stands me up against the wall to kiss me one last time and feels me falling as I lose my balance. It's way past midnight and it's been quite a night.

'You're just like a little girl sometimes,' he laughs, and stands me up straight.

He goes into the night. It's windy out there, fresh wind from the river, but not very cold.

'The moon is full, kiddo!' he says, as he walks up the slope to his car.

He's gone now. I feel full and satisfied and ready for bed, to catch as much sleep as I can before five o'clock, when my body will wake up, used to being an early bird.

★ ★ ★

I ask Aaron: 'What's romantic?', because I know he doesn't like romantic.

He says, 'Romantic is all about *not* being here and now. It's about living in the imagination; twinkly eyes. It's not real.'

Well, that puts it in a nutshell. Other people would include things like flowers and chocolates, but these are so far removed from Aaron's values that he doesn't think of mentioning them. He'd rather give up his time to make my computer work better. He'd rather kiss me and feel how nice that is for both of us. He'd rather spend time sitting parked in a car near the ocean, watching the sky and the waves with me. Presence rather than presents.

'I think of you now and again and then I forget you,' he says, because he's always honest with me. He knows that I think of him often — as I go about my housework, when I drive, when I wake up in the morning and when I go to sleep.

'You're not the romantic sort; I know that much!' I laugh. I've never met anyone who makes less of an effort to make a good impression.

'Carla van Raay,' Aaron says, 'welcome to love. This is who you are! This is how a man and a woman should enjoy each other.'

Aaron's good at soliloquies. For instance, today he tells me:

'I'm yours, for richer and poorer, till death do us part. And I'm *not* yours, and *you're* not mine.

'We're separate.

'We're individuals.

'We have our own energy.

'We are ourselves.

'We do not own anyone.

'I keep telling you this — this is my message to you: we're together and separate.

'If we lose each other, or if one of us loses the other, we will know grief, but it will be sharp and clean, not clingy, self-indulgent or forever. Long-term grief is losing yourself. It's trying to live your life through the other person, forgetting that all you have is your own energy. Sitting in sorrow is losing your boundaries and your reality. Romance is about grief. Love is real.

'You're feeling who you are. I want you to be all you can be. That's what I can do for you: show you who you are and help you to become all you can be. If I have to come along with a two-foot dick and fuck you right up to your eyeballs for you to get the message, I'll do it.'

Silence. An essential pause.

Aaron continues. 'We've been very patient people. I've been very patient. And lonely. And then we run into each other again. It's all been worth it.'

'I know,' I say. 'I've been like that too, except I changed my loneliness to aloneness.'

'What would you have done if I hadn't come back into your life?'

'I don't know. Kept on the way I was, I suppose, getting kissed by life. I passed up opportunities for sex because I knew they'd lead to disappointment. I want *this*, this love we're growing each other with, not just sex and company to cover up feelings of loneliness.'

We lie in the semi-darkness, pleased with the way we can communicate with each other, pleased with the knowledge that, this time, we're not going to ruin everything with romantic or neurotic demands. Or not so easily, anyway.

'Isn't this love what all men and women want?' I muse.

'No, people want romance. They get jealous, and they stop caring when you no longer give them what they want. People want others to fulfil their dreams. They don't want responsibility and reality. They suffer and they don't know why.'

Aaron is speaking from experience.

'I had a dog once. Well, it wasn't mine to begin with. The girlfriend I was with wanted to have a puppy, so I relented and said, "Okay, it's your puppy and you look after it." Our relationship turned bad and when she left, she said, "The puppy's yours." So there it was.

A beautiful dog with a woman's eyes, all adoring, and a soft, shaggy coat. She became my best friend, followed me around, slept anywhere she wanted, including on my bed ... *inside* my bed. She did exactly as I told her. She loved me so much, was so loyal, came running as soon as I called her, no matter what she was into at the time. And she'd sit by a door and stay there for hours, just because I told her to. We had lots of fun together.

'Then I got interested in building a house, and it took up a lot of my attention — so much so that she started to miss me badly. She'd whimper because we didn't do things together any more and I didn't spend time with her the way I used to. Six months later she was dead. Got swiped by a car. Tore off her left leg and hip — the feminine parts. I reckon she killed herself; couldn't take it any more.'

Aaron doesn't say it, but this story mirrors the relationships he's been in: women who've loved him loyally like this dog; women who weren't able to do without him when he was busy; women who thrived on his attention and became needy for his presence. Women who didn't get themselves killed, like his dog did, but hurt *him* first to get his attention back, then hurt *themselves* more and more in desperate attempts to make him feel guilty and get him where they wanted him to be. He'd been patient with them, he said, tried to make it easier for them, but it had always ended bitterly. Aaron had become extremely wary of women.

After the last relationship, six years ago, he'd sworn to himself that he would 'never stick his dick in anything unsafe again', to use his own expression. He preferred to get all sexual attractions and arousals out of his system by masturbating them away.

'Women like me,' he says.

'Why's that?' I lie in the crook of his arm, feeling blissful. Instead of waiting for his reply, I try to answer myself. 'I know, for lots of reasons. Women sense your capacity for love, for starters.'

'How do they do that?' He's genuinely surprised by my words.

'They sense it in your energy. They also know that you can't be possessed, and that's a challenge to some of them — to make you change your mind.'

He considers this and nods. He knows this one, apparently. Bastard! He's doing it with me too.

'I'm particularly a challenge for the ball-breakers,' he says, with a meaningful look on his face. Ball-breakers won't have a chance with Aaron any more then, since he spots them from a mile off.

I decide to tell him all the good points I can. 'It's also because you're so present with people.'

He doesn't seem to understand this, so I explain that it's his ability to really give people attention, without self-centredness.

'But I'm extremely self-centred,' he counters.

Yes, of course he is, in the sense that he talks to women because he wants to, for the pleasure it gives him. But he isn't self-centred the way some men are, who want to manipulate women for their own ends.

He nods. Manipulation is the furthest thing from his mind, and the one thing he won't tolerate for a minute from a woman either.

I'm watching him do his thing on his computer. I've been sitting there for ages.

He turns around. 'Do you want to go to bed?'

I nod.

'Then why didn't you say so, instead of staying rugged up in that chair?'

The truth is that I wanted to see what would happen if I didn't initiate anything. Would he just let me sit there and then leave when it was time to go? Or would he want to be close to me for a while?

'You were so busy,' is all I say, but he complains.

'I need you to say what you feel ... communicate more, be more assertive.'

I'm aghast. 'I always think I'm obvious to you.' I recall times when he has surprised me with his observation of my body language, when I believed I was being enigmatic.

'I need to know what you think and feel,' he says.

It is then that I confide a terrible secret. Well, terrible and secret to me, as I don't realise how very common it is. I've only carried it recently as a secret, aware that Aaron constantly keeps all his options open.

'I don't speak up because I'm afraid of losing you.'

He looks at me with sudden surprise, then pulls me close.

'I didn't want to tell you, Aaron, because it sounds too much like attachment and you hate that.'

Aaron is silent for a moment or two. Then he holds my chin so my eyes meet his. 'I really want you to hear this.' He chooses his words carefully, words he means with all his heart: 'I like you, and I'm your friend.'

I look at him for a bit; I feel both happy and sad at the words. Happy to have a friend like him and sad that he isn't more than that. I don't know yet that, for him, to 'like' someone is a high compliment, something more solid than love. But what if he should move on for some reason?

'If I disappeared, I can't believe you wouldn't find exactly what you have now,' he says.

He's speaking for himself, I realize; if I disappeared, *he* would find someone else.

'I'd find sex like this,' I say, 'but not the energy that is you.'

That's the truth and he knows it. Only he can't understand what it is about his energy that is so attractive to me.

'It's your spirit energy,' I try to explain again. 'It's like my own. I see myself in you. We're the same. It's your soul, the quality of your being.'

I thought he had understood this. But men forget, perhaps.

I'm happy to lie next to him, but a sadness creeps into my heart. *This man is too young to understand.* I thought we had found each other at last: two pieces of one soul — soul-mates — but to him there's no such thing.

'We're individuals,' he says once more. 'We die alone. All I can take with me is my energy and what I've done with it, its qualities.' He follows this with, 'I'd like to have sex with you.'

I remove the clothes he calls Vogue Plate, although it's only a denim skirt over pantyhose. He's wearing a blue check shirt — a concession to the cold — over a white T-shirt. The colour of the shirt suits his eyes so much, the sight almost hurts. I have to look away because his exquisite beauty grabs my soul beyond anything I'm capable of controlling. It's a sure sign I'm in love; I'm not quite sane.

In moments he makes me melt. I'm ecstatic and he watches me with delight.

A recent detox diet has done something to his face: I swear he looks no more than nineteen. I can't take my eyes off his face; to look at him makes me swoon so much it's almost indecent. In the background Creedence Clearwater Revival is playing — music I haven't heard for decades.

'You're making love the way you used to thirty years ago,' he whispers. His hands have been loosely clenched beside his chest, but he takes my buttocks now, to move me the way he wants.

'But it's much more intense than thirty years ago.'

It was special back then, but not like this. I would never have let him go if it were; it would have been impossible. But I'll still have to let him go now, even if not yet. We don't know what the details are, but a feeling is gathering that all this will be curtailed; by distance, at least (his beloved house in Darkan is so far away), and by the myriad possibilities that can fill the spaces of time.

Aaron's fascinated by black holes. To him, they're a powerful symbol of hell.

'Only a black hole is singularly dark. Its attraction for anything that has arrived in its field is absolutely irresistible. The agonisingly painful reality about a black hole is that the offered attraction has no consummation. There's never, ever, any union. Time is literally stretched out to infinity, so there's no "getting there".'

Ah! Now I understand Aaron's fascination. This is what the misery of attachment is all about.

What's the opposite to this black hole scenario? Is it a white hole? But there isn't such a thing. No; the opposite must mean to give out, to radiate instead of attract. To radiate unconditionally, like the sun.

'I go into a black hole sometimes,' he says. 'Stay away from me when I do. I know how to get out of them.'

I most certainly will. I have no desire to go to the 'event horizon', as that wizard of physics, Stephen Hawkings, calls it, and get sucked in.

DON COMES TO VISIT

Any real ecstasy is a sign
you are moving
in the right
direction
St Teresa of Avila

 Lady Chatterley's Lover and DH Lawrence's other works were on the list of forbidden books when I was a nun in the convent. When I finally got to read the infamous story of love between Lady Chatterley and the keeper of her estate, I was deeply touched by Lawrence's descriptions of the passionate nature of real and total sexuality. I couldn't see why the novel had ever been called pornographic. Those critics must have had the stuffiest of love lives themselves to be so upset by the raw beauty of unfettered loving.

'What are people going to say about my book?' I ask Don when he comes to visit me. I've been showing him my notes now and again for this story I feel compelled to write about my relationship with Aaron. Before this, I was writing a self-help book for women who had been abused, but only weeks after meeting Aaron again, the reasoned style of the workbook had to give way to expressing in words what was going on inside me, because of the enormous change to my quiet life. For most of my life, I've journalled to get my emotions onto paper so I can make more sense out of them. Only recently have I confided to Aaron what I'm doing, and my feeling that our story may become the stuff of my next book. Aaron blanched temporarily, then dismissed his concern with the sensible thought that publication was very far away. Besides that, somewhere in his face I swear I saw a glimpse of a thought that this could actually be rather neat: himself, Aaron, in a book. Even so, he refuses to read any of my notes; a good move, I think, in case he becomes self-conscious. Even if he did read my writing and object to its content, it would be impossible for me to stop. I am obeying a call, an immensely strong pull to write what comes to me.

Nevertheless, I value the input of an objective reader and have emailed Don some chapters.

Today he comes to my house to give me feedback and to answer my question about how people might respond to my book. Don begins by telling me about a close friend who does lap-dancing at a club. 'When she first came to Perth she won a contest, because she was so wholehearted and open,' he says. 'She showed herself completely — physically and emotionally, unself-consciously and without limitation. People loved it. But she's no longer like that. She's become reserved — still provocative, but holding back where it matters most. A good performance, but not something that stops the heart with its beauty.'

Don hesitates a moment. Then: 'People want God,' he says. 'They hunger for what comes out of the soul. Look around you. How much writing is there, in literature, about great love-making? What you're doing with your writing is expressing your innermost soul, and it will be what people want. How to present it so it won't be mistaken for anything less will be your challenge.'

THE STUFF OF CRISIS

And truly I was afraid, most afraid.
DH Lawrence, 'Snake'

 It's Wednesday evening and I haven't seen Aaron since Thursday. Six days without any communication. He doesn't have a mobile, and there isn't a phone in his under-the-house room at his parents' place.

Aaron left his home in Darkan with the idea of becoming a teacher so he could earn the money he needed to renovate his house. If he hadn't come to Perth in January to study, we probably wouldn't have met up. Aaron spotted the article about me in his father's newspaper, but didn't contact me until after he'd settled down to his university routine. 'I had to psych myself up for meeting you again,' he said. 'I knew that my life probably wouldn't be normal any more.'

Aaron has suffered several crises in his studies. More than once he's been convinced he should give it away, except that his character isn't the quitting kind and so he continued with renewed determination.

He's sitting an exam right now. I've been sending him encouragement via my thoughts. For hours on end as I work, my inner ear listens to the music we've shared. In my imagination, I dance to our favourite tracks to increase the flow of energy towards him. This is a particularly difficult exam for him, to do with language.

'I have a reading problem,' he's said more than once. Apparently, he got stuck on a particular way of reading as a child; his study of how children learn has made him aware of it. Aaron is also predominantly right-brained. It took him a decade in three separate universities to complete his degree in architecture, the difficulty even then being his problem with understanding academic language. His brain copes very well with everything to do with imagination, spaces and materials, but just won't remember academic statements that mean nothing to him. Yet he still wants to be a teacher. He gets on so well with children.

I begin to notice a consistent study pattern in Aaron: he looks at a question and *guesses* the answer before finding the information in the text. This is the reason for his failure: he's trying to answer questions with what he thinks is the truth, when all that he's being asked to do is furnish his tutors with the information given in books and lectures, using the proper jargon. Finding information specific to a question, without having read the whole text first, can be infuriatingly difficult, yet that's what he's been attempting.

I advise him in my most earnest voice to read the text at least three times before attempting to answer questions on it. A lesser man may baulk at his girlfriend becoming his teacher. Not so Aaron: he kisses me fervently to thank me. 'How simply and elegantly put,' he says.

A strange thing occurs at 10.15 a.m. — so strange I make a point of looking at the clock. In the middle of doing my housework upstairs, my belly suddenly goes into turmoil and I feel sick. I immediately connect it with something going on with Aaron. I don't feel good about it; this feeling could be an indication of the wrong kind of attachment, one that could hurt me. Half an hour later, the sensation disappears. I am peaceful again and the inner music returns.

What was it about? Was Aaron upset about something; perhaps daunted by his exam? Was he attracted to someone, and giving her the kind of attention that could break the connection between us for that time?

I have to face the fact again that there is a large age difference between us. More than that, if Aaron successfully gains his teacher's diploma, he'll most likely go north to work in a remote Aboriginal community. That would really suit him: he'd delight in forging good relationships with the people, as well as getting the children onside. There'd be plenty of scope for his sense of fun and his innovative character. Roughing it doesn't bother him. At the end of a couple of years, he'd have the money he needs to finish building his house. The only thing is: there's no room for me in any of these plans.

At 8 p.m. Aaron rings, asking to come and talk to me. This is odd; he's supposed to be in another exam now. 'I'll explain later,' he says.

It's a different Aaron who comes in the door. His smile is ambiguous: he's pleased to be at my place again — such a peaceful haven for him, he says — but he's also just failed his course.

'The whole course?' I repeat, puzzled.

'Yep, this subject was crucial to me staying in the course, and I failed it.'

'Are you sure you failed it?'

Aaron pulls out some sheets of paper covered in his handwriting. I read them:

> *My mind has gone blank. I'm completely unconcerned about it. Nothing at all comes to mind that will help me answer my exam questions. I did all the preparation for it, to the last detail. My room is hung with papers, with all the information in logical sequences, with mind maps and references, and I can imagine going into my room but can't read anything from the papers, and I remember absolutely nothing from what I studied.*

I'm quiet. What can you say to this kind of thing?

'I left the room so my confused energy wouldn't affect the other students,' Aaron says. 'They were all going at it as hard as they could. I cried on the way back to my car. I'm so glad I was alone then. I kept crying as I drove here. My plans are in ruins. I can't be a teacher. All I wanted was to work in the outback with some Aboriginal kids, watch the landscape, live in a simple house, but I'm not made for this academic stuff. I think there's something wrong with the wiring of my brain, or else there's emotional stuff there getting in the way of my succeeding in this.'

'It could be a bit of both,' I say.

'I feel like a little boy again,' he says, 'hating to go to school because he gets teased by the same bullies, year after year. My parents don't understand how horrible it is for me to go to school. I can't get it right. The teachers tell me I'm no good. I can't do it the way the other children do.'

Aaron's talking in present tense, as if he's that little boy right now. He moans, and puts his head in his hands. He's so willing for me to see him in this utterly vulnerable state.

'You're a good listener,' he says. 'I'm visual. All my life, I've encouraged my visual ability. I did architecture, which is a lot about visualising and drawing spaces, and I watch videos instead of reading books.'

He's also got a great understanding of physics — I've noticed this from the conversations we've had. A visual/scientific mind not suited to remembering a whole lot of academic data for reproduction in an exam.

'Reality's setting in,' he says grimly.

I finally have something to say. 'In spite of what it looks like just now, this event can't be all bad. I even sent you some special energy this morning, and then again at six o'clock this evening.'

He jumps at that. 'So it was you! You did that to me!' He's not accusing me, although what I did had an effect and not the one he'd wanted. But I have implicit trust in the divine intelligence that directs such love energy. It must have been the right effect somehow.

He nibbles at my brazil and almond nuts until they're all gone. Then he eats two pears, an apple and a banana. He's not had dinner; he'd gone to his exam without any food in his stomach.

'Can we lie down and cuddle?' he asks wearily.

I take him to my bedroom and lead by removing all my clothes. He's relieved that I do this, loves being comfortably naked. We cuddle and kiss and soon he feels better, though still shocked, still numb, still liable to slide into depressive thoughts. I witness the whole emotional spectrum.

He finally laughs. 'This is such a humiliating experience! I had such grandiose thoughts about myself, even that I was special.'

Now I know what made me feel sick this morning. It wasn't merely that his connection to me had been broken; he'd lost his belief in himself. He'd fallen for the idea that he couldn't do the exam, couldn't pass the course, and it had been like falling into a vortex of negativity. Once inside the exam room, he sat in the eye of the storm without any part of his brain moving.

'You might have the new experience of being ordinary,' I say.

Aaron tells me about the three months he spent in therapy. The therapist asked him about his father: what characteristics of his father's made him angry. Aaron came up with sixteen traits and expressed huge anger. But the thing is, he didn't get rid of his anger about his father's negative traits; he just realised that he didn't want to be like his father.

'Well,' I say pragmatically, 'it's too late. You're like him already.'

Aaron looks stunned, but it must have been obvious to him too that this anger hadn't had any positive results; he just needed a person like me to say it — 'the emperor isn't wearing any clothes' kind of revelation.

Two weeks later, Aaron has a different attitude.

'I'll do anything to heal what's inside me,' he says. 'I know that my memory loss in the exam was to do with stress of the past, with stress of performing to get my father's approval. My father was a teacher for forty-three years. I thought I could be like him.'

It's a very long and complex story, this father–son dynamic.

AARON'S PLACE

On the Sabbath try to make no noise that
Goes beyond your house.
Cries of passion between lovers are exempt.
St Thomas Aquinas, 'On The Sabbath'

My friend Virginia lives in a street adjacent to Aaron's parents' place. She's totalled her car and I offer her a lift home at the end of an evening course we've both attended. She gives me a pamphlet titled, *Brain Mechanics: How the brain works*. I think immediately that this information would be great for Aaron. The pamphlet is like a good omen: it gives me enough courage to go to his place after dropping Virginia off, even though by now it's past 10 p.m. and raining.

My heart beats faster as I turn into the familiar street. It's been thirty-one years since I was last here. Aaron's described to me where he parks his car: down the slope of the lawn, behind some grass tree plants. I can see the grass trees — huge old things — but no car. Aaron's out. There are lights on in the house, however, so, clutching the pamphlet under my coat to keep it dry, I go up to the front door. Timidly, I knock on the glass window. I catch a glimpse of a woman making a startled move, then she opens the door. It's Aaron's mother and she immediately knows who I am.

'Aaron's not at home,' she says.

'It doesn't matter really,' I cut in, heading off whatever else she is about to say. 'I've got this pamphlet for him and just wanted to drop it by. I was in the neighbourhood and it's rather late, but I hope it's alright.'

She doesn't want me to disappear into the night and invites me in. She offers me a cup of tea and a home-made-looking biscuit. 'But it isn't,' she says, 'it came out of a packet. Have another one – you look as if you can do with feeding up.'

As we chat, I take in her presence. She's an elderly woman with a certain prettiness still about her face. She's short, her hair's white and curly, but her eyes are bright with intelligence and interest. I recognise Aaron in the shape of her mouth, her chin, the roundness of her eyes. I call her Mrs Walters. If anyone did that to me, I'd ask them to use my first name. She doesn't. It emphasises the age gap between us, although, in fact, it's probably not so many years.

Twenty minutes later, Aaron arrives back and knocks at the front door. His mother doesn't get up straightaway. I think I sense her weariness, or is she waiting for me to answer it? I'm sitting nearest the door, after all, but this isn't my house. Then she gets up, opens the door and Aaron bursts in. He walks straight past her to give me a kiss.

'What about me?' comes his mother's furious voice. She's still standing at the door, unbelieving that he would ignore her upturned, expectant face.

Aaron walks back to her. 'You're second, Mum,' he says as he kisses her. 'You're second.'

He sits on the couch opposite me and she has to take that in as she makes her way back to her chair.

'Do you want a cup of tea?' she asks him, knowing he'll say yes. 'Well, make it yourself,' she adds. 'I can't be bothered getting up again.'

Mrs Walters remembers the reason for my visit. 'Carla's got a leaflet for you; it's on the dresser.'

Aaron finds it and has a brief look. To me, it's awesome divine intelligence that has arranged for this leaflet to reach Aaron. He needs to understand how his brain works right now.

Cup of tea finished, Aaron takes all the dishes and puts them in the kitchen, where he knows his father will eventually wash them, then invites me to come and see his den, his study, his cave, his room under the house. He takes me through the kitchen and laundry onto the dark verandah. 'Hello!' he says, and gives me a proper kiss and hug before leading me down several irregular steps to his domain.

I like it immediately: a cosy, extremely well-organised, neat space. It smells of fresh air — inevitable really, since the door is simply a thick curtain moving in the night breeze. There are shelves groaning with books and files built around most of the walls, a large table with two computers and a tangle of things electronic, plus a pair of speakers. A rack of clothes to one side of the room, and his bed — a single, iron-slung bedstead — to the right as you come in. There are two office chairs, one with arms.

We sit down and we talk about yesterday, about that strange and completely new experience Aaron had of brainless peace.

'You stopped thinking,' I say.

'The peace was indescribable,' he tells me. 'I was so unconcerned; the world was removed from me by miles and yet someone was sitting at the desk right next to me. There was silence, nothingness.'

What's going on with him? He talked to a counsellor at college today, and she was a good listener and understood a lot, he tells me, but she couldn't go where he wanted her to. He'd wanted her to see that this expansive experience is linked to a darkly knotted part of himself that remains from a long time ago.

'I've experienced so much trauma in my life,' he says. 'I've loved too much.'

It's true that Aaron is the rescuer type. He's proved that in his relationships with women over the years. Now, though, he feels that his compassionate nature has been through the wringer so often that he's had to shut down and become numb.

'Still, I'm not in bad shape, considering what I've been through,' he says. 'That's what my friends tell me.'

'I want you to enjoy this attachment,' says Aaron. I'm lying in his narrow bed, fully dressed except for my coat and shoes, as he is, and my forehead is against his right cheek, while his arm circles my shoulder. He moves the hair away from my forehead now and again, kisses it. 'I don't want you to get hurt.' He's said this a few times now.

A dim light is on above us and music softly fills the room. It's my music; Aaron has stored some of my CDs in his computer. It's strange to hear my music in his room. His recording system has more high fidelity; the sound is so much purer, so much more refined, so much more what it should be. It's as if he's made my music his own and improved on it. This is what Aaron does, I muse. He takes in what he loves, then lives it even better than its originator.

'The part of me that deals with relationships has really grown,' he mumbles to me with his eyes closed, his voice reverberating in his chest. 'I was a taxi driver for ten years and I experienced forty relationships a day! Forty bubbles of relationships. People who came and went in my life, people I got close to who then disappeared. I learnt to let go all the time. I also had attachments to girlfriends, deep loves, and in the end they all turned out bad. I really know what I'm doing now, when I'm in a relationship.'

Well ... does he really? Is this a credible explanation for why he sometimes doesn't contact me? Do I have to believe all this guff? Or isn't it guff? It's hard to tell with Aaron.

I watch his profile as he speaks — his mouth, his lips. His detachment has the effect of somehow firing my attachment, and he knows it. He knows it all.

He's taking his clothes off now. I take off my own as quickly as possible, because it's cold, and duck under the bed covers.

'I know you want to touch me, but my dad sleeps directly above me, so we have to be good.' Aaron points up to the beams of his ceiling. His father's — hopefully sleeping — body is literally a couple of metres away.

He kisses me back when I lift my head to his mouth, but it's a pouty kiss.

'What's with the pecky kisses?' I want to know.

'I'm keeping you cool,' he says. 'I'm retraining you to stay calm in my company.'

'It was *you* who was all on fire last time,' I retort.

He smiles. 'I was getting rid of a few years of pent-up energy then. It's not like that now. I'm getting older.' Then he adds, 'But I want you to know that I belong to you.'

He looks at me to see the impact of what he's just said, but I have no words; I'm floored.

I suddenly notice that it's way past midnight. 'I'm leaving in five minutes,' I warn.

'No, you're not.' He's quietly firm. 'You can leave when you've had a bit of sleep, but not in five minutes.' There's a pause. 'When I leave your place after a little sleep, I'm happy,' he says, 'and when I drive home, I'm happy. Then I get into my bed, and continue my sleep, and I'm happy. Be like me.'

I stay, but don't sleep. I'm too much in love. I want to drink in this moment of resting near him like this, so peacefully, even if he does snore, even if he seems to have a light form of sleep apnoea. Eventually, I get up, and he does too, putting on his socks and sneakers and joking that it's a bit of a change to see *me* dress to go home. He shows me to my car with the help of a torch and opens the door for me.

'You're a gentleman, Aaron.'

The rain has stopped. He gives me directions. It takes me half an hour to get home. Only then do I notice that it's nearly 2 a.m.

A 'sex-man' Aaron calls himself one evening. 'I'm so glad that I can just be a sex-man with you. I've had so much criticism for loving sex.'

Not that he's fixated on his penis. He has attentive hands, is even touching my breasts now. He probably does it because he can tell I like it so much, not because they turn him on. It's a wonder, though, that he doesn't clue on to the fact that I would be wet in seconds if he touched my nipples instead of trying to turn me on just with kisses.

Aaron asks whether I'll still be interested in sex when I'm seventy-five or eighty.

I laugh at the thought, at the same time starkly aware that seventy-five is only ten years away. 'I'll only be interested in serenity by then,' I venture gaily.

'Tell me ... does your age, the sense of your mortality, make the moment more intense?'

'Yes, it does. I'm aware of how short-lived everything is.'

'Good!' he says. 'That helps you to let go when you're having sex.'

He catches me again some time later, asking the question in a slightly different way. 'For how long will you be sexual?' he wants to know.

'Hmm, I don't know, maybe another ten, fifteen years.'

'Keep my name in your address book, will you?'

I can't believe he's serious. But he is.

A woman who wears black clothes, he says, wants to attract sex. Black absorbs, it doesn't give out. Women who know they are sexy, and exude it, don't need to wear black.

'What a load of codswallop,' says a Melbourne friend of mine who loves wearing black.

Aaron has a theory about women's shoes too. High heels are off the earth and are about uneasy control. Low heels, he says, are on the earth and allow the earth energy to flow up the body.

My friend has to agree, reluctantly.

WHAT IS LOVE, THEN?

Romance is a simple
mistake
Nirmala, untitled poem

Denise and I have been friends for about twenty years, even though we're very different in our lifestyles and tastes. She's a pretty brunette of forty-six, and her romantic style of dressing suits her. She has a sweet smile and a lilting voice. A perfect hostess with great cooking skills, she's also extremely well informed about health, and successfully runs a business based on water filtering systems. I'm her occasional cleaner, as well as her friend; I'm good at this job and enjoy it.

Today, I'm visiting to retrieve a book by Dan Brown I lent her. As usual, Denise's cheerfully chatty. I look for an opportunity to mention that I have a lover, after twelve years of celibacy. When I come out with it, I immediately regret it.

'Ooh!' Denise coos. 'Just like me! I met Alan two months ago. We can't keep our hands off each other!'

My heart sinks at her frivolous attitude. Is this what love is? Can't keep our hands off each other? In spite of the passion Aaron and I share, we're not like that. My heart is sorry for Denise, who has had a string of attachments that have all ended with her heart badly broken. She doesn't seem to need to know anything more about my relationship and I'm relieved. I eat some of her excellent home-made soup and go home. I can't stop thinking about the idea of relationship, though.

Everything ends, I remind myself, and that reminder stops me from losing my centre. Denise's relationship will end. My relationship with Aaron will end. It's forever changing; already the shape of it is dying, even at this moment, and a new shape will freshly appear.

Oh, my Beloved! I silently address the only One who never changes — my Self, to whom I can be faithful unto death, and death will not part us but will instead remove any idea of separation that ever existed. It is the only constant; everything revolves around it. The relationship can change, even drop away, and I will still have my centre, my Self.

'I'm committed to my Self and that will never change,' I said to Aaron once, only days after our first love-making. Aaron didn't hear the capital 'S', of course, but he did understand that I wouldn't lose myself in him and try to live my life through him. He was pleased about that. Aaron definitely doesn't want the responsibility thrown on him of having to save a heart from being broken.

It's been days since I spoke to Aaron. I miss him. I'm miserable. Where's all my talk of not needing him? If only he'd phone, just to let me know how he is. Finally, I allow myself to whimper. My whimper becomes a wail. I sound like a dog abandoned by its master. Tears run down my face. I sob.

There. My soul is laid bare. I feel like a severed electrical cord, unravelled. I can't look forward to our meeting again; it's this moment that's painful, because there's been no communication. No feeling in him is strong enough to make him go to the phone.

Another wail goes up, interrupted by a sudden need to evacuate. Ah, well, at least I have the presence of mind to thank the Infinite for my healthy bowels as I flush away the thick, smooth stools, long before breakfast. Such a change from being constipated as a nun in my convent days.

I feel the need of Aaron, but it's okay. I'd rather need him than not. I'd rather be raw than smug. I'd rather be too sensitive than dull; rather have tears than dry up. My body's not on a rack like it used to be in my younger days, when I was jealous. This is a sweeter pain, just the other side of pleasure.

I sense that the price of my passion will always be pain. But even as I think this, pleasure returns. Are all emotions illusions then? They do seem to share an illusory quality.

I think of the movie *Troy* I saw recently, and that one line by Brad Pitt's character that made this Hollywood excuse for bloodthirsty machismo worthwhile for me: *The gods envy us because we are mortal.* The Greek gods live forever, but we humans die a thousand deaths every day and then die for good. Is this why, when we experience the greatest pleasure, we think of death?

Unlike the gods, we can't be complacent about our loves and passions. The price we pay for not seizing the moment is the sound of time ticking by.

Contrary to Aaron's expectations, he hasn't failed all of his exams, and he's working hard again. I've come to visit him in his study; he's had his face down in his books for over an hour now. At last he comes to join me (already snuggled in his narrow bed), keeping his T-shirt, socks and underpants on, same as me. It's long past the bedtime deadline Aaron's given himself. He wants to be up bright and early tomorrow morning, for his third day of teaching practice. It's taken all this time to complete the preparation, and I admire the discipline and concentration he's put into the task.

He whispers, since his father, Rick, is upstairs in his room. We hear him shuffle about, and then the bed creaks above our heads as he launches himself into it.

'Your dad's deaf, though,' I say.

'Isn't.'

'What?'

'Isn't!' he says emphatically.

'So he pretends to be deaf, is that it?'

'Mm.'

Interesting. Maybe it is a strategy Rick has adopted to create distance between himself and his wife. It doesn't work. She feels even freer to give voice to her feelings, releasing them into the common space, while he simply keeps silent.

Aaron didn't formally introduce me to his father; instead, he swept into the house and left me at the door with Rick. He didn't extend his hand to me but I didn't take it as a sign that he didn't want me there; more that he has become extremely rusty when it comes to expressing cordiality. It was difficult to see into Rick, because his eyes wouldn't meet mine.

So we whisper in the semi-darkness, Aaron and I. The only source of light is from the computer at the end of the room, which is also the source of the soft music wafting over us. What can we do in this confined space, with his father's ears above us?

We start by discarding pants and socks; they fly through the darkness. We keep our tops on for ease of dressing later. I make a reluctant move to turn my back to him; he knows why — it's the most practical position in the circumstances — but he asks me to face him.

'Can I enter you from the front?' he says.

I nod, turning towards him. But how is he going to manage it?

Penetration is just too difficult because of the confined space. I decide to sit on top of him. There, the perfect position for a cramped space. It gives him more control over what's happening than when he's on top, with his weight causing the wire-slung bed to make terrible creaking noises. Also, with me on top, our weight is more evenly distributed, keeping the bed from sagging as much. He drapes the thin white doona over my head and shoulders to keep me warm. He pulls the doona — and me — towards him, creating a tent-like space. The scent of unwashed bodies wafts up — neither of us has been near a shower since this morning.

'Excuse me, won't you,' he says, and collects some spittle to put on our genitals.

My vagina envelops his penis and I'm at once in that indescribable place. He's concerned that I'll make a noise.

'Take it steady — like this,' he demonstrates, taking me by the hips. 'Stay still; let me do it,' and he moves my body up and down with his powerful arms. He relaxes against the pillow, keeping up the steady movement, eyes dilating in the darkness.

He doesn't know how beautiful he looks when he makes love, but I tell him. The last time I said this, he made movements with his hands to indicate that what I was saying was giving him a swollen head, but I told him it had nothing to do with him. He remembers this when I say, 'You're beautiful, and don't take this for your ego.'

It seems to be a time for compliments.

'You look so young when you make love,' he suddenly says.

My face is different, flushed with the heat of rapture, and I acknowledge his words with my eyes.

What he says next seems out of sequence. 'I will die alone,' he whispers intently, as if informing me of something he's known for a long time. 'And when I die, I will know that you love me.'

His hands have abandoned the doona and are around my shoulders as he says this. I take one of them and lay it against my cheek. It's so warm, and the energy from it so gentle, so masculine, so much the touch of what I remember from thirty years ago, I'm ready to die myself — from sheer emotional overload.

I'm in your life because I want you to be all you can be. That's what love is.

'Together and apart,' I hear him say, telling me once more of his fear of attachment.

I kiss him, and he asks me to stop.

'It'll make me come.'

'No, Aaron, don't do that!' I'm thinking of tomorrow. He'll need his energy to be bright and vital when he steps in front of his class. And so we stop moving and spend time just being with one another, with me still sitting on top of him. In a while he takes me again, keeping me at a perfect distance to prevent too deep a penetration. I admire his skill and strength.

'I've had lots of practice,' he quips. 'I know some party tricks, like you do.'

'Party tricks?' My elbow is on his chest, my face close to his. '*I don't have any party tricks!*'

He sees my serious face and laughs. I don't like the sound of 'party tricks' at all. So cheap! He makes good a bit later with a stream of compliments. He times his words with our rhythm and they come out staccato:'I . . . love . . . having . . . my . . . dick . . . inside . . . your . . . vagina; can't . . . think . . . of . . . a . . . better . . . place . . . to . . . put . . . it. I'm . . . so glad . . . you . . . love . . . sex . . . and . . . you . love , , , me . . . and . . . I . . . could . . . have . . . you . . . like . . . this . . . all . . . night.'

I bend down to kiss him again.

'How did you survive without kisses for *twelve years*?' he wonders.

'I had angel kisses,' I tell him. I think he knows me well enough now to understand.

'You're so good to be with,' he whispers. 'I love fucking you.'

It's the first time he's used the 'F' word. It's strange how this word can be totally inoffensive and deeply erotic.

'I love being fucked by you, Aaron.'

And the words take us deep into a state of hypnotic arousal, our whispering giving them an extra charge of intensity. I feel the juices inside me well up; no need for lubricant of any other kind tonight.

Aaron is compelled to tell me what's so important to him. 'With you there are absolutely no politics. You love me and want me, and you let me know it, and there's not a hint of manipulation anywhere. I'm waiting for that to change, and it doesn't! I know now that this is who you are: simple, direct, no games.'

He eases off when I ask him and I think that I'll soon be getting off him and the bed and leaving to go home. But before I make that final move, he resumes thrusting, knowing that the sensation will be more intense for having waited. Once again he wants to see the swooning on my face, so helpless, so gone and so silent, clamping down on the desire to wail; instead, with my throat closed, hearing the sound somewhere in the ether. He finally lets himself go.

In the midst of our gentle coming-down, I think back to an exchange we had earlier this evening, when he'd conjured up Kate Bush's picture on his computer.

'What do you see there?' he asked.

'A luscious woman,' I replied.

'Luscious? How?'

'Luscious mouth,' I said.

'You know that's mainly make-up, don't you?'

I shrugged my shoulders and continued. 'Gorgeous wild hair, beautiful dark eyes, lovely face.'

'She's the kind of woman that has no time for you,' he said. 'If you did anything she didn't like, she'd spit you out. No hesitation.'

I looked at her again, at that coolly self-possessed expression. Maybe he was right; he was talking from past experience of falling for irresistibly beautiful women who wanted to possess him the way Kate Bush was proclaiming in her painfully tragic and bitter songs. *Why did you leave me, just when I wanted to possess you?*

Aaron is desperate for some normality, some dependability.

'I see dysfunctional relationships everywhere,' he says. 'I look around and see a lot of very lonely people. You and I have learnt to be alone, and we could get along without each other and still be happy. Our togetherness is a bonus.'

The next evening I'm at Aaron's again. His homework's finished and we snuggle up in his bed.

'You were my first love,' he says, 'and I've looked for you in every love since then. Your love became a reference point for what was true and what wasn't. I know that now. I've yearned for you for thirty years.'

We'd both fallen in love with something so pure in one another that we would never forget it. Back then, we couldn't have appreciated the rarity of this meeting of souls; only time would teach us this by way of other experiences — also wonderful and truly loving, yet not encompassing that unique, pristine quality. That quality was like a peculiar kind of music, reverberating forever after in the ether.

I didn't speak these words; I just thought them. Words come out of Aaron's mouth so confidently, so gracefully, but I tend to stumble. He looks at me and smiles, knowing I have this limitation when making love; my verbal brain switches off when awash in ecstatic hormones.

Aaron suggests putting pillows on the floor so we can make love and allow deeper penetration on the more solid surface. I consider this, but tell him what he knows already: I'm likely to shriek with deep penetration. So we don't. Besides, it's cold out there. So I decide to sit on top of him again.

During our love-making, when I'm lying on his chest, Aaron loses it. He suddenly becomes anxious and tells me to roll off him, *now*! It takes a few moments for my brain to respond to his urgency and then I flop unceremoniously beside him, head on my elbow, eyes asking, 'What's the matter?'

He's listening to sounds and I realise he's expecting his mother to walk in, even at this time of night. She'd come down unexpectedly earlier this evening to offer him the upstairs dining table to work on, since upstairs is nicely heated and Aaron's den on the cool side. She'd noticed my cold fingers when we'd held hands to say grace together before dinner and scolded Aaron for not looking after me.

'So what if she comes in?' I'm unmoved by his concern. 'If she wants to walk in on us, she'll get what she came for. Who cares?'

He relaxes, and says, 'You're right, I'm not a thirteen-year-old any more. Come to think of it, neither are you.'

He wants me return to our previous position. I say no, and get up to get dressed. Aaron sees me to my car. It's about 10.30 p.m., a bit later than planned, but not too late for both of us to get a good night's sleep, ready for a working day tomorrow.

He tells me more about his mother. 'She loved me coming up from Darkan to live at home. She could get back into the mother thing and look after me. Since I've met you again, she knows she's not the only woman in my life. She can't control me either, and she doesn't try. We sit and talk, and lately she's been telling me about her teenage years. Why would she be doing that? Maybe she's reviewing her life as she gets ready to die. She's been sad and angry for years, always wanting to be loved by my dad the way he never did love her. I asked her, why look for love where you know you won't get it? But my mum and dad are in a rut now and they'll probably never change.

'She can't quite place you,' he goes on. 'You're older than me, but not as old as she is. She's really old.'

'How old is she?' I ask.

'Seventy-five.'

I thought she'd be older to be 'really old', but she sees me as a youngster. '*Take care of that girl,*' she said at dinner. '*Her hands are cold.*'

LET'S MAKE A PACT

. . . feast on this
feed the deepest longing
drink until thirst is a distant memory
Nirmala, untitled poem

 It's early in the morning, about five o'clock. I've dreamed about Aaron. I can't remember the pictures, just the feelings: heavy feelings. Feeling that death is not far away — not mine, but Aaron's. Not so long ago, Aaron dropped a bombshell. 'I'll die at fifty-four,' he said. 'I had this intuition when I was only six and asked God how long I had to stay on this planet.'

My breathing is quite shallow, I notice. I get a pen and paper and write to Aaron.

Today I know that you will die way before me. You said yourself, months ago, that you had an intuition you'd die at fifty-four. Are all your warnings for me not to fall in love with you meant to prepare me for that moment?

My love, when we die, let's decide not to come back to this plane of existence again. Let's decide this together. If we come back, we have to go through all that suffering of forgetting again, before waking up once more to who we are and spending many years searching for each other. Look how many years it took this time! Look how few years there are left, if it's still years we can count on.

I've seen your death in my dream. I've seen those lips so dear to me; that mouth, silent, without breath, without the ability to feel or respond. I've seen your eyes closed, no longer able to look at me. Although my dream didn't reveal how it was you died, I wasn't far away. You died on your own, knowing that I love you, just as you yourself predicted. My grief won't be helped. It will create a wail in heaven no soul can ignore. But you must learn to listen and not hear. You must know that this time, grief will be a very short song, and your decision to stay around me out of compassion part of a long, long history. I don't want you around, even if my whole heart longs for your presence.

Instead, let's make a pact. Promise, once the angels have taken you away from the immediacy of this plane, not to hesitate to enter the Light. The opportunity will only present itself for the briefest of time, if I'm to believe the Tibetan Book of the Dead. Only the soul who knows surrender will take oblivion.

Isn't it you who are teaching me not to get lost in you? Well, my love, don't you get lost in compassion. I need you to lead the way. Let's have enough of to-ing and fro-ing and stay with ourselves for ever.

In the meantime, let me dance for you. I dreamed that you died before I did this dance, so you must sit and be entertained. And after that, listen to the song of grief and longing that will reverberate through the heavens after you die. Listen to it now so you will recognise it and not be moved by it. No song is the truth. This song will die.

I would sense it if you decided to stay around in ethereal form. Then you would be a guide to me until that form, too, dissolved and you were finally laid to rest.

Consider well what you truly want, my love. Perhaps it's no big deal for you; perhaps it's only my own heart I'm addressing: the challenges that would face me, were I the first to go. But I know that it will be you.

And now I'll just stop all this. It won't do to get maudlin, after all. The dramas we cook up for ourselves! My heart is breaking already. I went to a funeral yesterday, you see. A sister of a friend died at the age of fifty-two from deep vein thrombosis. Her daughters spoke about their mother, and her husband let his words be spoken by the celebrant. 'You were always keen for us to use the correct word,' she read, 'and for us to know the meaning of words. Now, I know the meaning of the word grief.'

You're not here, so I can't dance for you just yet. You wanted to go to your nephew's birthday party and make him a card. That's exactly how it should be. Your nephews and nieces are lucky to have an uncle so genuinely interested in them — the best uncle alive! That pun makes me smile and eases the pain. It's no use thinking that we'll be apart for an eternity and make that a reason for being together. Just live one moment at a time, being an uncle, being a lover, being a son, being whatever the moment calls for.

Let me be in peace.

I am speaking to the pain in my chest. Oh, I hope that tomorrow I'll breathe better again, after a different dream.

This same evening, Aaron comes around after leaving his nephew's party. He's just been with a lively group of youngsters and is beaming. As for me, I've just come back from a Pilates exercise session and am glowing with vitality. He gazes at me with admiration, remarking on how well I look. I look at him strangely; I am seeing someone alive who has been imagined dead. It is such a joy to see him. I now understand how people feel when they have anxiously awaited news of a loved one when he or she may have died overseas — after the bomb blast in Bali in October 2002, for instance. To see a daughter, son or wife, husband or friend, alive at such a time is like a special bonus. Life suddenly becomes more precious. A person's presence becomes profoundly appreciated.

'I want to dance for you. Sit there, Aaron, and watch.'

I put on Emma Shapplin's music, and take on a pose electrified by her passion. Music makes my body fluid. It can do things in response to music that it can't do in the gym. My spine loosens up, my head comes undone from its rigid hold, and my hands, arms and legs become like flowing rivers of energy. My whole body becomes alive with sensuality. I can forget myself and immerse myself in this indulgence of delight in moving ...

I don't get very far. Aaron's eyes light up and he just can't help himself: he gets up, comes in close, and wants to join me in the dance. If only he'd move freely in his own space! But no, he grabs my hands and wants to dance in tandem. Aaron has no sense of rhythm and his feet are slow. The effect of this is that he stops me dead.

I frown at first, then have to laugh. I forgive him: after all, he's just a hopeless admirer. His face glows, oblivious to the fact that he's just killed off my dance. Who cares anyway? I can dance by myself tomorrow, as I often do, by way of a work-out.

After Aaron leaves, I lie down on the floor with my feet propped up on my wobbler — a machine that wobbles the feet sideways and allows the spine to follow with a pleasant sway. If being soul-mates means anything, this relationship must be it, I muse. Not because we get on so well, which is what people imagine about soul-mates, but because we seem to be different aspects of the same energy — energy differentiated into male and female but with a common core.

And then I remember my dream, and that I wouldn't finish a dance for him before he died.

Tonight, Aaron has come to share his thoughts about the funeral he attended this afternoon — for Bill, a distant friend from his rebellious hippie days. No longer a hippie himself, Aaron's friends stay in touch and he respects their loyalty. It's strange that both of us should be at a funeral the very same week. It's a bit like the way he injured the ring finger on his left hand two days ago and today I cut mine on the right hand. He put his hand against mine: we mirrored each other!

Bill's funeral affected Aaron in an unexpected way. There was no funeral parlour, no speeches, just a rent-a-priest ceremony for a man, aged seventy-two, who had mostly led a destitute life. The coffin was very small. 'He must have shrunk,' Aaron mutters.

'There were about forty people there,' Aaron goes on. 'All hard faces. Samantha, my old girlfriend, was there, with her no-good boyfriend. They kept complaining about each other like they always do. So I said to them, "Why don't you get yourselves some nice person to have a relationship with, both of you, and leave each other alone!"'

'What did they say?'

'They said, "Where do you find nice people?" They don't have a clue! I realised I'd spent years living in a really crappy world like theirs. You live in such a different world, Carla. It's so simple, your world. And so good.'

I look at him and sense the weight in him of years of rejecting the society he was born into, which he sees as lacking in every good and worthwhile value. He joined a crowd whose rejection becomes their badge of honour, without realising they're hurting themselves in the process with their sarcastic, caustic criticism. It fills them like a sickness.

Aaron confesses that he feels depressed. I nod, noticing the greyness of his face, the lack of humour in his eyes. I ask him what kind of thoughts he's having. He says his bright plans of becoming a teacher and getting a well-paid job so he can build his house are coming to a grinding halt because he just can't go on with his studies. 'My life's gone down a big hole,' he says. I've heard that phrase a few times now. It's time to challenge it.

'Is this true?'

'No, it isn't true,' he says. 'I don't know. I'm just being depressed.'

I ask him who is doing the depressing.

'It's me, only me,' he admits. 'I just don't know how to think other thoughts. My brain is terribly fatigued.

'Do you know what I'd like?' he asks.

I can't guess, of course, so he launches shyly into describing an imagined scene.

'I'm relaxing in a cane chair, surrounded by trees and shrubs, and there's no sound except some bush animals here and there, and the feeling of the breeze on my face. No traffic and no music. It's sunny, very bright and warm, and you're in the background, walking about in the house, doing things.'

He looks at me.

'Nice picture.' I briefly cradle his head in my arms before I open the fridge.

His scene is a picture of healing. In reality, he's living the opposite right now, although in Darkan he may have close to what he imagines. He'll go there soon, to feel the healing influence of nature. His soul longs for it. Only I won't be there; I have things to do that will keep me in Perth. That part of the picture will have to come later.

I place sticks of celery, cut into strips, on the table, and a newly opened jar of tahini. 'Organically grown and very sweet,' I tell him about the celery, enticing him because his appetite is low. He has already knocked back my offer of soup. We talk; he mentions his coming exam. Yes, he wants to re-sit the one he recently failed, and study for it every day so he won't have to cram on the last day, as before. The celery is demolished, then a pear and an apple. We each down a glass of stout.

I've developed a taste for this dark beer lately, and drinking it is helping me put on weight. I can't drink wine; it makes me woozy immediately, destroys my brain cells. This sweet-tasting stout is without preservatives, full of healthy vitamins and does me good. Last week, after giving a talk at the Bunbury Golf Club, I requested a bottle as a thank-you gift, instead of the proffered bottle of wine. I should have done this long ago; should have told people that I'm not a wine drinker, thanks very much, but some bottles of stout would be lovely.

Feeling slightly better, Aaron takes himself off to the bedroom to lie down and rest. I follow. It's no good him wearing his tracksuit under the doona, or for me to keep on my corduroys, so we take these off. Aaron keeps on his underpants and T-shirt, and I my white sockettes, panties and a singlet. I take off my bra — the thing with falsies that I'm ashamed of. I keep my distance, knowing Aaron's not feeling romantic, but he puts his right arm under me and pulls me to him. I lie on my side with my head close to his while he stays on his back. And so we rest, legs loosely entwined. I make not a single move to change his mood, respecting our agreement and his need for recovery.

Aaron turns to plant kisses on my head every few seconds, then returns to his thoughts, or to semi-sleep. I notice when his breathing changes, indicating sleep, but he doesn't go far enough down to really sleep. He moves to take my head in his hands and kiss me. I return his kiss, but let myself sink back in repose. Aaron removes his remaining clothes, throwing them at a chair not far away. I'm comfortable with mine on and keep my eyes closed in rest while he's undressing.

It's Aaron who languidly starts kissing me, again and again, until I raise my head up from the pillow to kiss him properly. Our kissing excites both of us. I can feel the fluctuations of his penis against my leg, but it's only a temporary excitement, not something urgent or fully sexual. I feel comfortable kissing him with relish, fully, with heart wide open, enjoying him for this. Then I feel him pulling at my panties, playfully tugging the material against my clitoris. I feel sexual and it's nice. I relax.

Before Aaron arrived this evening, I'd been reading about the healing properties of sexual intercourse in Mantak Chia's book *Healing Love Through the Tao; Cultivating Female Sexual Energy*. He describes postures in love-making that produce energies for specific areas of the body, for both the female and male. An idea enters my head.

'I want to sit on top of you,' I tell Aaron, 'and you're not to do anything except tighten the muscles of your anus while you send energy to your liver and kidneys.'

Aaron agrees. He's intrigued, but doesn't feel the need to ask questions.

I grope for my socks and throw them into the distance, followed by my panties. I get on my knees and reach for the lubricant, applying it generously to his half-flaccid penis and my genitals. I know he likes me to rub the tip of his penis against my clitoris, so I start to do this, slowly, rhythmically, with all of my attention. When his penis becomes erect enough to insert it, I bring it into the first folds of my vagina and move only over the tip still, without any hurry. When this results in a full erection, I slowly bring myself over his penis completely and rest on his abdomen. I can't feel him well this way, but that's not the point. I keep moving myself up and down his shaft, halfway, then all the way, varying the length. With my right hand, I feel his balls and then manipulate them gently.

'Are you pulling at your sphincter?' I ask.

He nods, his hands in fists beside his torso, his eyes glowing, his face coming alight. His penis grows inside me and I moan to feel it excite my vagina. Aaron involuntarily lifts his buttocks to push his penis up further, making me gasp with sudden pleasure. He relaxes again, takes it all in, occasionally repeating his brief thrusting.

'Are you thinking of your liver and your kidneys?' I ask.

'I'm enjoying looking at your face. You glow when you make love.'

I remember from the book that this is what is supposed to happen. 'Yes, that's part of the healing; enjoy!' And I keep up my motion, growing into the pleasure of it, my eyes and face swooning, hoping that this will be part of his healing.

I take off my cotton singlet, deciding not to hide any more what he knows I'm not comfortable with. He does what he's never done before, something that makes me cry out in sheer surprise: he pulls me to him so he can fondle my breasts and nipples with his mouth. I hold on to the top of the bed to balance myself while he turns from one breast to the other. Small, deformed breasts, I call them in my mind, and even now that's how I think of them, but it makes no difference to him. He can see the honour it does me, and he fondles them again and again.

I straighten up and think of resuming my activity.

'Carla, stop!' he says suddenly. 'I want to get on top of you.'

I object.

'No, it's what I really want to do,' he says. 'I want to give *you* something.'

Our roles are reversed. I'm not prepared for what happens next. He enters me gently, then pulls the pillow out from under my head. It lands on the floor. I laugh, knowing that this changes the angle of the vagina. He knows it too, but I notice the intense seriousness on his face. Aaron bends his face to mine. His kisses are tender and total, his body bent to meet mine so our cheeks are together as he moves. I'm not to do anything but receive. He holds me close like this, our bodies together so his gentle thrusting doesn't separate us.

'Close your eyes,' he whispers.

I obey, and sink into what's happening. What I begin to feel breaks my heart: this energy that is Aaron is so loving, so sweet, that the pleasure of being in it mingles with the pain of not being able to feel all of it. This love has no boundaries.

I cry, and he holds my face against his and stays silent. He holds me so close, for so long, that I can't help but get it: he loves me absolutely, generous beyond all bounds, for eternity. He stays like this, clasping me closer and closer, his arms around my body and head, my arms around his torso. Sometimes I use my arms to pull his buttocks closer to me, and he uses this as a guide for deeper thrusting. I can't tell how long we are like this.

'Carla, close your eyes!' he orders again when he feels my eyelashes brushing his cheek. 'Feel!'

And I do, and for the first time in my life I feel beyond a threshold I didn't know existed. I allow myself to receive this energy that is Aaron into a deeper space within me, and at the same time

I give up any role to play for him. I just let it happen; I surrender to him. And I'm taken where no man has taken me before. I lose consciousness in some way. He's taking me to a space where I clearly know myself as Woman, ultimately honoured for her female energy, where she can clearly love her man for the purity of his masculinity. And the taking goes even deeper. At a certain moment, even the concept of Woman and Man recedes, and there is only an infinite feeling of spaciousness. He kisses me and I cry with the passion of it, the pain that mingles with pleasure when the senses are finally stretched to their limit.

'I want to come,' I hear Aaron saying. His voice is wistful, soft, full of fire, but not at all out of control. He's distanced himself from me a little so he can focus on my face.

I open my eyes in panic. 'No, don't!' But he smiles. 'Do you know what you're doing?' I'm partly accusing. He knows what I mean: is he now going to squander his energy? But I realise he knows exactly what he wants.

'Close your eyes, Carla; feel!'

I do, and as he comes I feel the fineness of the energy that now ripples through my body; it's like the gentlest of light explosions and this light is made of pure love. Aaron's body is back in close contact with me. 'This is how much I love you,' he finally says, lifting his head so he can see into my eyes, 'and it has no romantic connotations.' I swoon again.

Later, I will remember that there was no music of any sort in the background to influence our mood, nothing to induce romance. This is what making love is all about, and I'd only half-known it in my lifetime. My gratitude to life for giving me this experience knows no bounds.

Aaron finally lifts himself to a kneeling position. He's smiling; today, something has happened that has changed our relationship into a 'forever thing'.

'I'm not coming down in the usual sense,' he observes. 'I still feel sexual.'

Astonishing! He doesn't break from me until the fluids want to escape onto the sheets, then he makes a wad from a few tissues and hands it to me.

Once he's lying next to me, he wants me to know something. 'I came here with the firm knowledge that I would not have sex with you,' he begins. 'I'm learning to do only what I want to do.'

At least this is one positive result from his having gone so heavily against the grain in undertaking his studies.

'All I did was because I fully wanted to do it. You wanted to sit on top of me to heal me. It was a completely selfless action. You wanted nothing for yourself. It made me want to give to you what I did.'

I look at the peaceful, radiant face beside me. 'Are you still depressed?' I ask, knowing the answer. 'That depressed person isn't you.'

He puts a finger on my mouth, stopping me from becoming the therapist in this precious moment.

'I'm no longer depressed,' he says simply. And then, 'Remember this. Remember this moment, Carla.'

His words carry the weight of an admonition, a foreboding — or maybe not. Maybe he's simply saying, Remember this, because this is how you can always love.

I move to rest my head against his chest. I will remember. I can't possibly forget. This is a gift that will last for eternity.

'I loved someone else like this once,' he says.

I know that what he is saying must be significant; thoughts produced so close on the heels of our most intimate and sacred love-making.

'We were close, just like you and me, and we lived together for seven years. She hasn't spoken to me for twenty years.'

Aaron lived with her for seven years! That seems phenomenal. He's brought up the subject of his great love before — the story of a ring given him as a treasure that turned out to be a trinket — but he has never told me what actually occurred. I ask him for more details.

'Something got out of control,' he says.

'What?' I want to know so my imagination won't have to fill in the gaps and perhaps create an image worse than the truth. But he won't tell me. Whatever it is, it's not only painful but shameful, and too highly personal to share with me now. So I don't probe for an answer.

'We both made a terrible mistake and I left when it became too hard to live with.'

So it was he who left her.

'It destroyed both of us.'

His deep sense of regret is evident. He isn't looking at me as he speaks. He lies beside me, occasionally wiping a hand over his face, as if to wipe away dried tears.

'Well, she might feel that you're thinking of her,' I say, 'and you might meet up again one day. Do you know where she lives?'

No, he doesn't. 'I hear she's around, but that's all.'

A cognition drops into my soul. It's this re-experiencing what he's had before that will bring the past into focus. His past might have an opportunity to be healed. He might meet her again, and there's a chance that her hatred will have changed into what it really is: disappointed love.

'She only hates me so much because she loves me,' Aaron says wistfully, as if reading my mind.

Will they eventually get together again? This much I know: their relationship now has a chance to be healed, even at a distance, and there is a possibility that they will at least become friends.

Will I lose Aaron then? No chance of that, I tell myself — not even death would make me lose him. He might no longer be my lover, but that's not the same as losing him, although my body and mind might try to tell me this for a while.

We're already 'together and apart'. The apart bit has to do with the fact that in spite of our closeness, we know we're individuals, incapable of total union with the other as such. Love and sex bring us as close as possible, then take us beyond ourselves, to a place where our minds don't know who is what any more, before we subside into individuality again and have to live our lives from our own energy, not that of the other. At least, this is what I am beginning to learn. It takes experience and many choices for a small knowing to ripen into wisdom.

A QUESTION OF CONTROL

Give me your foolish thoughts . . .
you don't need them anymore
Nirmala, untitled poem

 Aaron is healing me of the habits I developed in the love-making of many years ago. When I started my career as a sex worker, I was motivated to make up for the incredible suppression of my sexuality during my time as a nun and reclaim myself as a woman. My sexual contact with clients who were appreciative and who flattered me with money and compliments went some way towards achieving this. I flowered in an essential way, enjoying my sexuality and giving sexual pleasure to others. I lost my inhibitions — or so I thought. But inhibition can be subtle. As a prostitute, I had to be always in control of the situation; I could never lose myself completely. Part of me hung on; hung on for dear life, in fact. I didn't want to go where I seemed to have no control.

With James, the man I married when I was thirty-two going on seventeen, I had friendly and clean sex. It was alright, but it didn't engage deep parts of me. I married James because he loved me, and although I tried to crank up loving feelings for him, it was a strain.

It was different with Hal, because I was in love with him. Hal, who was a virgin when I met him, studied up on love-making and developed some excellent techniques. Our bodies and sexual energies matched well, and it was with Hal that I experienced earth-shaking orgasms. I felt close to him during our love-making and far apart when I was out of his arms. Hal wasn't good at communicating verbally, and neither was I. We didn't think of brushing up on our communication skills, and after a few ruptures that resulted in one of us leaving, then returning, then leaving again, we parted. Hal later declared that he had never loved me. What that implies is that his love-making was all about lust and technique. I don't really believe this. I believe Hal had to convince himself that he never loved me in order to feel better about getting married to a girl he met who was twenty-three years younger. But there it is.

With the other love in my life, George, whom I met in the little town of Denmark — well, that certainly was different. With him, I felt the way I imagine women might have felt with Rasputin, the Russian monk who exuded an animal magnetism. Rasputin was a healer and so was George. He was charismatic, and physical contact with him somehow healed the spirit. I was madly in love with sex when I was with George. It was simple for him: he put out phenomenal energy and I would get lost in it. He used his sexual prowess to enthral me, until he saw that I was hopelessly attached to him. That's when he started to withdraw — his body, his presence and his conversation — and left me to sort it all out. George was afraid of intimacy. He just wanted a nice friend to fuck, without any relationship responsibilities. As for myself, I didn't know how to keep my centre with him. He loved my sex and wanted my friendship. I wanted more, but never looked hard at what it was I wanted. I wanted to be *adored*, to be *the only one in his life*, and to *live through him*. No wonder George didn't want any of that. Too bad for both of us that we weren't able to recognise then what was going on. It took a lot of growing up on my part to even begin to see the patterns operating in me. With George, I experienced letting go to a degree I hadn't done before, but I was still holding back. And my holding back had to do with not knowing who I was. I hadn't gone to the innermost parts of myself, so I couldn't share them or enter into the ecstasy of sexual abandon. All I did was get lost in George, give myself to him as much as I could to please him. This looked like total sex. I know better now.

'Shh, Carla. Close your eyes. Feel!'

I listen in deep silence while we make love, so I can feel myself and feel him. And when it's over and I share what has happened, he tells me that all I've experienced is *myself*.

'This is *you*!' he whispers emphatically. 'I want you to know who you are!'

'But it's *you* who takes me to this experience of myself, Aaron.'

'Yes, alright,' he concedes, 'but what you're feeling are *your* feelings.'

OK, I get it now. My feelings are my feelings. They aren't his feelings and he didn't induce them. What he did was to bring them out of me.

This is what Aaron does for himself. All his attention is with me as he loves and he feels *himself*.

'I'm forever in you, and you are in me, because of my love for you and your love for me,' he says. 'That's how the two become as one.'

'*Say I am you,*' the Sufi mystic Rumi said to his dearest friend, Sham. '*Say I am you.*'

'What does my penis do to you?'

Aaron asks confronting questions. He looks at my face, waiting intently for my response.

I could just say, *I'll answer that another time, thanks*. Instead, to please him, I shut my eyes and say what comes into my mind.

'I get filled up with the sense of you; you become my whole universe and I surrender to you. It's utter bliss when you thrust me further and further away from my sense of where and who I am and my mind stops thinking anything.'

I hear him breathing. He says nothing, so I open my eyes.

'All that, eh?' he says, awed.

I somehow wish he wasn't so awed, that it was an experience he himself had and that his comment was, *I understand exactly what you mean; I do the same.*

Instead, he says, 'I used to be able to feel; now I'm numb. What's happened to me?'

I've learned to take Aaron's words at face value. What he says is true for him today, perhaps wasn't yesterday, and probably won't be tomorrow. He's comparing himself with me in this moment and feeling inadequate. It's what he does sometimes. He feels out of sorts today. The pressure of study and meeting deadlines is over temporarily and all he can think of is that he wants me around.

'I've gotten used to you.'

'I miss you too, Aaron. Where's this all going to go?'

He's known unrequited love, he tells, me, waiting around for Rachel – a woman who took five lovers in three months after she rejected him for admitting he sometimes thought of other women. She'd been a fiery lover, and he felt that she just thought of pleasing herself. One night, Aaron had enough of his agony. He looked around for a symbol of his connection with her and decided on the telephone — a symbol of communication. It was winter and a fire blazed in his hearth, so he threw the telephone into the flames and watched it slowly implode. It was made of bakelite so it took a while; Aaron stood there, fist on the mantelpiece, cutting the connection that had held him in thrall . . . the umbilical cord. Finally, it was done and he went to bed, free from the attachment that had made him crazy and anorexic for three months.

In the early morning, he was awakened by a tapping at his window. It was Rachel, hair dishevelled, looking haggard. 'I couldn't sleep all night!' she said. 'It's got something to do with you. What's going on?' And it was then she knew that she loved him. But it was too late.

'Too late for you to change your mind?' I ask him, and freeze at his answer.

'There was nothing left,' he said. 'The severance was complete and couldn't be reversed.'

I look at Aaron's profile as he lies there telling me this story, and sense the strength I first admired in him when he was nineteen and already possessed what my then husband did not.

'Now I know what has made you into a man,' I say. His strength and this emotional scar are both indelibly etched onto his psyche.

Aaron wanted to honour Rachel for the brazen passion she embodied. That's why he wears that silver ring in his right ear — in her memory. It's a mixed-up story, this one.

LOVE PAIN

What a hideous dream
it was — thinking
those things were
needed to be happy
Adyashanti, *Emptiness Dancing*

 This morning I feel my heart breaking. My chest is tight and my belly's in turmoil. I can't afford to cry: I'm attending a workshop all day. But as it happens, the workshop provides the perfect opportunity for me to break down and cry. I am learning the Emotional Freedom Technique, a system based on the one thing that has healed so much in me in the past: self-acceptance of the terrible, unrelenting kind. That's why I trust this method to do something for me in my present situation.

'I deeply and completely accept this part of me that is afraid.'

I repeat the phrase over and over, the words themselves begging for acceptance into my subconscious.

'Accept, accept! Don't be too proud to feel fear and sadness, to feel your heart break. Accept that you feel this way. Accept the part of you that feels this way. It's part of you, *part* of you, therefore not the whole of you. Embrace, embrace, embrace!'

I repeat the words as pain distorts my mouth and tears roll down my face.

Warren, another participant turned facilitator for this exercise, stays with me, seated in a chair opposite, encouraging me to keep going. I can't believe the depth of my pain. I can't believe that this part of me is so wounded. It's also incredible that another part of me, much larger, it seems, is guiding this part, is doing the accepting, is taking it in as if into a large heart capable of healing anything that enters it.

Gradually, the sharpness of the pain in my chest and heart eases into a diffused, softer feeling encompassing my belly. Gradually, the pain subsides. Gradually, a feeling of peace takes its place.

I've done an Aaron thing, I realise, but in a few minutes instead of a few hours. I remember how Aaron let go of his love in one bitter night of detachment. During that night he developed a protection for a hurt heart, and in the morning no feeling of love was left. I am doing more than that: I, too, am detaching from what hurts me, but I won't love less. In fact, this will leave me free to love even more recklessly! Pain will no longer dominate me. Pain will come and go. It may come as a result of pleasure, and one could be as great as the other, but both will come and go. I'm intact, and soft.

My inexperienced facilitator is very concerned, but is reassured by Peter Graham, who leads the workshop. Warren fetches me a cup of tea and has some questions for Peter.

'How do you manage not to get entangled in your client's emotions?'

Warren is a Hare Krishna devotee and has a gentle heart. Strangely enough, it's not Peter but me, with barely dry eyes, who answers him.

'I read my client's energy, but it doesn't affect me,' I tell him. 'I remind myself that even though the pain is real for my client, in reality he's suffering an illusion and he'll come to realise this himself.'

There. I've just described myself. My pain was so real, but the fact that it has subsided into peace has shown me that peace is the greater reality, encompassing pain.

And what is this pain? It's the thought that this relationship has nowhere to go, and I want it to go on forever, just as it is. It's an impossible desire, but so strong that I can't drop it. There's also the realisation that Aaron is essentially a hermit, a person so independent that he doesn't know how to sustain a deep connection any more; communication and initiative will have to come mostly, if not all, from me. It's not what I want. I want an equal relationship. I want to be desired the way I desire him. I want him to feel passionately, the way I do.

There's more — new pain. I want to be young again, to start a life of young love, two people living together in a free and passionate style, the way I know Aaron did when I was a nun in a convent. All these thoughts are being mashed into one big, poignant pain. It racks my body with fierce waves of grief. I've experienced nothing and I'm in grieving! I don't know if any of what I am saying to myself is true, and I'm in anguish!

At the next session at Peter's workshop, I keep tapping on my misery, not letting anyone know where this agony comes from. My facilitator squirms in his seat, overflowing with compassion. I have my eyes closed as the tears flow down my face, which is contorted in grimaces of unbearable pain.

'Even though part of me feels this pain, I deeply and completely accept this part of me,' I say over and over. 'Even though part of me thinks it's impossible to get over this problem, I deeply and completely accept this part of me.'

My facilitator asks me to describe where in my body the pain is manifesting.

'Well,' I tell him, 'it's in my belly, where it's a churning, upset feeling, and it's constricting in my chest, and the pain is in my heart.'

Right there and then, the pain also comes to my throat, constricting it so I can only speak hoarsely. We tap and tap and endlessly repeat the redeeming phrases of acceptance. Gradually, but surely, the feelings subside, along with the physical discomfort and the tears. Only a feeling of my emotions being massaged to a point of tenderness remains. A peaceful glow enters the spaces previously occupied by racking pain. But the work is not complete, far from it.

When I get home, not knowing what Aaron's plans might be — but suspecting that he'll be preparing to go to Darkan without warning me first — revives the pain. I ring him.

'What's up, babe?'

'I want to know if you'll come over tomorrow at about two o'clock.'

Silence for a moment. Then, 'I was going to go to Darkan this evening. I've been expecting you to turn up so I stayed around the house, but you didn't. Something serious going on? Heavy?'

'I want you to know what's going on with me,' I say. 'You can do with it what you like, but I want to be heard completely for once.'

'Sounds heavy,' he says. 'It must be important; I'll come over.'

I explain that I tried to phone him early in the morning, before going to the workshop, to let him know that it wouldn't be possible to drop in, but no one picked up the phone. Aaron lives downstairs and his parents stay in bed until late in the morning.

Love pain. Will it ever end? I write out what I'm going to say to Aaron, revise it twice, no, three times, sure that it's going nowhere. I won't be able to remember any of this stuff when I'm with him. The power of his energy takes over, makes my mind go blank. Must try, though, to stick with what's in my mind and get it out.

'So,' says Aaron, 'what's up?' And he sits down on the pouffe in the lounge room, elbows on his knees, looking intent. I'm on the couch, feeling self-conscious.

'Come on, spit it out!'

It's up to me to say it now. 'Do we have a relationship?' It's only later that I realise the terrible denial in my words.

Aaron rocks back on his seat. '*I* do! Do you?'

'You once said you couldn't see yourself as the love of my life. What did you mean by that?'

'I can't see myself as the love of *anyone's* life,' he says. 'Life is always changing. We don't know how long a relationship lasts. I keep telling you: relationship is about exchanging energy. Is this the woman who wrote to me about "this is how it is, until it isn't any more"?'

I remember that piece, the very words. Words, I realise, are cheap, however inspired; they have to be lived in order to become real. I have my opening now, a way to confront him with my real issue.

'Relationship is also about communication.'

'Sure it is,' says Aaron. 'All the time.'

'But it's not all the time when I don't hear from you for three days in a row!'

'I hate the phone,' he says. This is supposed to clear up everything on that topic.

'The phone is better than nothing, surely!'

'Carla, I don't have the need to talk to you every day. If you need that, then it's up to you to connect with me.'

Bastard!

'It's so hard to phone you, Aaron! You don't have a phone in your room. You're dependent on your parents to call you upstairs to the phone, and they don't answer it until late in the morning, and can't answer it when they're out of the house. How can you put all the responsibility on me? Why can't you take it into consideration that staying in contact is important to me?'

Aaron can't believe this is about phoning.

'I hate the phone,' he says. 'I hate talking to an electronic thing. If you want to talk to me, hop in your car and come to see me. Even if it's two in the morning, that's alright with me. If you need me, get yourself over to me.'

This conversation isn't going where I want it to. I could get uppity now and call him an arrogant bastard, but something in his body language tells me he's trying to get something across to me, even if it's in a confronting way just now. He can see the strain on my face. I've relaxed a little just from seeing him, but my expression is hardly soft or easy. I've tried to hide the fact that I look pale and haggard by putting on layers of tinted moisturiser, without much effect. Strange, how my face always gives me away. I'm such a poor actor. I feel obliged to act normal, and acting makes me feel insecure. Aaron notices my body language. He knows how I feel. I know he knows how I feel. It makes me even more insecure. What will he think of me being so insecure?

'I've seen your insecurity from the first day,' he says, reading my thoughts exactly. 'I spotted it in your body language: the little girl inside you, wanting to please everybody. It's not who you are.'

I don't know what to do with myself, want to curl up and die. And then I know I'm not being judged. A friendly voice inside reminds me, *He didn't reject you back then, and doesn't now either.*

'You're in love,' he tells me. This conversation is definitely not the one I planned. 'You love Aaron, and have started to live in his energy. You've lost yourself in him. You imagine you need my presence now to be happy. You have to have my attention. You have to know that I'm thinking of you.'

'I'm addicted, Aaron . . . No, listen: I'm addicted. To you, to sex, to this relationship. I'm looking at it head on. This is how it is right now.'

'That's a real confession,' he says. 'Do you feel better now?'

'I do,' I say, realising it's true. 'It's good to have someone close to you that you trust, so you can communicate everything you feel.'

'Then that's more important to you than it is to me,' he says. 'I don't know if I'll be different in the future regarding more contact.'

At least he's heard me, and understands my best reason for wanting to be in contact.

I have another important thing to tell him, something about himself.

'When I'm close to you, I feel your pain.' He knows what I mean; I've said this to him before. 'When you were a little boy, your mind helped you to numb it out; that's how your mind protected you. Later on, when you had pain in your relationships, you also numbed it out in order to cope. Your mind is that suppressive device, right?'

'Right,' he says. 'So where's this leading to?'

'You've told me that you're very clever and can work out from one session with a therapist how to do this process yourself. You're going to use your mind to fix your mind. Well, it just can't be done.'

I want Aaron to admit that he's avoiding issues, but I may have underestimated him, judged him according to my own ways.

'I go inside to face myself,' he says. 'I do this every day — go through my insecurities and fears. They come and they go but they happen every day. In Darkan, I can face myself more intensely. I let whatever wants to come up come up, and I watch it, and that's how I learn.'

'What I want to say next —'

But he's had enough of this. He doesn't want to argue the point any more and caving in is not his style.

'Carla, words don't do it for me. Forget this. Do you want to be with me this evening, or shall I go?'

I look at him. He doesn't appear to be angry, just determined not to go down this road. He's even inviting me to enjoy him. I have to be content that he listened to me. Aaron opens his arms and smiles wryly. He takes two steps to my one and wraps me in his arms. 'I'm in-your-face Aaron, if you haven't noticed. I make no pretence of having good manners most of the time.'

'How will you die?' he asks me later.

'Alone,' I reply.

'Do you realise what you've just said?'

'Yes. I'm learning.'

'I didn't know I had all this insecurity inside me,' I confide out loud. 'I had no idea. I like to think of myself as stable!'

A few days ago, when I asked Aaron if he ever worried about the way I felt, he'd said no; he felt I was stable and not about to freak out.

'I like the way you come out with it,' he said. 'At least you don't come at me in a fury, accusing me of having neglected you, or accusing me of not taking care of you, or accusing me of being careless and thoughtless. You just state your case and you don't make it heavy for me.'

So I'm insecure, but stable all the same, I think now. I imagine the scenes he's alluded to: hysterical women trying to drum into him how they want to be treated by a man with such phenomenal energy — who keeps it contained.

'I wouldn't have this energy if I gave it away through concern about what people think of me,' he says. 'I want *you* to be like that. Piss people right off, if you need to. Do what Carla wants, without excuse for being yourself. People will love you and will hate you, but you will like yourself, and that's the only important thing. Put that in your book. Write about it until you know what you're writing about.'

I take him up on that. 'It's going to be a hell of a book.'

He turns slightly pale.

'You've gone all shy,' I say.

'Well,' he says, 'I am ... shy.'

And he smiles and turns up his face, and love drips all over him from my adoring face above him. I love this man so much, I think it's impossible to love more — until the next time we're together, when the boundaries will be pushed even further.

WHY, LORD, WHY?

Our greatest fear is not that we are inadequate.
Marianne Williamson, *A Return to Love*

 Lynda and I meet up with Laura, a mutual girlfriend. Laura is facing a spiritual challenge: how to be in her own energy — the same challenge I'm facing. She feels a lack of intimacy with her husband. On the other hand, she loves her lifestyle and her two sons, all supported financially by him. She's a very well-informed, spiritually inclined, strong and talented woman who is skirting the issue of taking the next leap in consciousness. She's afraid of being all she can be. I wonder what it is that keeps us so afraid of our light?

My own fear has to do with this. Aaron keeps on saying, 'Be all you can be, Carla,' but I really feel this would be the end of our relationship as we know it. It could mean entering a lifestyle he wouldn't want to share. The irony of the truth of this is exquisite. Aaron's already seen this; Aaron who wants me to have it all.

'I hope that whatever happens, we'll still have our special moments,' he said a while back. 'Bring your man, if you want, but come and be with me.'

There's nothing like a love affair to pull you off your centre.

Lynda tells us how she deals with desire. She loves her ex-husband, Don. Lynda and Don are extremely good friends, and that's all that Don wants, although Lynda would dearly love to be together with him again, or else just enjoy more physical relations with him.

'Constraint creates more passion and more love,' she says. 'What we do with sex and love — such important aspects of life.

'So I go to my meditation and sit with the desire,' she continues. 'I'm fully in the feeling of it and I accept it. I accept this desire with all the exquisite pain of not having it fulfilled. I accept it as what is in life. This is how it *is* and I don't run away from it.'

'Does the desire go then?' I ask her. 'Or do you feel that what this desire represents, you have already anyway?'

'Yes, it does,' she says, answering the first part of my question. 'And no, I might not feel that I have this already. I might, or I might not. In any case, it doesn't matter. I've surrendered.'

Then she adds, 'And this is the only time I believe we make a clear choice. At all other times we think we make choices, but all we're doing is following a program. Most of the time we're on automatic, acting out a script, following a program. It's only in those moments when we completely accept what *is* that we make a real choice.'

Lynda's telling me something I glimpsed in a poetry book by a teacher called Nirmala. Poetry is my preferred way of learning matters of the heart. I've also read about it in Eckhart Tolle's book *The Power of Now*. Somehow, it's a bigger deal for me today. A kind of Satori experience. The only real choice we have is to accept.

Lynda is the deep sort. It's worth listening to what is true for her.

'To accept reality is to alter the course of history,' she boldly asserts. 'It alone has the power to further evolution, so to speak. We can't do anything to will ourselves into being; only acceptance of what is does that. Then we become more present and we have more energy. Energy keeps building this way until it collapses once more into unity, when all is finally accepted.'

She's talking about the whole of mankind at the end of the path of experience on this planet. I remember a phrase about 'being lived'.

That makes more sense to me now. It seems we have the choice to be lived by life, or to struggle. We can be breathed, or breathe with stress. We can surrender, or suffer. We can rest in the arms of the Beloved, or forever break our hearts searching for love and peace.

Wow, Lynda! You're more capable of living this truth than I am.

Once more snuggled up to Aaron's chest, I burst into tears. He wants to know what's going on this time. So I tell him.

'I'm crying for the beauty of what I feel here. I can feel your heart; it's so wide open and beautiful. I can feel its purity and its great capacity for love ... and its *pain*.'

'My pain?'

'Yes, I can feel enormous pain. Maybe it comes from your childhood, maybe from more recent events, but it's there and it makes me sad.'

For once, Aaron has no words by way of reply. Behind closed eyes, he's getting in touch with what I've just said.

'I'm an energy. Everything can be taken from me, but this I will take with me when I die.' Aaron is apt to utter his deepest wisdom in the post-orgasmic state.

'A relationship doesn't complete you! It doesn't give you a life! You have a life first, then you add a relationship. You get into trouble if you think of yourself as a halfful cup that needs half of another person to fill it. That's the way people end up depleting one another very fast.'

'Miss me all you want when I go away, but realise it's yourself you're missing. There's no one else to miss. Call yourself back. Be with yourself. Then your Beloved will kiss you.'

I wake and feel my breasts: they're very tender this Monday morning. I massage them, as I do these days, to make them grow. I'm sure it's working; for a couple of weeks I've been feeling growing pains. The nipples have been so sensitive that it hurts to touch them unless with wet fingers or hands. Today the sensitivity is back to normal; alright to touch lightly, squeeze between index finger and thumb and feel the direct line of sensation to my vagina. This sensation makes my vagina come alive, and I talk to Aaron through the ether, because I'm alone, in bed, and not feeling so well.

'Am I really not going to see you till Wednesday? I'm so wet!'

I'm surprised at the wetness because I have a temperature — the flu, most likely. Where's all this energy coming from? I feel inside my vagina: it's dripping. I bring some of the juices to my clitoris and labia, and soon all of them are drenched.

'Look how my vagina wants you!' I continue my one-way talk with absent Aaron. 'Watch how my clitoris is swelling, and how my breasts are growing, while I think of you. My labia are so wet, so welcoming of this pleasure. Look, my pelvis is opening and rising towards you, wanting you, rising up further and wanting you, wanting you, WANTING YOU . . .!!!'

My orgasm is loud and sweet and a release of tension I didn't know was there. This masturbation was different from others I've had alone — the ones I used to have, sporadically, before I met Aaron. This time, connecting to another person has made the difference. It's a few minutes before eight; I'll ask Aaron later what he was doing at the same time.

It's only Monday, and I won't see him till Wednesday — that is, if he can even make it then. I'm listening again to Emma Shapplin. I play this music often and it never fails to move me. *Je suis à toi*. I weep to it, my heart soars to it, I dance to it the way no one should see me do, and I don't get enough of it. Why am I listening to it today, when my heart feels not altogether whole?

All of a sudden, I know. In a moment of utter clarity, I know what must be obvious to anyone else who knows us: Aaron doesn't feel the way I do. His feelings just aren't capable of responding like mine. In his own words, he's numb. Because he's numb, he can't appreciate what I feel, and he can't appreciate what he would lose if I left him. That's why he can say, 'If you leave me, I'll just find another Carla,' and say this three times in as many weeks.

He loves being loved, there's no doubt that his ecstasy is a lot about that. He owns the passion of sexual sensuality, but what about the passion of love?

He's been hurt in the past and has said to himself, *Never again. I'll never love so much again that I'll hurt when she leaves me.* It's made him strong, and it's also made him impervious. Aaron will never give himself the way I do; he would call that foolish; he would call that losing himself. He's seen me lose myself in him and he doesn't like it. 'Love me to bits, put me on a pedestal if you want, but stay with yourself!' he tells me.

Stay with yourself? How dare he use my most sacred words? He would have a right to, if he knew how to give himself and stay with himself at the same time. But he doesn't give in the first place. He gives me his penis, his sensuality, his kisses, his admiration, his appreciation, his words — ah, such magnificent words! The words of a poet, whispered intensely, calculated to infiltrate the heart. He doesn't say he has 'party tricks' any more, not since I wrinkled my nose at that, but perhaps that's what they largely are: party tricks; the words he knows will turn a woman on and make her feel good about herself. Ugh, it makes me feel sick.

Am I perhaps doing him an injustice? His words have come from his heart many times, surely? Yes, surely. And yet his actions belie his words. If he could feel like me, if he could appreciate the passion directed at him, he would make this relationship a priority. He would realise, like me, that what we have is rare, that time is short for everyone, but especially for us because of our age. Life may very well make us part in the future, even if we don't want to.

But no, his priority has been to study, when he knows he won't stay at college anyway. Not even for an hour or two, but whole days at a time. Complaints mean nothing. He stays away. He says that I can come over and hang around if I really need him.

My cheeks burn to see those words on paper, written in my journal. My eyes are always damp these days, and right now they're brimming.

Carla, it's reality time. You've been in love with Aaron's potential: what you can see in him that he can't see himself. It's time to look at what is real now. How big is the gap between his potential and the reality? The gap, dear Carla, is a *gulf*.

Emma's words are suddenly my own. She's crying to heaven: *Signor, perché? Why, Lord, why?*

Aaron talks to me about my insecurity. This is a topic very close to his heart, so his voice is earnest. 'I want *you* to know the way *I* know. I *trust* that you *can* know. Overcome this insecurity, Carla.'

He's been hurt many times by seeing his girlfriends turn on him when they couldn't 'possess' him, as he calls it. Aaron the Independent; Aaron who nevertheless chooses women who soon can't do without him. Aaron who has learnt to protect himself and may not be able to imagine the effect his wariness has on others, including me.

'Neglect brings out the worst in women,' I tell him. 'I can understand how your women would have gone crazy with you not communicating to them and sitting in your ivory tower, smugly arrogant in your detachment. It would make them raving mad with fury!'

Aaron's not about to throw away his grievances on account of my little speech. He cites the viciousness of some of his exes. It still seems to me that it takes two to tango. Aaron is also not about to experience any deep realisations about this. He's keen to continue to educate me about 'his way'.

'You want me to talk to you every day. That's not my way. If I want to know how you are, I get a picture in my head, and I know how you are. It works; check it out.'

'Bullshit, Aaron! If you'd done that only once last Sunday, you'd have come over. I was desperate then.'

'What happened?'

I have his attention now. He's no longer arguing; he wants to hear what's been going on.

'I was feeling bitter grief about the way this relationship isn't going to work,' I begin bravely, exposing my weakness that he's so afraid of. Keeping it secret is worse. If Aaron's going to reject me because of my insecurity, he might as well do it sooner rather than later. 'When I was doing the workshop at the weekend, I was breaking my heart for a future that didn't exist yet. I know that was stupid and I learnt from it. I won't do it again, but it was a horrible time for me.'

'*How* did you learn from it?' he asks.

'I let the feeling have its way with me while I tapped on the acupressure points Lynda showed you.'

I have a vivid memory of how waves of pitiful grief washed over and through me that day, and how the tears flowed from my broken heart.

'I don't think I'll ever need to do that again. I faced the worst, and dealt with it,' I say.

'We're attracted to each other because we each want something from the other,' Aaron says, as if pronouncing his conclusions. 'You want to be independent, like me, and I want your passion.'

I sigh with relief. 'Well said, Aaron.'

'It's not going to come from *me*, what you want, Carla. You'll develop this in yourself through contact with me. Sex is a great way of exchanging energies. We really get each other when we make love.'

I know from what he's saying that things will get better between us. He needn't spell it out. He'll come my way, if I'm prepared to learn more of his way.

'You want my confidence in myself,' he says. 'You want to get rid of your insecurity. I can never give you this confidence, and you can't live through me, but you can sense it in me, you can taste it, you can know it and bring it out of yourself. You'll find yourself behaving like me.'

I listen to these prophetic words. In spite of the residue of emotional damage that's making Aaron choose to be reserved and cautious, this sounds like wisdom distilled from his life experience.

It's a night for straight talking, and Aaron's doing most of it.

'I can see how vulnerable you are when you love me one hundred per cent. I will never want to hurt that. I want you to be the Carla you can be — so happy with yourself that you are immortal, indestructible, unbreakable in your sense of your self. You're regaining the supreme confidence you had when you were a child. Your father saw that in you and couldn't stand it. He had to take it away. Ever since then you've walked around with feelings of unworthiness. You always had beauty, but you couldn't see it. Now you're beginning to realise that you can be yourself again, and have it all. You're waking up to yourself, and I'm here to make that happen for you.

'You're wanted!' he suddenly says passionately, just when I've given up on ever expecting reassurances again. 'You're wanted! Not just sexually, but I want to feel the way you do!'

I look at him, tenderness welling out of my eyes. He returns my gaze and we sit there for a while, lost in each other's sight, savouring what has been said, sure that we're growing in a way that some divine intelligence, which Aaron calls the Cogs, has organised. My heart is so wide open that it hurts, but I wouldn't want it any other way. The hurt I feel is always the same: it's the intuition that it will all end one day.

'This is how two people become as one,' he says, breaking the silence. 'You will bring out of yourself what you love in me, and I will bring out of myself what I love in you. Don't be insecure, Carla. We were apart for thirty years, and we've found each other again. What are two days, five days, two weeks? Trust yourself!'

AARON'S SPACE

One day, your soul will hoist a white flag
on your behalf.
You will know what this means.
Robert Rabbin, 'Humility'

 We're both on the way to Aaron's house in Darkan. It's about 11 p.m. and we're driving through misty valleys, looking out for kangaroos on the roads. The trees lining the road to Darkan are like strong-limbed angels, nakedly beautiful in the headlights. I'm awed by their presence. Whatever Darkan has not, it has the most beautiful trees in the world.

I've driven the first half of our trip, but I give the wheel to Aaron so he can navigate the unfamiliar roads and his town in the dark. He points out the shadowy buildings as we pass. 'That's the town hall, the biggest building, and now we're coming to my shed.' Its high walls and large round window are visible above a fence. 'And there's the pile of sleepers ... remember, I told you about them.'

We enter his driveway. It's so quiet. He fumbles for the house key and turns on lights. I'm grateful to see a flushing toilet not too far from the house, with green outdoor carpet generously spread between it and the little back verandah. I soon discover that the toilet has a wooden seat. This touch of quality is not a rare thing in this place of make-do. Everything has been made from recycled material — from what other people throw out, mostly — but it's all been so deliberately thought through.

Our few belongings go into the house and in a few seconds a kettle is on the boil for a quick drink of Milo and a couple of hot water bottles.

Aaron makes his bed. A sheet from a single bed will have to cover the sheepskin that stretches across the bed that is almost, but not quite, a double. A pile of doonas goes over that. It's important to get to bed soon, since the temperature is below zero and we're tired. Two hot water bottles are tossed between the sheets. I clean my teeth, undress as fast as possible and climb in. Aaron hangs my newly acquired, voice-activated tape recorder from the end of the brass bedhead near his pillow. He wants to know what his snoring sounds like.

It's snuggly and special being in Aaron's bed, in his own house. He's so pleased that I've come here. This is a baptism of sorts, a sealing of a friendship, a validation of himself. It's late, but we make love with a passion fuelled by Aaron's appreciation of my presence in his bed. It's hours after midnight when we settle down to sleep, me with earplugs.

Aaron slips into sleep easily. I'm awake for a long time, enjoying the closeness of his body, breathing with him and listening to his snoring. Mostly he breathes normally, until the breathing gets somehow diverted. Then it stops altogether, as his body tries to control something. For five or even ten long seconds, his breathing is suppressed until one violent snort releases it. 'My disturbed subconscious,' he calls it. 'I don't want you to have to listen to it.' But he does, really. He must know that I won't judge him.

Aaron awakens briefly and kisses me. 'Was I snoring?'

'Yes, you were, but it's okay.'

'She doesn't mind my snoring. Something's wrong!' he mocks, and falls asleep again. I sleep and wake and sleep, and feel myself in heaven.

* * *

It's 11 a.m. He's still in bed. Doesn't want to get up. Doesn't know
what to do. I've been pottering around since eight in my dressing
gown: cup of tea, wander outside, oat porridge breakfast (not for
Aaron, who hates porridge), wash up, read.

This house is like no other on earth. Every available shelf is piled
high with things collected from the roadside or from the tip or
bought at bargain prices. There's not just one frying pan but seven;
not just one salad bowl but every size imaginable, including giant size;
not just a few boxes of tissues but a whole wall of them. Aaron's a
compulsive collector. The whole house feels crowded — hardly any
room to move. There are no easy chairs. The bathroom hasn't been
cleaned for years, if ever. The floor gets wet every time someone has
a shower. It's the house of a man who only has need of the basics.

I decide to join him under the blankets in my dressing gown and
ask what the matter is. He doesn't know, he says, but when he turns
to face me, our eyes meet for a moment in a question, and the answer
is a thought-free desire to embrace and kiss.

His hands want to feel me through my clothes. I struggle to pull
them off — dressing gown, nightie, knickers and socks put on as a
buffer against the crisp morning air of wintry Darkan.

Once naked and under the pile of doonas, warmth is guaranteed.
Aaron's hands are greedy and strong. I'm helpless when his
masculinity takes over in such a firm, yet gentle, way. He knows what
to do with me, and how to pleasure us both, but all of it is so simple.
It's the passion that flows between us and out of our hands and eyes
and skin that transforms little gestures into torrents of pleasure. It's
soon too hot under the covers.

I am lying on top of him, open to the cold air and spread-eagled,
when his hand reaches over my buttocks and two fingers make
their way unerringly to my clitoris. My already aroused body
electrifies. I squirm to disperse the energy building there, but his
fingers follow my movements. Finally, I roll off him and he is

immediately on top of me, his head above my chest, his mouth rapidly attacking my nipples. My fingers take over from his to stimulate my clitoris. Aaron's eager mouth and tongue flick from one breast to another, holding them with his hands. My heat builds and I stop stimulation to let waves of it radiate out, then resume, and do this rising and stopping until my body can take it no longer, erupting in a volcanic explosion. My throat opens to a high scream, flowing like the note of a song, penetrating walls and gardens. But my mind is not on passers-by. My scream is so prolonged that Aaron's hand finally goes up to try and block it, but it's just a reflex action: he knows it's no use.

It's been weeks since I had a clitoral orgasm; most of my peak experiences originate in my vagina and cervix. A clitoral orgasm expends a lot of energy and I indulge in it only seldom, but there's a right time for these things and this morning is it, in Aaron's bed, in his house, in Darkan.

I sink back in utter contentment. I feel the complete pleasure of perfect balance in every part of my body. All of it has been bathed in energy, warmed by the expansiveness of this orgasm. Every organ is alive and singing. I can especially sense how good my bowel feels. The very centre of my belly radiates contentedness.

'Were you always as sexual as this?'

Aaron's questions are never casual. He looks at me intently; he's been wanting to know this for a while. I sit next to him on the edge of his bed, considering my answer.

'I think I always *wanted* to be as sexual as this,' I say. 'I had the feeling in me, but it never came out like this before.'

'What stopped you?'

'I never found my equal, until now.'

'So that's what it is. We're two of a kind. We both love sex to excess.'

'It isn't just that —' I say, but he interrupts.

'I know. It's other things as well, but apart from all that, it's that we can be completely sexual with each other.'

Later, he sees the cup I'm using and reprimands me. 'That's my special cup! No one but me uses that one! And while I'm at it — that one over there is Carol's, who lives next door, and that one there is Eddie's. You can use any of the other ones.'

Aaron continues to instruct me in the way his house is kept. I get that one obeys. To do otherwise would be to interrupt the usual and make life more difficult. Oh well. This house is Aaron's castle.

It has a friendly feel about it. Everywhere there are sentimental reminders of the past: photos, bric-a-brac — full of stories, all of them. But I couldn't live here, that's plain. I couldn't even stay longer than one day and a night.

When the jobs that needed doing have been done, like taking umpteen computers apart to salvage the bits that only Aaron could think of finding a use for, and raking the leaves in the yard — I duck under the doonas again. That's where Aaron finds me.

'What am I good at?' he asks, as I pull the covers over both of us.

'I think you're a naturally brilliant architect.'

'Why do you say that?' His voice comes to me muffled from under the sheets.

I tell him. 'You're practical and intelligent, and you think outside of the box. You have solutions for people who present you with building problems. You have a great mind for remembering what's relevant to the job. You just can't remember academic stuff that deals with ephemeral concepts. You're a hands-on person: you love creating things with your hands.'

Does that say it all? No, there's more.

'I saw how competent you were when you explained the design of your house to me, and what you did to put your amazing shed together.'

It's a shed like none other. After it was approved by the local council and built, someone realised the staggering size of it and officials came around to ask Aaron to make it smaller. They had no chance!

Aaron's a natural problem-solver when it comes to house design and he does it in a totally creative way. Why does he have no confidence in being successful as an architect? It beats me, but I guess it has something to do with being too left field, which means too anti-establishment and irreverent, too *not* like the image that architects like to project about themselves.

'Thanks for saying that,' he says, taking my head in his hands and kissing me, 'but we both know that jobs aren't exactly waiting out there for people like me to snap up.'

Conversation over, he flips the blankets off himself, undresses by chucking his clothes roughly in the direction of the nearest chair, and turns back to me.

It's after dark when we head for Perth again. It's Aaron's preferred time for travelling: the roads are by now clear of kangaroos, there's little traffic, and the air is cool and sweet.

I've survived the Darkan experience. 'How did you like it?' Aaron asks. Later, he confides that he didn't believe a word I said.

MISSING WARDROBE

If any of these were the real world
they would never disappear
Robert Rabbin, 'Reality'

 It's 3 a.m. I wake up in my bed, moaning from a nightmare. In the dream I was a nun, a member of a community, and happy until the thought occurred that I was deprived — chronically deprived of a wardrobe! I became depressed and hid under my veil. No one could see my face under there, but I became more and more miserable until I slumped down on the table I was sitting at, right on top of some sacred objects — a bowl and ashes and oils for a ceremony. The sisters gasped. I didn't care. I moved away to sit on a bench against the wall and still kept myself under my veil. When I peeped out, I saw a wardrobe in the doorway, coming towards me. It must be for me, but nobody said so, so I didn't want to believe it prematurely and kept hiding.

I came to bed last night with frayed feelings. Early that day, I'd suddenly become aware of a pulsing in my vagina, as if some version of Aaron's penis had penetrated me. The sensation was strong and unmistakeable. I got up to write about the sensations I was feeling and, as I did, an orgasm swept through my body. Waves of sexual energy travelled from my toes to my head, making me inhale sharply and stretch my body to help move the energy. I spasmed and gasped, vagina throbbing, yet I hadn't touched any part of myself.

I imagined that Aaron was stroking his 'happy dick', as he had called it, but not that he was masturbating. Surely not, since that would interfere with his energy for our love-making! I noted the time and, when I went to see him in the afternoon, asked what he'd been doing then.

He knew exactly what he'd been doing, he said: masturbating to get rid of an erotic image he'd carried forward from the day before, when he'd spotted some 'healthy breasts' on a female student at college. They'd reminded him of his mother's breasts when he was a boy and she was bathing with him in the same tub to save water. His mother caught his stare and jumped out of the bath in a fit of modesty. Her embarrassed reaction had reinforced the erotic quality of the incident, which was never to be repeated and never erased.

Somehow, this masturbation of Aaron's — as a result of being so powerfully aroused by someone else's breasts — disturbed me deeply. I looked at him; he was yawning. 'It's been a busy day,' he explained.

Yes, it had been, starting with a huge expenditure of energy before breakfast. I asked him if he knew how to divert that energy to his heart.

'Yeah, yeah, but I didn't want to walk around with this image all day, distracting me.'

I didn't pursue the subject. Instead, we stood in his tiny space and hugged. His hands went up my body, as a man's hands do, and stopped at my breasts — only they weren't real. He was touching my falsies — empty space.

And so I came to bed last night with a feeling, not fully acknowledged, of deep sorrow about the state of my breasts. As soon as my head lay on the pillow in the dark, it became all too obvious what my feelings were and the thinking that went with it. Aaron wasn't turned on by my breasts; in fact, most of the time he ignored them, and I was grateful for that, feeling that if he really noticed them he'd be utterly turned off. He loves me sitting on top of him when we make love, and that puts my breasts right in front of his vision. When my back is straight, they look like reasonably normal, very small breasts, but when I bend forward — which happens a lot — they become empty sacks, hanging like rubber funnels with a nipple stuck to the tip. Pathetic! The best I can do is try to forget them, but of course I seldom do. I wonder if I *ever* do. Isn't it true that I am *always* aware of the fact that they're inadequate, less than sexy, the supreme and impossible-to-hide symbol of my advancing age? Oh, the pain of it! The pain of losing my sexual identity!

My dream spoke to me of my shame: my longing for a 'wardrobe' — looking 'right' — and of feeling like a nun because of my inadequate breasts, my loss of womanhood. How can a woman be sexual and sensual and not have breasts — *the* symbol of her sexuality, and the thing that turns Aaron on?

Right now, I feel like I have no sexuality left. I feel like phoning Aaron to warn him not to expect sex if he comes over this evening, because I'm feeling miserable. This is how the conversation runs in my head:

'Hi, how are you, babe? What's up?' (Aaron always senses when something is on my mind.)

'Aaron, I feel ratshit. I don't feel like having sex.'

'Well, I won't come over for a while then.'

Silence.

'Babe?'

I put the phone down just as a suppressed sob threatens to break into the space. And he doesn't phone back. He hates histrionics. He's had a gutful of them from other women. He wants to believe that he's safe with me, that I'm stable and won't go into weird places that make him feel responsible.

So what's true here?

I start having a look at myself and my feelings. For one thing, I have to face the awful fact that I've identified with this body of mine and that I'm grieving its gradual breaking down. For another thing, I've been feeding my ego with Aaron's appreciation of my sexuality. I've been foolish enough to make these things all-important. I've let sex and Aaron's idea of me become the most valuable things in my life, instead of the peace and strength of my own centre. I've wanted the gifts of life for my own gratification, for my ego-image, allowing my sexual prowess and relationship to build me up as a more worthwhile person than I was before, when I was celibate and mild.

It's now 4.30 a.m. I have the good sense to turn on some familiar music. The purity of Mozart's notes from Zaide again fill my heart like some forgotten truth, relaxing it the way Aaron's hand does when he touches my face. It's not enough, though. I mustn't let myself get seduced either by music or by love-making. Music comes and goes. Lovers come and go. Lovers love what they see, what they experience; they love being loved. It isn't an ultimate thing, this loving, and this music — or is it? It isn't and it is. I have to feel what's true here, and not destroy it out of pique.

Essence is so delicate; a rejection by way of a complaint destroys its integrity.

My soul gives me to understand that complaint destroys the integrity of love. So what if my body isn't perfect? How many bodies are? So what if my man is hung up on full breasts? It's up to him to respond to what he sees when he's with me and, so far, his response has been magnificent. He has been there for me to pour out my love to ... and while it poured in utter gratitude, it was true and completely satisfying. As soon as my loving became a *concern* about how it was perceived *as a body-package,* I was no longer with Aaron-as-my-Beloved; I was with my head, looking to see if I measured up, if I was making the right impression. God! It isn't my breasts that are pathetic, but this concern of mine. How my vanity can get in the way of the sweetest love! How easily my mind can ravage, with its ideas and concepts, what is beyond the premise of mind altogether.

I'm more astonished than ashamed. How tricky the mind is. But now I'm aware more than ever of how it works: whenever I entertain a *complaint*, I can be sure that the slaying mind is at work.

I feel my face relax. I haven't had much sleep, but I feel refreshed. My muscles ache, especially in my shoulders and back — signs of the tension held there for hours by doubt. Yes, doubt: doubt of my Beloved, of God. I have no control over my body's shape as it is now. It isn't *my* body. It isn't *my* sexuality. It isn't even *my* breath. I'm being breathed and lived, and the only full joy there is is to surrender. No more doubt. Peace. Tears of gratitude fill my eyes.

Inwardly, I declare my ultra-sensitive nipples to be OK for being so incongruously attached to breasts that look like little rubber funnels. That's how they are. That's the given in this moment, the gift. Of course, the greatest gift in my rubber funnels is the opportunity, in the early hours of this morning, to dis-identify from my body as a reality apart from my Being.

My heart sings with the music. Mozart must have been in touch with this. The essence of this music is eternal, as is the essence of my love and my lover. I'm more open to love than ever before, yet there is no Aaron in my arms. I've once more surrendered to Life, my Beloved, and regained my sanity.

It is around 3.30 p.m. when I have a strong impulse to phone Aaron. I set aside the thought that this isn't wise, that he'll read this as a desperate woman wanting to be near him all the time.

He's just arrived back from a shopping trip and is very pleased to hear from me.

'What's up?' is his question, and I say I want to work with him, to be his therapist for a bit, to deal with the episode he told me about from when he was a taxi driver.

'Come over,' he says, and when I arrive, he tells me how he's just had an incident with a guy at a computer shop. He feels miserable because of the way he was dealt with. Aaron is ready for some work. He's grateful for my presence and we don't waste any time.

The counsellor in me comes to the fore. I pull his chair towards me and take his hands away from his face. He's crying and doesn't want me to see it.

Oh, the steps we take are so gradual! His pain is so deep, his hidden tears so vast, that he won't let go except a little at a time. He knows that the morning's painful experience is only a trigger for the pain that has been there since he was a child. As a taxi driver, he was accused of behaving in a sexually harassing way, and instead of simply paying the fine, he spent thousands of dollars in futile attempts to prove his innocence. Everyone involved was interested in proving him guilty, since they all stood to gain from his conviction. 'Everyone in that court was getting paid for what they were doing. I was the only one paying,' was his way of putting it. In his eyes, they were the evil-doers.

Aaron digresses to talk about what happens in a war situation. His preoccupation with the last world war and all wars is this very same thing: evidence of how evil humans can be, what they do to inflict horror on each other.

'The Russian soldiers invaded Berlin near the end of the war,' he tells me. 'They were more ruthless than the Allies. Their commanders sent them into battle to be cannon fodder. Wave after wave got mowed down by the Germans, until the Germans ran out of bullets. By the end of the war, five million men had been sacrificed this way. A Russian soldier wasn't able to say no. If he turned away, he was shot immediately. The Russian generals fought a war of attrition.

'The Allies, on the other hand, thought it was a good idea to blow Dresden to bits from the air, even though the war was nearly won. They used incendiary bombs to obliterate the population. The heat was so intense that the charred bodies had to be scraped off the bitumen.'

He looks at me. The immense sadness in his eyes tells me of what he suffers. This story is symbolic of the charred remains of an innocent child in his psyche. The stories keep the pain alive, so one day it can be healed. What takes away his hope is his core belief in the irredeemable nature of evil. It also keeps him in perpetual victimhood and perpetual blame. When will he be ready to face all this?

Aaron fights to stay with me, but he puts his head in my lap time and again, hands over his face, unable to go into the abyss any further. I beg him to do just one thing for me: to look at me without thinking any thoughts, to just be here and feel his feeling.

Face to face, he manages this for a minute or so. 'This feels better,' he says. I ask him not to think or say anything, to just be here. He manages another minute before breaking down again. I know that this is as far as he will go today. He looks so exhausted.

'When are we going to have a cuddle in your bed, under this doona?' I ask.

He smiles, takes off his jacket, kicks off his slippers and dives into bed on the far side. I join him. His head on my shoulder, he soon falls into the grateful oblivion of sleep. I am tired and follow him, sleeping lightly and sweetly, so happy to have my love by my side.

I'm in the area after an afternoon's workshop with the National Speakers Association and could easily call in on Aaron, but decide against it. I don't feel a particular pull to go and see him. Also, I was there only yesterday.

Better make myself scarce, I think as I turn for home. He wouldn't want to see me again so soon.

At home, the blinking on my answering machine tells me there's a message. '*Aaron here. Listen carefully. Kiss, kiss, kiss, KISS!*'

I have to laugh — with a painful heart. I keep underestimating this man, and keep being delighted by his quirkiness. I listen again, just for the sheer joy of it, then sit down to figure out how to transfer music CDs onto my hard drive, as he showed me. I can't manage it, but won't ring up. It will have to wait.

There's a knock on my door and there's Aaron, holding an ergonomic keyboard that he's just found.

'I've come around to tell you how much I appreciate having you as my friend,' he says, stepping inside and giving me a kiss — no, three kisses in a row.

'It's four,' I say, and receive another one from his soft mouth.

Aaron heads for the sink, where he finds a brush to clean the keyboard. He often restores things people have thrown out and makes them useful. I've wanted a keyboard like this for over a year! Aaron's so skilled at finding exactly what he has in mind that it's becoming a series of little miracles. In a yellow skip he recently spotted a pile of slate that was perfect for his bathroom in Darkan. 'God is pointing me to things for my house,' he says cheerfully, indicating that maybe God is willing for him to get started on building it in the not-too-distant future.

After a few more kisses, he takes apart the keyboard and removes every trace of dirt and dust. I cook dinner and we talk. He finds the time to show me how to transfer my music to my computer, and this time I write down the instructions. More kisses, then he pulls me to the bed and throws me down. But only for a cuddle and a few more kisses; he's got to get up early tomorrow.

We manage to be good, even if his wicked self can't help telling me how much he enjoys having his dick in me and I go mad with a fit of desire. We eat dinner and he skilfully reassembles the keyboard. Our observations about how nice it is just to be together, doing things, evolves into a conversation about how it would be if we lived together.

'That's a scary thought,' says Aaron. 'I've never done that without things going bad in the end.'

'But you managed to keep it harmonious for years on end.'

This isn't taken up.

'All the women I ever lived with didn't know how to have a life of their own,' he says, 'except one. She told me one day that she wanted to leave me and have other relationships. I accepted it and told her that's what she should do if she didn't want to stay. What's the point of doing anything else? I took myself off to a dark room and missed her sadly. In a couple of days I got over her.'

This is Aaron. His life experiences have taught him something that he's now able to slowly teach me.

'I feel safe with you, because you've learnt how to have a life for yourself,' he says. 'You love me, but you have your own core.'

'You value your freedom above all else,' I add. 'So do I: we're two of a kind.'

Aaron replies, 'I value being myself. If I compromised on that, I'd start to live someone's story. That's what most people do. Then they lose the ability to exchange energies. They take from one another instead of exchanging. Then they treat nature and the planet the same way: take without thanks, without consideration.'

There's no more talk of our living together.

I think of the time, not all that long ago, when I lost my core. But I dealt with it. I went into that feeling of insecurity without resistance and accepted every nuance of it and of myself and of the situation that triggered it. And I became stronger. If Aaron can transpose what he's learnt in this area of his life to all other areas, he'll heal himself. Maybe that's what I'm here for, to help him do that.

Meantime, the fundamental lesson of staying with myself never lets up. This seems to be the lesson of my life, and I expect Life to do everything it takes until I learn it thoroughly. It's still a scary thought: I know that the test for this might be the loss of what I hold dear. If not now, then in death, when all will fall away to slime and bones and nothing will be left. Better to die in every moment then, than be in a space of resistance when the time for letting go comes.

'Every time you think of me, you leave yourself.' Aaron breaks in on my thoughts. 'And that's okay, provided you go back to yourself.'

He smiles up at me from his task at the now new-looking keyboard. 'The answer is not to love less or to restrain yourself, but to be willing to own it all, all the time. Be in love with me as much as you want; sweat over me every minute of the day; but know it's all you — your own feelings.'

If love is letting another be who they are, then Aaron loves. Having experienced manipulation himself, as a horror of disrespect and mistrust, he's not capable of manipulating someone else. But no one can manipulate him any more, either.

* * *

Pen in hand, I sit up in bed. Early morning is one of the best times for writing.

> *I'm learning, learning, being pulled by the scruff of my neck. How to go into the centre of the nectar and not get lost there? How to be there as a free being, not seduced into addiction by being absolutely loved, every cell bathed in delight, every nerve soothed by sweetness? How to be there and know that it is all yourself, your Beloved Self? How to be grateful instead of needy, grateful for this validation of what Love can be like? Even, how to know that this love, however great, is only a shadow of the Love that we are?*

As I write, sobs of gratitude are wrenched from a depth thus far untapped. My soul is prostrate in a boundless feeling of gratitude. By some incongruence, I remember the vow of chastity I once made in an attempt to be free from bondage to sexuality. How far removed from truth that was! How utterly insane to cut oneself off from physical love in order to be free! How can denial serve what has been denied? How can un-love serve love? How can physical detachment lead to understanding of full human and spiritual love?

It can, something tells me, if that is what God arranges for a soul. I made the decision to take a vow of chastity out of ignorance, not because it was plain from my physical, or other, condition that this was asked of me. And yet it was correct, so correct for me to have done just that. My condition was one of extreme ignorance, and convent life provided me with the protection I needed until I had grown and come to myself.

Tears of gratitude again fill my eyes. The wisdom of divine intelligence is so profound, so loving and entirely beneficent, that my heart breaks with recognition of the way I have been loved. *This is how much I love you*, says Life, and I surrender in deepest tears, now that I can see it.

The embrace of Life is all around me, enveloping my body like the arms of a lover, enveloping my space, entering every moment and everything in my life, from the glass of water on my table to the computer I write on, to every soul and everything on this planet. It is all my Beloved, and all is a stage on which I can to relate to this mysterious Self. I can never lose my Self, my essence, the energy that infuses all shapes and people, and brings Aaron into my life, then takes him away when the time comes. Nothing stays, and nothing gets lost. Love continues even as our hearts get broken, because being human means to feel loss even as we know we are not losing anything. That's the paradox. No wonder it takes a brave soul to be fully human. It's the greatest joy and the greatest pain.

The gods envy us, because we are mortal. We mortals have time, we have space, we have change, we have one day and not the next, one moment and not the next. Our Now is rich. Our ignorance is our delight when we become wise. It is only the ignorant who become wise, after all. Angelic beings do not have to become wise, and they cannot experience despair. We are privileged to suffer.

Oh God, can I take more of this?

MIRRORS IN OUR LIVES

Join me now
here
where we have never parted
Nirmala, untitled poem

Gustav Mahler's music fills my room as I read in bed. Dawn is only just breaking; I can't see it, but I can visualise the light that begins to stir the shadows. The Vienna Philharmonic is playing the Adagietto, the same piece that was played at Robert Kennedy's funeral.

I'm reading *Constantine's Sword*, a book by James Carroll about anti-Semitism in the Christian churches. The chapter that stuns me right now is the one about Abelard and Heloise, who loved each other in the Middle Ages. He was a semi-cleric and her teacher, and she was a brilliant student twenty years his junior. Theirs is one of the greatest love stories of all time, although they were physically separated for so much of it. Alas, Abelard's scandalised students punished him for choosing love when he was supposed to be choosing philosophy by castrating him!

The part that fascinates me most is Heloise's love for Abelard. When they separated after the brutal incident of his castration, she became a nun and an abbess. In a letter to him shortly before his death at the age of sixty-three, she wrote: *God knows I would not have hesitated to follow you or to precede you into hell itself if you had given me the order.* That's strange enough, but then she goes on: *My heart was not my own, but yours. Even now, more than ever before, it is not with you, it is nowhere, for you are its very existence.* Later in the same letter, she states: *Truly, I reserved nothing for myself but to be yours before everything.* (Heloise, 'Letters' 2, *Patrologia Latina*, PL 178, 186–7; quoted by Etienne Gilson in *Heloise and Abelard*, Académie Française Library Vrin, 1938.)

I know the temptation of losing myself in another, but Heloise could not have been referring to that. If so, how could she have survived being apart from Abelard? How could their relationship have survived his castration? And yet their relationship never lost its ardour and she *completely* surrendered to him.

The paradox that constantly turns up when the centre of truth is touched turns up here — so deliciously that the feeling of it floods my chest. Heloise no longer had any physical relations with Abelard when she wrote those words: *my heart is not with you, it is nowhere, for you are its very existence.* Heloise saw the very existence of her own heart, her love, as his. She was truly one with him, in the sense that all is One. Fortunate is the person who can find that oneness reflected in a so-called other and have absolutely no hesitation in surrendering to that other. That surrender is a surrender to one's own heart. Her phrase, *my heart is yours,* has two meanings. In the West, it means that the person gives his or her heart *to* the other; often giving up their autonomy. Heloise, on the contrary, knows that *her* heart is *his:* it's a recognition of the oneness of their being.

Some awakened souls seem able to feel this with everyone, even if they dislike a person's character traits or behaviour. They can still feel that they are one with that person's core, their heart. Most of us have glimpses of this, but the thing that can give us tremendous insight into that love is the presence of just one special person with whose heart we can identify. This person is somehow the perfect mirror for us; he or she speaks the right language, has the right symbolism. That's how it was with Heloise and Abelard. Will it ever be like that between Aaron and me? Is the potential there?

I come out of my reverie and reach for my pen. For me, writing is a clarifying process. I write what I have just realised about Heloise and Abelard. Surrender to the truth has become more of a preoccupation since I've been in this physical love relationship with Aaron. For decades I've asked friends, strangers and wise people, *What is surrender?* So far, I've understood it to be about staying with myself, faithful to my innermost truth, whatever that is from moment to moment.

Life seems to use all our decisions and mistakes as fodder for the end plan. As all the dramas of my life play out, I'm constantly being steered back on course, as if there's a gravitational pull I can't escape. My conscious self has nothing to do with that divine intelligence. I can only surrender to it. *And that's what I've done.*

The me I call Carla cooperated with life whenever she surrendered; life took over and brought me back to myself each time, until I learnt to surrender to myself more and more. Hmm, shouldn't that be 'surrender to *life*'? No . . . well, yes, because it's the same thing! This isn't confusing to me in this moment, when the rising sun brings light to the ceiling of my room. I realise I basically have only one choice: to arrive at my destiny either sooner or later. I believe that no one can escape this.

God's Callgirl had a long and very interesting detour. Life is like that: colourful and dangerous — and in the end, we emerge from the tunnel of horrors and light-shows and step into the soft, bright light of truth.

My heart still clenches at the thought of 'losing Aaron'. Yet that's exactly the kind of thought I need to relax. *How?* I wonder. And the answer comes: *Rest in the arms of your Beloved, your Life, and expect nothing — even as you can expect* everything. You have the right to expect everything; everything your heart desires. Life is magnificent; magnificent and overflowing with possibilities and offers of realities — *but* leave the shape of this up to life. Don't demand that life continues to give you Aaron for any length of time at all. Give him up NOW! Let nothing keep you enthralled. *Be Mine.* The written words come as if spoken. *Be Mine, and that way I can give you all you want.*

Gustav Mahler's music ends. It's time to get up.

I watch Aaron walking about the room. It's a delight to see how his body moves without a hint of self-consciousness. Not like me — struggling with how I present to him. I know he watches me. His eyes are soft, non-judgmental, but I know he notices the awkwardness I feel as I sense him looking.

It's gruesome, the way he can see me so clearly. I can't hide from him. He reads my energy and doesn't get fooled by pretence or attempts to cover up — mine or anyone else's. My programmed response is to escape my apparent nakedness. It's no use! He calls me over and puts a kindly arm around me. I *detest* the way he smiles so knowingly! I'm supposed to be the mysterious female here, not an open book that he can read so easily. I'm not used to being upped by a man, someone who is my lover, someone so much younger than me!

But I needn't worry. Aaron loves me, just not in the romantic sense that a woman like me might dream about. Reality doesn't upset him — the reality, that is, that I'm flawed from just about every angle. He doesn't mind being my teacher of sorts. In fact, I'm beginning to realise that he thinks of himself as someone who has something to give me, and it's more than friendship or love or sex or a good time. It's the growing up of Carla in the areas where she's been stunted by her own opinions of herself. 'I want you to be Carla,' he says earnestly, taking my shoulders in his hands. Looking at him, I get a sense of what he means. Aaron's schooling me to be true not to him, but to myself. I'm wild with love for this gift!

Aaron's kind of love breaks my heart wide open and he loves what he gets back.

'I love the way you can enjoy me,' he says simply. 'No one's ever enjoyed me as much.'

He's Aaron, and not like anyone else on earth. He doesn't play the game of behaving to please or impress others. People just love him or not. Usually they do, because he's so humorously uncompromising. He is what everyone around him wants to be: just happy in themselves. His big energy affects those around him without words, but he loves words.

'I own the energy of who I am; that's all I've got. I don't live off anyone else's energy, and they won't be able to live off mine. I leave if someone doesn't like that. I stay if they can be themselves with me.'

I'm so amazed at his own positive appraisal of himself. It has nothing to do with pride. It's just healthy. And it feels like fun to be in that space.

'Things have gone up a notch,' Aaron announces on his way back from the bathroom, as if he's had an inspiration while sitting on the toilet. 'I used to like you,' he says, sitting beside me at the computer, 'and I don't say these things lightly. When I say I like you, I really mean it. But now I want to say that I'm in love with you.'

I lean my head on my hand, elbow on the computer table, grateful for the support, since I feel faint.

'Am I hearing you right? Did you say you're in love with me?'

'Yes, I did.'

I watch his face, all lit up with something deep within. But I'm cautious. 'Isn't that a no-no in your life, Aaron?' I remember the many comments about romantic, 'unreal' love.

'I'm in love with you and it's not romantic,' he says, slightly impatiently.

It's a pity I didn't take his declaration at face value. I should have known that caution was unnecessary, but somehow I needed time to let his announcement sink in.

He explains. 'It means that you're always with me. I carry the thought of you around. I feel you constantly. You're the most important thing in my life. You're deeply in my system now.'

This really does change things. It introduces a level of familiarity that wasn't there before, a new intimacy. It also puts us on an equal footing at last, I think.

He sits there smiling, waiting for my response. He looks so relaxed, so pleased with life, himself and me.

This is a moment so simple and profound that it will stay with me. Lord knows, I may need moments like this to stay with me. Always there is a sense of foreboding in my heart, this Romeo and Juliet feeling that some disaster is going to overcome our relationship and end it. It never leaves me, and while I haven't the slightest idea of what it means, I don't think it's just a neurotic feeling.

'Now you know how I've been feeling about *you*.' Instead of more words, I lean over to kiss him.

The tenderness coming from his mouth melts my body. He's depressed, though, from the thoughts that have haunted him today, and I sense he wants to take time in my safe space to recover. I chat to him as I cook.

'I listened to that teenybopper album this morning, while I cleaned my verandah,' I say. 'It's all about romantic love — the stuff of broken hearts!'

'Don't deny young people their romantic love, Carla,' he butts in earnestly. 'It's the way they learn to look for love. You have to want love to start looking for it. They're learning to find themselves through contact with others and experiencing pleasure and pain. That's how it should be. It's when they don't wake up to what's causing their pain that the trouble stays; then they don't grow up.'

I'm humbled by his non-judgmental views of heart-sick teenagers (and others) screaming their disappointment and longing through a microphone. Suddenly, I experience their music differently; I have what practitioners of Neuro Linguistic Programming would call 'a rapid reframe'. It's all become much more acceptable. The music is actually very sexy, I notice, when I play it again later.

CONSIDERATIONS

God's reckless wobble.
Galway Kinnell, 'Oatmeal'

 My friend Susan has successfully undergone different types of plastic surgery: lifts and stretches and breast implants. She looks fantastic, and I feel compelled to investigate these procedures for myself. I visit a woman plastic surgeon. As she talks, I become convinced I'll be one of those few women whose bodies reject an implant as a foreign object. Besides, I can't imagine putting up with the pain of having a breast muscle split to make room for the implant. It is heavy as well, even only in a B size. How on earth do women cope with D-cups?

The surgeon is kind enough to point out that my breasts are already nice: firm, symmetrical, not droopy, and not nearly as small as some she's seen. Her words do something huge for my breast-ego. Evidently, the natural remedies from the Menopause Institute have done a great job in dissolving most of the lumps in my breasts; only the left one retains a single lump, and that's no longer visible.

I decide against breast implants, but do sign up for a reduction of my eyelids. I have my mother's droopy-eyelid genes, so much so that it's becoming more and more difficult to open my eyes in the morning. The operation is a great success: I really like the refreshed look I see in the mirror. This was a good decision! Even so, the pain is unexpectedly fierce and long. Pain can be an ageing thing in itself, which is another reason I wouldn't go for anything more complicated.

Aaron's always so delighted when I turn up unexpectedly. 'A girl stays at home and waits for visitors,' he once said, 'but a woman goes after what she wants!'

I head for his place late in the morning, after having my hair done. I get it coloured and cut every six weeks. I don't know what I'd look like if I didn't do this. Some women get away with nothing but an occasional trim; I'm one of those high-maintenance women who have to do a lot to look as if they do hardly anything.

We manage to get away from Rick and head for Aaron's den under the house.

'Stay warm,' he says, holding his heaviest, thickest jacket over my shoulders. 'No, get your arms in there. Trust me, it makes a difference.'

It's not only winter; here, in this room without a door and no windows, it's freezing cold.

'I need something over my knees,' I say. 'When your knees are cold, your whole body's cold.'

'I'll go and get a hot water bottle,' he says.

'How have you been this morning?' I enquire, once I've got a hot water bottle on my knees, with a jumper to cover it up and keep it hot. He sits down at his computer again; it seems the tasks related to it are endless.

'I'm giving up the course,' he finally says, wrenching his eyes from the computer screen. 'I had a discussion with my dad, told him I was thinking of giving it away. I was so relieved when he said he understood. He said that he himself had always experienced stress as a teacher, which really surprised me. He said he hadn't wanted to interfere with my wish to become a teacher, but he doesn't expect me to go on if it doesn't suit my nature. I never expected my dad to be so understanding.'

Aaron swivels in his chair, moved by his father's generosity. 'I've got to tell my mum sometime today. I wonder what she'll think.'

'She loves you. She'll just want whatever makes you happy.'

He has the chance to find out when his mother comes downstairs after lunch. He makes her sit down and announces that he wants to tell her something. She sits on the edge of his bed, mouth prim, hearing aid turned on.

'I talked to Dad this morning and told him that I'm quitting the course,' Aaron begins. His mother, who now wants me to call her Beryl, is impassive. She waits for more. 'What do *you* think of that, Mum?'

Aaron's mother is a person who's reluctant to give straight answers. But the occasion is serious and she simply says, 'It's your life, Aaron. I gave birth to you and raised you, and what you do with your life is your affair. I only hope that in the end you won't think you have wasted your life. What are you going to do now?'

It's the question he was waiting for.

'I'll look for work,' he says, ignoring her insinuation about wasting his life. 'Did you hear on the news how they're short of workers in the wheat belt to get the harvest in?' This job, he's already explained to me, is 'back o' Burke' — if not literally way off in the desert wilderness, still many hundreds of kilometres away. The thing is, it's good money. 'If I get the job, I'll earn $800 a week,' he says. 'I want to get enough money together to build my house. I reckon I need about $20,000 to do it.'

'What do *you* think, Carla?' Beryl turns to me, unexpectedly.

Well, my opinion is that I hate seeing him stressed, and I say so. I've been puzzled and dismayed by Aaron's determination to stay with a lost cause until it is completely dead, as now. It occurs to me that he has treated his past relationships the same way: hoping against hope they would survive, loyal beyond reason. What's finally put Aaron off his dream of becoming a teacher isn't the study demands, but the bureaucracy within the education system and the cold knowledge that this job would demand he attends work every school day. Being told what to do against his better judgment, filling in papers, the constant demands on his attention — all these factors would send him crazy.

Aaron is an eccentric, and much of his charm comes from that, but I find myself wishing that he had a good, steady job and that he was, by now, financially secure.

Beryl is actually relieved that her son is choosing to give away this study, which becomes obvious when she launches into stories about relatives who suffered dementia as a result of stress, or died from heart attacks. 'There's a gene in the family that can't take stress,' she says emphatically, 'and I reckon you've got that gene, so you do what's right for you and give it away.'

Both Aaron's parents are on his side. He was worried for nothing.

When we're alone again, he turns to me; he knows what I am thinking. If he works for $800 a week till he's saved $20,000, that's half a year! But the wheat-harvesting season isn't that long.

'I know you don't like this idea,' he says.

He does know me now. It's a comfort, but I know him too. I know that he'll do what's right for him, without letting his desire for my company get in the way.

'Trust that you're always with me,' he says and smiles.

My only comfort is knowing that he may come as close to missing me as I will him. My heart clenches: 'together and apart' may soon become 'apart and together'. I have to be able to *live* this. But am I ready? It doesn't feel like it.

'I've known for some time that your life will take you away from me,' he says, suddenly turning the tables on me, making me realise that he's been through exactly the same dilemma as I have, but without fanfare.

'As this world crumbles,' he goes on, holding my eyes serenely, gently in touch with me, 'people will hunger for what gives them hope, for a reality they can live from their hearts. I've seen for a long time that you can offer a different view to those who want to hear. I know that what you have to do will take you away from me.'

Haven't I had the same thought myself, but forgotten it in the face of what Aaron might do? In a way, this life has already begun. My talks are more and more in demand. I may have to travel. My recent interest in plastic surgery was all about being more presentable in a world where first impressions count.

I remind him that he has the option to go back to taxi driving, although he would have to overcome his disdain of the industry.

'I might front up. And if they're nice to me, I'll go for it. And if they make things difficult for me, I'll leave,' he says, with a definitive wave of his arm. Taxi driving is evidently still too hard a thing for him to think about realistically.

'How do you think you've changed?' Aaron turns to me from where he's seated at my computer.

It's quite a question. I *have* changed. But how have I changed? Well, for starters, I'm not beating myself up the way I used to.

'I don't let my mind run away with negative ideas so easily,' I say. 'I catch myself when I start imagining the worst, and bring myself back to centre.'

He nods, waits.

'Actually, I think I've changed a lot, but it isn't obvious at first look.'

He still waits.

'I'm more content with what the moment brings, instead of hankering after something that isn't there.'

All this seems important, but the one thing that makes most sense to him is, 'I'm more grounded. My feet are on the ground and it feels good.'

'Good!' he says, like a teacher giving me a mark.

I look at him and wonder if he's noticed how much *he's* changed. I've taken it for granted that he has, but until now, I hadn't really thought about it. Later that evening, he tells me, after love has satiated us and it's way past midnight and we sleep and wake every few minutes to caress, kiss and talk again.

'I feel strange these days,' he says in a drowsy voice, lying on his side. 'I'm not my lonely self any more and I'm not used to feeling this way. I used to be more in control.' He's used to being wary with women, protecting himself from being exploited or used. 'Blokes are so simple, but women complicate things in no time with their demands for what they can't have.'

I know the stories. I have an inkling of what Aaron's exes might have gone through before they started tearing his (and their) hair out.

'I think it might have been your strategy of being aloof and being the observer, rather than being committed and out there,' I say. 'You've gone past that lately.'

And it's true, I suddenly realise: he's become unreserved now when we're together. He just gives, the way he sees me do. I love to love him; I feel it's an utter privilege. There can't possibly be a strategy attached to this, and he's doing the same. But Aaron's gone further than that. He has no caution; he's become reckless, unreckoning, giving all of himself and wanting to give more. He's become undone, in the psychological sense.

'What did you say about women finding me attractive because I was reserved, or something?'

I recall the words. 'Some women will want you because they are attracted to what is not attainable.'

'Well,' he says, 'I'm not available, because I belong to you!'

He's lying on his back now, and I can make out his profile in the semi-darkness. From anyone else, such words would sound normal. You can expect a man to say *I belong to you* when he loves you, but from Aaron this is definitely not normal! As a matter of fact, he's used the very opposite words, emphatically: *I don't belong to anyone but myself.* Does he realise how he's contradicting himself? Apparently not.

Oblivious, he continues, 'This is the closest I've ever come to being married.'

He sounds as if he's talking to himself, deliberating, not in his right mind, half in alpha, half in theta, his brainwaves evidently not engaged in what would normally put him on guard. I'm riveted! What's the matter with me that such little words make so great an impact on me?

It's because Aaron is making strides he's never made before. I'm identifying with his process, and proud of him.

Aaron turns to me, and his eyes are not what I'm used to. They're like *my* eyes, expressing a wonder and tenderness that belong to *my* soul, and now I see this expressed in his. His hand reaches out to stroke my face.

'I love the look of your face. You're so beautiful.'

All such ordinary words, spoken with such passion! They're new words — new, because this is the first time he's uttered them to me, and new because they come from a different, fresh place. His kisses are like mine now, unrestrained and full of desire to convey deepest love and wanting.

'I'm frustrated,' he says at last. 'I'm frustrated because no matter how hard I try, I can't be you. I touch you where we meet and melt, and then I come back to myself.'

'But the core of you is the same as me, Aaron. We're the same when we forget who we are.'

'We're like two pages in one book,' he says, because he likes to talk in pictures, then asks, 'What fonts are we?'

'I'm a Times New Roman font,' I say without hesitation. 'And you're Middle Earth.'

'Middle Earth? What font is that? Oh, maybe that's Gothic.'

'Yep, Gothic.'

'Why are you Times New Roman?'

'Because it's the most recognisable font in the writing world,' I explain. 'It's simple, unpretentious, elegant and universally readable.'

I don't know if that describes me, really. It's so down to earth, and that's not how I have ever described myself. But this is a time for change. 'Down to earth' could be an adjectival phrase I may wear as a badge of honour, after all.

'Why Gothic Middle Earth?'

'Oh, because I watched *The Lord of the Rings* recently, I guess.'

But he has his own idea. 'It's otherworldly, that's what it is. It's not used in legal documents. It speaks of undercurrents and history and the mystical.'

'The writing's different, but the paper's the same.' I go on with the analogy he's begun. 'The imprint is on the same stuff that we're both made of.'

'That's true. We're both the same stuff, somehow.'

Where we meet, we know each other to be the same. Maybe it's this sameness that has to do with who we've been over many ages; that's what it feels like.

'We go back a long way, you and me.'

Aaron is voicing my own thoughts. We go back not just thirty years, but to God knows how many lifetimes and adventures together. Middle Earth — that's where the mysteries might be recorded; but it doesn't matter, we needn't know. To enjoy the depth of our friendship is what matters. We're trusted, inviolate friends, and are lucky to be lovers too.

My face is above his now, as we talk. I am overcome with the in-loveness I see there, the sensitive traits of guileless youth on the face of a mature man.

'When I see you, I see my own innocence.' My words come tumbling out, meet his eyes and his heart. The only answer is an embrace of utter thankfulness for this togetherness. Skin upon skin, my softness against his strength, my face against his, breath mingled.

Maybe it is only those who've experienced guilt and shame in their lives who can dwell in such ecstatic innocence. It's the advantage of age, of maturity, of having faced the demons, reaching compassion for others instead of condemnation, seeing the beauty in the moment because life is now shorter, more compelling and immediate.

We untangle ourselves from our love-making and face each other, hunched on our knees. We look at each other as if we've never seen one another before. We must go into some kind of trance, because time passes and still we do nothing but sit. Tears quietly well in my eyes. I am vaguely aware of the sting of salt collecting there, yet still make no move. Not even my eyes are moving. There's no thinking. I'm not thinking about Aaron, whose face is now in shadow so his eyes are barely visible, and I'm not thinking about myself. There's no thought, no concept, nothing but wonder. Wonder, wonder but no thought, no question and no answer. Gratitude. True passion is priceless, in that it demands no price at all.

Aaron breaks the spell by slightly moving his hand. I blink. He takes his hand to his face to wipe it. We lie down silently and he pulls the doona over us. It is only then that I see his face glistening near his eyes. Aaron in tears? Really? We say nothing and lie close for a long time.

Later, he wants to know what went on in me. He props his head up on his right hand so he can see me. I look at him nonplussed: how do you describe those kind of feelings without sounding sentimental or, worse, corny?

'Describe it as a picture,' he says. 'Let a picture come to mind. It doesn't matter if nothing comes.'

I shut my eyes and wait, then describe the image that presents itself.

'It's like the ocean,' I begin, keeping my eyes closed so I can hold the image. 'At the top of the ocean the water is moving around in great, powerful, noisy waves, and at the bottom of the ocean the water is still, and it is totally quiet. In between is a broad sweep of slow-moving water, which is pulled about by the top layer of waves, like in a dance. That's it.'

Aaron's impressed.

'That's good,' he says, 'you can make feelings into pictures. You're becoming like me.'

DOWN IN THE VALLEY

Down in the valley, valley so low
Hang your head over, hear the wind blow
Traditional American folksong

All day, I've felt a nose-cold brewing and now, at the end of a National Speakers Association event at a venue near Aaron's place, it's full-blown. He's expecting me to call in on him, but I phone instead with the news that I'm not well.

'I'm homework bound anyway,' he says.

I'm floored. He's doing homework for a course he's abandoning?

'Come around for a cup of tea,' he suggests, and I agree. Ten minutes later I'm in his room. He gets up from his chair in front of the computer to welcome me.

'I'm worn out,' he warns me. 'Have no energy for a cuddle in bed. Do you want to sit on that chair?' He's relieved when I say okay. 'You look ratshit,' he says. 'You look sick.'

'Well,' I say, shrugging my shoulders, 'it can't be helped. But I feel okay inside. How much work is there left to do?' This work has taken days already; it's the same task I helped him with last week.

'It's this loyalty thing,' he explains. 'I don't want to let my two co-students down.'

I listen with complete astonishment. 'Why are you rescuing those two?'

His brain has become so tired that direct questions like this only make a dim impact. His mother comes down and suggests I warm up in the bath upstairs.

While I soak in the blessed heat of the soothing water, I think of our situation. The love he feels for me isn't the kind that makes a priority out of our relationship. He'll do homework for others instead, wearing out his brain because he finds the work so difficult.

A week has passed. It's Sunday morning and I'm once more in Aaron's room, my critical thoughts of last week a dim memory.

'Tell me what you're thinking,' he says.

I'm sitting on him in his bed, not thinking at all. I switch on my brain to make words come, then tell him, 'I respect you.'

I see him do a double-take. Respect? He doesn't really get how I respect the beauty I see in him.

'I respect your sweetness, your simplicity, your directness.'

The love on his face transforms him, or else the love in me is tricking my eyes.

And then he comes out with a remark he'll regret. Maybe it's because he finds it so difficult to accept compliments. He even smiles as he says it. 'Carla's done a dumb thing: she's chosen Aaron for a boyfriend.'

A brick drops into my belly. A flash of fury sweeps over me, but the feeling quickly changes to sadness and a sob rises from my chest. Aaron sees his joke go horribly wrong, but just paraphrases what he said. 'Carla, you've made a really dumb mistake. You've chosen Aaron for a boyfriend.'

The tears flow hard for a moment and Aaron reaches for the tissue box. I blow, and toss the balled tissue, aiming vaguely for the rubbish bin.

'That's the way to treat tissues,' he says. He's still treating this as a joke.

He suddenly realises that it may not sound funny to me at all. He soothes me with his warm, gentle hands. Wanting to reassure me that this meant nothing, he starts to undress me. 'You want to make love tonight, don't you?'

Part of me is still in disbelief. I can't really believe that he meant what he said, but why then did he say it?

I'm undressed before I can think of an answer. He enters my naked body the moment it is laid on his bed, and all thought leaves me as sensations take hold of my body. Aaron pauses again and again to control the eroticism that surges through him. I try hard to smother the sounds that escape from my throat, thinking of his father asleep in his bed right above us. Aaron can't control himself for long. I can see it and whisper urgently, 'Give it to me, baby!', making the most of the inevitable.

'You've got it,' he says ruefully.

It's over. He's so tired now. We don't get back into bed.

I get dressed to leave and he accompanies me to the car. Aaron's got something on his mind, something he hasn't been able to say all evening. Now it's got to come out before I go home. It's a question, and I can see from his hesitation that he's thought about it quite a bit.

'Do you think you're committing self-sabotage by being in a relationship with me?'

What? Later it'll sink in that this question links to his 'You're dumb to choose Aaron' statement. He must really feel inferior, and is seriously doubting himself as a suitable partner for me.

My answer, unfortunately, is hot and immediate — an attempt to make him feel better while ignoring the pain I still feel.

'No!'

The force of it makes him wobble. I take his stubbly face in my hands.

'This is the man I want!' I tell him. I kiss him. 'I want you, Aaron!' And I kiss him again. His lips try to respond. They're soft, but he's not there with me. He's obviously moved, though.

He shrugs his shoulders as I get into my car. 'What can I say?'

'Say it to me on Wednesday, Aaron.'

It's only Sunday; Wednesday is three days away. What if three days of separation, of having no contact, of reflection, changes things again? Human nature can be treacherous. The best woman in the world — me — can also be treacherous. Or else her mind has been deceiving her up till now, and coming to her senses will look a lot like treachery.

It's Wednesday evening; I don't expect him so early. Aaron comes in clean-shaven and light; he had gone to college to say goodbye to the lecturers and students and they had been gratifyingly sad to see him go. He couldn't have left his course on a better note, knowing that he can return next year if he wants.

He's also pleased because he's found a computer case for me: an old but sturdy ex-industrial unit that fits under my table. It cost only $5 at his 'special shop', the Dalcatta tip.

He's come to sleep with me, he says. He sure needs to sleep; he seems exhausted. I'm fairly tired as well, after travelling to Mandurah and back to give a talk to a group of women of all different persuasions and backgrounds. They were mostly very welcoming, just a few who were quietly hostile. I had no proper lunch and no break at all. Going to sleep is an attractive proposition. Can we manage to just sleep and do nothing else?

It's good how comfortable we are with one another now. We get into bed and talk from our pillows. Aaron talks about possible options for his future. One of them is to go back to his beloved house in Darkan, his number one project.

'Would you ever come to Darkan — not to live, but to visit?' he asks.

'Of course I would.'

'Will you be very sad and pine for me if I leave Perth?'

Since last Sunday something in me has strengthened. My answer's not the one I would have given a week ago.

'No way. If you leave me, I'll find another boyfriend.'

Aaron doesn't quite like my words, but he can hardly object. Don't they sound like his own, spoken three times in the past? *If you leave me, I'll just find another Carla to love and to love me.* But he's not taking the bait. He feels that my words are just a defence against getting hurt.

'You're in love with me; you're attached and might feel distraught.'

Now he's given me the perfect chance to tell him how I've changed these last few days. I haven't seen him for three days and I've been very happy with my own company.

'I've pulled back, Aaron, since what you said last Sunday.'

'What was that?' he asks. Has he no idea what I'm referring to?

'You said, "Carla's done a dumb thing. She's chosen Aaron for a boyfriend." You said it *twice*.'

Aaron makes a move as if to take back those words. 'They were meant as a figure of speech!' he blurts. 'They belonged to the moment, not to forever!'

'They were spoken in a very serious moment. I was crying at the time.'

'You were crying?'

Does he really not remember? Doesn't he remember that I was sobbing into his neck, so forlorn about my love for a man who'd go away because his priorities don't include what we have together? It's possible that he doesn't quite remember. It's possible that because his mind was so fatigued at the time, what happened has become a blur.

Our conversation turns to other things, interspersed with casual caresses. In spite of our weariness, we suddenly get so aroused that in moments his penis once more reminds me what it can do to make a woman feel balanced and glowing. I break away, though. We talk again, but once more passion overtakes us, or rather, Aaron.

'On your back, kid!' he says. 'I want you!'

We're on top of the bedclothes. He pins back my arms. 'You're on the ground,' he whispers, 'the grassy ground. The air is kissing you. The air is kissing you and I'm the earth, and the earth is making love to you.' The imagery is so simple, so basic to our senses. It's also erotic, and the surge that overcomes me surges back to him.

'Your loins and mine are made for each other!' he asserts, and he becomes reckless. 'I want to waste all my energy! I want to take you all night! All night! Time and time again!' He moans as his semen erupts, helplessly.

We get back under the bedclothes and he laughs. 'We're doomed!' he says. 'We can't stay away from each other. We can't be close to each other without having sex.' He sighs, mock sad, a look of contentedness on his face that gives him that angelic look I can't help loving.

We sleep. We wake up with me tucked in behind his back. He brings my hand to his penis. It's hard, with a man's morning hard-on. It doesn't mean he's aroused, but it means that he would welcome my admiration and touch. 'Please hold him.' He turns onto his back so I can reach him better.

'Don't kiss me,' he warns. 'I've got very bad breath this morning.'

I believe it. I'd have the same, except that I've already scraped my tongue with a narrow blade I keep for the purpose.

I touch him languidly and he loves it, reaches to put his hand on my vagina, puts one finger, then two, inside it. 'It's a miracle that there's a hole in you, so I can put my dick right inside your body,' he says, apparently overcome with the thought. He takes the tube of lubricant and applies it to me so his caresses can be more fluid. Then he takes a good look at the tube itself. 'Good stuff,' he says, 'bloody good stuff. The best.'

Eventually, he gets up, cleans his teeth, decides not to shave since he did that last night, and gets back into bed. Neither of us has a busy schedule today. It's the first day in a long time that Aaron hasn't had to think of study.

'You know, I was going to get a dildo before I met you,' I tell him. 'That's why I got that lubricant. But I never bought a dildo.'

'That's because I'm your dildo.'

He gets up on his knees, pulls back the doona and examines my vulva. 'Researcher from the Dildo Department here,' he says, approaching my vagina with his erect penis. 'We're going to find out what is the right fit for you, madam. Customer satisfaction is of the utmost importance to us. We believe in quality as well as size, and the ability of the dildo to reach all the right spots in your ladyship's pleasure zones.'

By now he's 'experimenting' and 'demonstrating' and 'getting feedback for our records', then suddenly says that he wants to show me what else it can do.

'No!' I yell at him, raising my head and shoulders. 'Don't!'

He returns to his normal frame of mind. 'Why not?'

Has he really gone mad? 'You need your energy back. You're still recovering. Keep it!'

Thankfully, he has the sense to pull back and out. 'If madam is satisfied, please consider buying,' he concludes.

It's midday by the time he leaves. He wanted to teach me how to burn CDs and I'm a slow learner. Before he leaves, he makes an observation. 'You're so confident in lots of things, but when it comes to learning about computers, you have this nervousness and this attitude that you can't do it well. I think it's got to do with your father.'

Yes, it has to do with my father. My father, who first sexually abused me and then almost killed me when I was six to silence me. I became a nervous wreck of a child who lived in a fog, not sure whether I existed in a dream or in the real world. My father used to scoff at my deplorable absentmindedness, and I often wept at his derision, at least deep inside, in my wounded heart.

'I was so often in terror about getting things wrong,' I muse, surprised that I've known this for so long yet haven't connected it with my reluctance to learn new things.

'You're still nervous about getting things wrong,' Aaron says, standing above me as I sit huddled in my office chair. 'And so eager to please. You need to deal with it.'

I know he's right. I am much too eager to please.

'When you deal with this, you'll be a different woman,' he continues brightly. 'You'll be much stronger, much more your own person, no longer the little girl with a finger in her mouth.'

I can feel both ways now. I can feel my diffident child-self, and also the woman who is waiting in the wings; the one who knows what she wants, can do anything she wants to, and won't even think of apologising for mistakes.

A KNIGHT TO REMEMBER

Keep looking.
Keep looking until you see the mystery,
until the mystery sees you.
Robert Rabbin, 'Mystery'

Aaron's forgotten that I'm going out this evening. He's also forgotten that I was free all afternoon. He phones after five and asks me to come over and hang around.

I remind him that I'm going to my girlfriend Kate's fiftieth birthday party tonight. 'She's putting on a tango lesson.' I'm torn, feeling that he really wants me to come over, but I decide to keep to my plans.

'Come over afterwards, if you can,' he ends.

I think, What a good idea, but don't say so. I'll 'do an Aaron' and surprise him. Besides, I easily get bored at parties and always want to leave early. Talking to strangers you're not likely to see again about nothing in particular seems a terrible waste of time to me.

I arrive at the party at the same time as Tom, a friend who was once a mentor to me when I was new to the public speaking game. He catches up with me as I cross the road towards the venue.

'Hello, Carla. How lovely to see you here!'

167

Tom used to have a suave manner, which worked for him for years in the public relations industry. A recent marriage break-up has seriously eroded his polish, however, and the chipped article now striding beside me, speaking in his Scottish accent, is a pleasure to be with. I'm happy at the prospect of a good conversation with him.

We head for a radiant Kate to congratulate her on turning fifty. We deposit our presents on a table set aside for the purpose so Kate can enjoy unwrapping them all later.

Tom and I try to be sociable and join others at a table, but they ignore us, one and all. I've experienced this before at parties where most people know each other; it's a strange phenomenon that normal people can become socially autistic. One fellow leans across our table to talk to someone, his butt almost sticking into Tom's face. The man doesn't notice his rudeness and stays that way for quite a while. Tom just smiles and we talk about our relationships, his in particular, the one he no longer has and why it is so.

Then it's time for the tango lesson. Much as I like Tom, I don't want to dance with him because he's so much shorter than me. 'I'll go find a taller partner,' I say with a flourish, 'and find one for you as well.'

Confidently striding across the room, I head for the tallest beau, only to be pipped by another lady.

A guy nearby earlier caught my eye — so intriguingly handsome that I'm sure he's there with a partner. But no, he's standing by himself, quietly surveying the scene. I decided to burst in on his pre-choice musings.

'Do you have a partner?' I inquire, smiling as charmingly as I can, hoping he'll notice my nice dress. It's dusky rose with black lace, a tight bodice, a full, irregular skirt — some would call it a gypsy style. In any case, it has a dark and brooding air that relates to Argentina and the tango.

His eyes steady on me, he answers, 'No,' to which, of course, I immediately add my question: 'May I be your partner then?'

To my relief he replies with a good-natured, 'Yes, okay.'

Having secured my own partner, I go about looking for one for

Tom and soon find a lady suited to his size. He smiles his thanks broadly from across the room.

I turn my attention to my dance partner.

'My name is John,' he says politely.

'Carla,' I introduce myself in turn, and briefly shake his hand, asking if he has any experience with this dance. This is purely a conversational question; somehow, I know this man is a *dancer*, and that he's here because he knows the tango back to front, upside down, inside out.

The music starts to scratch its way out of the speakers and we take on the pose as instructed. My right hand finds itself gently enveloped in John's left, while the other softly lands on the upper part of his right shoulder. I catch him stealing a glance at the ring I'm wearing on the hand he's holding; it's my silver dolphin ring, the one I purchased for myself three weeks after leaving the convent. I feel him smile and bring his eyes back; I know that I'm not supposed to have noticed this. It tenses my body, but I consciously make it relax. You're not here to make an impression, I tell myself. You're an older woman who is going to have a delicious tango lesson with a sensual younger man who knows what he's doing.

John shows me how to lean in as closely as I'm comfortable with, and we start to walk. Walking is mainly what the lesson is about this evening: the man leading the way, the woman yielding constantly to his direction. I decide that the best thing to do is to close my eyes so I can better anticipate the subtle movements of his body. I sense him observing my movements even though the lashes of my eyes rest languidly on my cheeks; I am so tuned in that I can't help it.

The top parts of our bodies move well enough, but our knees keep hitting.

'Are they supposed to touch like this?' I ask.

'No,' he says, and I realise that my step backwards isn't long and bold enough.

Our next try is more successful, but then our instructor changes plans. We're to walk with the woman holding both hands against her partner's chest. I watch while the experienced Argentinean and his partner perform the steps. John, in the meantime, explains the dance to me.

'The tango,' he says, 'is one of the most sensual dances on earth. It is *the* dance. The man makes love to the woman while he has her in his arms, and then he lets her go [he bows, and moves his arms in goodbye as he speaks] and thanks her. The woman follows his lead; she surrenders to him for the duration of the dance. It's a three-minute love affair.'

I look into his eyes, eyes partly hidden in the folds of his face, but very steady.

'I'm a healer,' he says, apropos of nothing. 'I work for the government full-time as a computer person, and I also do massage. In massage, I approach the person gently. I place my hands on their body so they can get acquainted with my energy and there's no shock to their system.'

Now I know what he's trying to say. His approach to dancing is the same as to massage: he does it very consciously. He takes a woman's hand to make contact, not just to get it into position.

'I also do tai chi,' he says, demonstrating a couple of fluid poses. His movements are sinuous, tantalising and pure, without apology for their sensuality.

The dance begins. I lean into John's body, pushing it away; alternately taking strides backwards to accommodate his coming forward. Once again I close my eyes, and ignore my beating heart, to concentrate on the movement. I feel our bodies jarring at first, my legs doing a self-conscious thing, then the movement gradually smooths out and enters brief moments of fluidity.

The music stops. John compliments me. 'That's good,' he says. Then adds, seeing my slight blush, 'No, I mean it. I should know. You're a natural dancer.'

I have a great sense of rhythm, and love how this dance only comes into its own when strong masculinity takes the lead, and the woman has the opportunity to yield, as if in a sexual embrace, right there on the dance floor. But how can John know me so well in so short a time? The delight of being seen like this sends a thrill through my body. I'm flabbergasted. How can I spend decades without meeting a man that sees me, and, now that I have Aaron, meet another so easily?

Does John also feel that I know him for his exquisite sensuality? I only half dare think it, but the idea of making love to this man is as natural as it is to make love to Aaron. It's a shocking thought. Am I still that promiscuous person I was so many years ago? No, I wouldn't do that to Aaron, but the amazing thing is the possibility. I can understand how it is that a man or a woman truly in love, even committed to the other, can nevertheless have an affair with someone else. I've thought of Aaron and me as having a depth in our relationship that is unique and irreplaceable. I suddenly realise this is not true. Cruel thought. We *do* have something special; and yet it's not unique. There are others who can match my sexual passion. There are others who can see me. There are others who know how to love, and who love with much more consideration than my Aaron does.

John decides to ignore the tutor's lengthy instructions. He pulls me in close and teaches me the swing — moving gently from one foot to the other on the spot, perhaps moving in a circle, so that he can take off again in a different direction. We practise, interspersing the walking step with deliciously quiet moments of swinging.

'I take my cue from the music,' he says. 'Did you hear when it changed?'

But I didn't. I wasn't listening to the music at all.

'I'm concentrating on *you*!' I say, my cheek against his, my voice right next to his ear, and I sense a slight shock in his body. Now he knows what he has here.

Next, he teaches me the slide. Our first attempt is a failure because the movement of his leg, responding too late to the music, is abrupt. The next attempt is more graceful. I could have slid down and down and landed on the floor and had this man on top of me, and . . .

I find myself asking about lessons. He gives me his card and promises to email me details of when the next beginners classes are due to start. The lesson ends. I rejoin Tom, who is happily effusive about his experience. When I tell him I'm getting details regarding classes, he asks me to send them on to him.

It's nine when I stand up and put on my coat with a large gesture, meant to attract attention. I know John will notice, as I have been aware of his glances during my chat with Tom. I turned around once and caught him slightly off guard as he danced with Kate, whose birthday we're celebrating. It was too late for him to pretend he hadn't noticed me looking. I turn again as I leave the room and he smiles his goodbye, hands clasped together in a movement half towards me, half away, that says, *If you'd stay, I'd dance with you again.*

But I want to be with Aaron.

I sit in my car, incredulous at what has just happened. Never before, in all my life, have I come across someone so aware of body language. I learnt it myself during childhood as a self-protective device: I had to be aware of what my father might be about to do — fly off the handle, approach me to deride or hit me, whatever. When he came to me in the night, I learnt about raw, nervous sexual energy. As a callgirl, this knowledge made me a good judge of whether I could trust a man or not.

Now I've met a man who is like me, but unlike me. There was nothing about John that suggests he's been abused. I asked him for his birth date because I dabble in numerology. The number six shines large and luminous, representing sensual pleasure, love of harmony and beauty, music, food, dancing, healing ...

Never before have I been so sure that what I am reading in a man is also being read back to me, as if he can read my mind. The realisation makes my knees weak. And never before have I come across a person as non-cynical, clean and open about his sensuality.

John is a fair few years younger than me. Probably in his late forties.

'Does your husband or partner dance?' he asked me. 'No!' was my straightforward answer, knowing that this was his way of finding out if I was attached. I asked him the same, and he said, no, he didn't have a partner just now. But I already knew that.

I turn into the darkness, heading for the freeway.

It takes me half an hour to get to Aaron's place. He's at the computer, of course. His finger is poised on the print button as I enter his room. He switches his attention to me and gets up.

'How sweet of you to come!' he says, genuinely pleased to see me, and gently takes my face in his hands to kiss it. 'Shall I clear that chair for you? What do you want to do?'

I am in no mood to sit in his cold room watching him at his computer, so, pulling the bedclothes apart, I say, 'I want to snuggle with you in your bed, nice and cosy.' And I take off my coat and shoes and hop in, dress, pantyhose and all, with no plans for anything but a cuddle.

'I've missed you, Aaron!' His face is beside me on the pillow. I lean over to kiss him. 'You haven't bothered to shave!' The words come out involuntarily and I hastily add, 'But you didn't know I was coming, of course.'

It's too late; he's been hit by my remark and is weighing up the hurt against its reasonableness. The stubble is two days' worth, I guess. He seems to decide that I have reason to complain, but he's not going upstairs to shave right now; he's going to stay with me and kiss me with a lot of care, so his face doesn't rub against mine. *She's missed me. I need to address this.*

'I *love* missing you,' he says, trying to smile into my serious face. 'I miss you when you move away from me, even into the next room, and it's nice to miss you. I miss you for half an hour, a day, four days; it doesn't matter.'

The rogue!

'It matters to me,' I say. 'Five days is not at all the same as five minutes to me.'

We've had this conversation before. Aaron takes the lead this time.

'It's so beautiful and so tragic,' he says, 'the way you love me.' And he wipes my hair from my forehead as he speaks. 'Carla has to learn a lesson, and it's going to be painful and hard.'

My heart squelches under these words, then suddenly bursts. I sob quietly into his shoulder. He pushes me back so he can look at me and I can see him. My tears just keep rolling. He draws me close.

'It's alright, Carla. Cry. You're safe. You're loved; cry.

'I glory in missing you,' he says again. 'The feel of you is so rich, so fulfilling. I'm so grateful for this. You've enriched my life, you're healing my aloneness. You're what I need and what I want.' He knows all the right words.

'Tell me what's on your mind,' he says now.

'I want a relationship that's more supportive in a real way,' I begin. 'Yesterday, I spent the whole day getting ready for a big speaking event and there was no one to share it with. I was so lonely. Laurian popped in, otherwise I spoke to no one.'

'You've said everything with those words,' Aaron says. 'I think I understand, Carla. You love, you hurt. The two things go together. You love and you have grief. G.R.I.E.F. Why are you so insecure?'

'I don't doubt your love, but I want your physical presence more — to talk to you, share my life with you more than this.'

'If I lost you, I would grieve for a day and a half,' he says, 'but I refuse to *agonise* over wanting what I can't have.'

'Why do you think you will lose me, Aaron?'

'Because I'm a poor bloke, no lollies, and you're going to be rich, and you'll meet a guy who's going to be able to give you what you want.'

Haven't I had exactly the same thought myself many times? The thought hasn't been comforting, because all I want is Aaron, but an Aaron who has fulfilled some of his potential, that's for sure. I realise that he's been grieving as well, knowing this possibility.

'You love me,' he says. 'You love me so honestly, so totally. When I come to see you, you have the face of a child. When I leave, you have the face of a child.'

'And you're all grown-up,' I add.

'I'm in your life for a reason,' he says, 'but I never imagined that I would have a relationship with you when I decided to contact you.'

What is he trying to say? Whatever it is, he stops talking and starts to caress my body through my dress. He moves his hand under the skirt, under the pantyhose and knickers, and feels me. I'm very wet. His clothes come off and I struggle with mine. He undoes the zipper from the back and I ask him to undo my bra.

'Hang on,' he says, 'I'm not an expert at this.' He fumbles, but it comes off finally.

'You smell of talcum powder,' he says.

'I don't use talcum powder.'

'But you do, you definitely smell of talcum powder.'

'Must be from my dancing partner then.' Or it could be Tom. Yes, Tom's the talcum powder kind of man.

Aaron's penis hardens only gradually as we kiss. I guess he's tired. I sit on top of him and move over his penis. This excites it into action. The tears come again as I feel him inside me. The feeling is searingly exquisite; the smallest move makes me gasp with the intense flow of energy. His penis subsides after a while. We whisper. When his face is on the pillow and he's making love, he can easily look nineteen again, so heartbreakingly innocent, so taken with the love that is shining back into his face. I bend down to kiss him. His breath is particularly sweet. His stubble is terrible, but he manages to save it from rubbing my face.

'Your lips are beautiful,' he says. Because his words are new, they turn me on.

> *If you miss me, close your eyes and think of me.*
> *If that doesn't work, get busy with doing things.*
> *If that doesn't work, get out the black tube of Bodyglide.*
> *If that doesn't work, you're stuffed, Carla.*
> *Well, Aaron, thanks for that.*

Only one day later, John phones. He wants to meet up for coffee in a 'neutral place', somewhere that's not his usual place, nor mine. He suggests the Boatshed in South Perth. It's new to me, this coffee shop, and it's raining and I get lost. I get there finally, pretty wet from the walk from the car park. John awaits me on the porch and guides me to a table.

He starts the conversation. 'I found out you're an EFT person, like me,' he says.

The Emotional Freedom Technique. He's done a course with a mutual friend, Peter Graham.

'I phoned Peter and told him I had this massive connection with a woman called Carla I'd met at Kate's birthday party,' he goes on. Peter said, "You mean tall, blonde, attractive Carla? She's a good friend of mine. She did an EFT course with me and we have our follow-up meetings at her place."'

Massive connection, eh?

I ask if Peter also told him I've written a book about my life and had it published. Of course Peter did, and I'm glad John knows about my background without me having to tell him. He hasn't been put off by any of it. Instead, he's here to honour the attraction he felt.

'We met for a reason, Carla. Whatever that is, I want to follow it up. This sort of thing doesn't happen every day.'

My body sings. Apparently this intriguing feeling is mutual. The connection is so unusual for both of us it has to be explored. The trouble is, what if he feels *exactly* the way I do? Then he'd want to say very little and talk with his body instead. I sense danger, but not the kind that frightens. I'm thrilled when he takes my hand. We sit there like that while the coffee gets served. He moves closer, so our arms also touch. I feel brave and use my free hand to trace a finger over his lips. John closes his eyes. Finally, he bends over to kiss me. We're oblivious to all the other patrons.

If I've experienced exquisiteness before, I tell myself, once safely home, I've only had an introduction to the possibilities.

This is what goes on in my wicked brain, my unruly body.

I feel the space in my chest open wide. From its centre, all the other feelings and sensations radiate. There's no doubt about it: even though this connected feeling seems to come from a high and pure space, I'm committing adultery the way it's described in the Bible. I'm already making love to this man, without touching him anywhere except in his energy field. I feel his energy field around me right now. My hands are stuck to you now. My fingertips have grown into your skin. Uh-uh! Can't get them off!

Is he feeling the same way? I can't explain the intense feeling of his presence any other way.

I want to cry. Why is this happening? What about Aaron?

I AM YOUR LADY

Let us be like
Two falling stars in the day sky.
Hafiz, 'The Day Sky'

 'You look pretty tonight, really young. Hardly a line on your face. Have a look in the mirror.'

We're in the bathroom. Aaron's having a shower, I'm cleaning my teeth. I'm still high from the talk I gave this afternoon to a large audience. When I present, I surrender to an inner guidance so the right words come out of my mouth to the right corner of the room at the right time. To do this work is my joy. I'm experiencing the afterglow, and that's what he sees.

We lie side by side, facing each other on our pillows, gazing into each other's eyes. He doesn't know it, but I've decided not to move until he does. He's got used to me taking the lead, always being the one to instigate our love-making. It's difficult for me to just lie there and not move to his lips to awaken them, but I manage. It's when he finally makes a slight move towards me that I can't help meeting him with all I have, and the roller-coaster begins.

He tries to enter me sideways as we lie together, and I rise halfway to a sitting position to accommodate his efforts. Then I sink back on my side again instead of sitting on top of him. The casualness of this embrace is especially stimulating.

'We're the kids from next door, enjoying each other,' I whisper, and he catches the erotic connotation in my voice. 'We've just discovered we can do this together, and we love it.'

'Tell me what I can do for you,' he says, uncharacteristically.

I take advantage of his offer, asking him to touch my nipples and squeeze my breasts. He's rewarded by an immediate, juicy response. But he can't feel what I do, so he doesn't realise that it hurts when, instead of squeezing, he rubs his dry palms over my nipples. They need his mouth or his lubricated touch, but the occasion passes too fast for a lesson in love-making that he will forget again next time.

'I'd like to call you "my man",' I say, looking at him as we relax after making love, his penis still inside me, my left knee tucked comfortably under his armpit. 'I like it better than calling you my "boyfriend". I like being your "woman" better than being your "girlfriend". Can you feel the difference when I say that?'

No, he can't.

'It's the energy here that matters,' he says emphatically. 'Not the words!'

'But the words *carry* energies!' I persist. 'They *evoke* them!'

That seems to make no sense at all to Aaron.

I want to tell him about John.

'I met someone at Kate's party who wants to take me out.'

I expect that he will have some questions, but he hasn't. He lies on his back and speaks to the air. All he says is, 'Now I have to share you with someone else.'

'I've had to share you with your other priorities for so long already,' is my riposte.

'This is a bit different. It's time for you to understand the word "no" now, Carla. Say no and mean it.'

He won't stand in my way, though. And won't say another word about it.

He asks if I'll go down on his dick for him again.

'Sure,' I say, 'that'll happen sometime.' I want to surprise him when I do it.

When I choose the moment, he's speechless with surprise and delight. As for me, I'm flabbergasted at the pleasure I get from this action. He knows that once, not so long ago, this was almost a taboo for me.

'Tell me how my dick feels to you,' he wants to know.

'It feels smooth, strong and sweet,' I tell him.

'Yeah?' He's surprised. And then, 'What you said is important to me.'

His hands are balled in fists like a baby, up by his chest. It must have been quite a revelation. What on earth did he think of his penis before this? That it was revolting?

It finally feels like the right time to phone John. He's pleased to hear from me, but what he says makes me incredulous. John, fifty-three years of age, supposedly wise and experienced, declares over the phone that he wants to be my friend, my lover and my partner, after meeting me twice. I feel wonder, then dread.

He describes how he felt as he drove home after our meeting at the coffee shop, his lips still feeling the touch of my fingers. He relives the touching again and again and lets his imagination go further.

'I was touching the gearstick and it was you I was touching. I waited at the lights and my mind flew to holding you and kissing you on your breasts.'

This isn't easy to listen to, but it must be even harder to say. John's breath is irregular, the passion in his voice so strong that it travels down the telephone wires, into my brain and body.

'How did *you* feel after we parted?' he asks.

'I felt confused,' I say, 'because the fact is, I'm with Aaron. And as a sexual partner, he's all I want.' I emphasise the last few words.

John hastens to explain.

'Yes, I know that he's your lover and I don't want to take his place. As a matter of fact, the sexual part is not so important to me; can you understand that?'

I'm trying to understand. This extraordinarily strong but detached feeling has all the signs of an unusual spiritual connection spilling over into a physical attraction. Is this a case of two souls wanting in whatever way they can to bring who they are to each other in whatever way they can? *If that's so, Carla*, says an internal voice, *it shouldn't be underestimated.*

I want to test John's outrageous statements a bit further.

'John, you barely know me.'

'I know; that's the scary part. My logical brain comes in and says all sorts of things, but there is spirit and this energy, and there is you and it's real.'

'You know that we can feel the way we do because of projection, or wishful thinking, or because of reminders of the past or whatever. This must have happened to you before, John.'

'A person like you has never happened to me before,' he continues. 'I've never before wanted to touch a woman's hand in public upon meeting her, to gather her in my arms as much as I could while I was sitting there at the table and, what's more, kiss her. And she is open and unembarrassed about it all.'

John pauses for a moment.

'All I know is that the energies are there, and I don't want to deny them. I want to hold you, kiss you and just be near you.'

I'm impressed.

I hear myself say, 'I'm open to that. I feel that if I'm honest with you and with Aaron, then it's clean and I'll feel good with it. Aaron keeps telling me to have it all, and he means it.'

Inside, I keep talking to myself. Aaron's a *man*, though, and he just might feel insecure. But he's very strong when it comes to relationships. He won't cut himself up about them.

As the words formulate in my brain, I realise that perhaps, for the first time in his life, Aaron may feel devastated if I left him. But the fact is, I don't want to leave him. Not at all. And I really can't imagine John taking his place. The thing that may happen is that Aaron opts out. That would cause pain to both of us. I sigh; it's a risk I'm deciding, right now, to take. 'I told Aaron about you,' I say to John. 'Not everything that transpired, but he's entitled to know.'

John doesn't know what to say to this, so I continue. 'I told Aaron that we'd meet regularly for coffee on Fridays and that you've got a ticket to the concert hall.'

I hear John suck in his breath. 'I know the plan, Carla, but can I tell you it's too hard to think that I won't see you till Friday. I want to be near you, touch you.' His voice wavers.

Damn, he's so disarming! There's nothing in this man that makes him want to appear 'cool' to me; he risks being rebuffed, rejected, or at the very least misunderstood. He's willing to put it all out there, rather than deny it or keep it to himself.

'You're an extraordinary person, John.'

We sit in silence on the phone.

'Is there anything else to say?' I ask.

'I'm just feeling you,' he says.

'It's such sweet torture, isn't it?'

Somehow, I can sense what he is feeling; energy surges through my body, turning it on like so many lights, making my nipples stand on end. But I'm not filled with the same extreme desire he is, right now, to be together; I'm the saner of the two here. My body is just responding to the ardour I feel coming through the airwaves.

I hear myself agree to meet him for lunch on Tuesday instead of waiting till Friday, and at my place instead of at a coffee shop. Am I mad? Overconfident? Silly? Probably. I'll still have time to reconsider after talking this over with Aaron.

Aaron and I sit across from each other at my dining table. It's been a disappointing evening for him. He's discovered that the motherboard I bought won't support my new video card. He hates hitches like this; says it's the fault of a friend of mine who came along on our shopping day, whose advice I took about which motherboard was best. 'A third person complicates things.'

We both avoid the topic of John, waiting for the right moment.

'Tell me how you've changed,' he says. He wants me to put him in a good light just now.

'I've become more of a woman because of you, Aaron.'

He nods in agreement, eyes alight, keen to know more of how my contact with him has had a beneficial impact.

'My sensuality has come alive in ways I didn't believe possible. I've blossomed and feel great about my femininity.'

He waits for more.

'I've learnt about "together and apart" from you. I've learnt the difference between hurt and grief.'

'Oh, how so?' Aaron's knees are crossed. One hand rests on the table and he's interrogating me, but I'm up to the challenge.

'Hurt happens when there's neediness, and expectations and demands that aren't met.'

He nods. 'Grief is unavoidable. It comes together with love, when things change and there is loss. Grief is about missing what was there before, but it isn't necessarily destructive. Grief can be clean, very sharp, and then be gone. Or it can linger and destroy you. I've done both. I've learnt my lesson! I've had pain, hurt, injustice in spades. Cruelty to myself, corrosive sickness, wasted energy.' He pauses, then his face lights up. 'Glorious wasted energy! Energy beautifully wasted because I grew from it.'

'All of life's experiences are our lovers and teachers,' I ponder.

'You've learnt well,' he says.

At the same time, he and I both know that words don't always reflect real learning. The acid test is life itself.

From my recent experiences with Aaron, I've learnt to step back from romantic neediness. I notice that the price I've paid is coming down to a reality that seems harsher and coarser. I now find myself beholding a man who isn't looking after himself the way he could. He not only looks awful in his perpetual tracksuit pants — which he

wears until they start to exude, well, not the freshest kind of smell —
but he's greying fast. The lines in his face have deepened since I first
met him five months ago. He looks permanently exhausted. His
breathing was always difficult because of his blocked sinuses
('consolidated tears, Carla'), but they are even more blocked now; this
affects his breathing so much that he practically snores at a low level
even when wide awake. I hear it on the phone: his every breath
contains a snort.

I know that when we go to bed, my view of him will change. I'll
be taken by his energy, that delightful core of him that exists in spite
of his carelessness. His lips will become full and luscious. The feeling
in his big, strong hands will electrify my body, and his penis will bring
all the ecstasy a vagina can bear. His face will reflect the youthfulness
I once knew in him. His beauty will become heartbreaking, because
it speaks to me of how he could be, if he valued himself more.

Yet it's not fair to say that he doesn't value himself; he does, but in
his own way. Valuing himself has been the opposite of what others
might value — such as image and prestige created by money and
success. He wants to be valued for himself. 'Who I am should be
enough.'

He has rare qualities: endless patience, humility, kindness,
compassion. He's extremely intelligent and has many practical talents.
A phenomenal trait is his astounding encyclopaedic mind full of
detailed and accurate information about the earth's geology as well as
the starry world of galaxies and universes. It reflects his love of nature
and of the earth.

His goal is to finish building his house, the ultimate expression of
his creative and inventive spirit. His rejection of society's values,
however, has made him too poor to achieve this, in all these years.
Somehow money doesn't want to stick to him.

Do I want to spend so much of my life with someone many would
call a loser? In the meantime, the universe has sent me John.

A FINE PIECE OF
CLASSICAL MUSIC

The subject tonight is love,
And for tomorrow night as well
Hafiz, 'The Day Sky'

 'John's in love with me, Aaron.' I tell him when we're both in bed and have made love again. It's become rather late. 'He's mad. He says that he wants to be my friend, my lover and my partner, and that's not logical.'

Aaron becomes unusually attentive. He turns his face to me. 'How long has he known you?'

'Two hours, maybe three in total.' It sounds ridiculous.

'This is a question of responsibility.'

He sees that I don't understand.

'You have to be able to take responsibility for your actions and for consequences. Make sure you know where your boundaries are and don't cross them. Make your "no" an absolutely strong one, one you won't violate.'

I don't know what he wants me to say no to, and I don't ask him, but there's strong feeling here.

'I was once in love,' he says. 'And I was miserable because she didn't love me any more. I decided to end it. I decided to say no to this pain and to this demand of my mind. Then when she wanted me to say yes again, it was impossible for me to do that. My no was total. The boundaries I had created for myself were so strong that I became strong. No meant no from then on. A no never becomes a yes again in my life.'

I feel a chill run through my belly. I hope to heaven I never get on the wrong side of Aaron.

'I've told John that I'm with you, and that as a sexual partner you're all I want.' But Aaron isn't assuaged, especially when I add, 'John wants to do the touching thing.'

'Do you know what you're getting yourself into, Carla?' he asks. 'Have you heard the term *playing with fire*? You're trying to keep lightning in a bucket.' He's seldom been this serious.

After a pause he says, 'You're going to have to turn into an Aaron.' He sees the big question mark on my face and goes on. 'You'll have to be very clear about "together and apart" with John.'

It hits me that this time it's John who's in love, not me, and that this time *I* have to set the boundaries. It is a mirror image of how things were between me and Aaron a few months ago. It's essential that I'm very, very honest with John.

I remember his words to me in the coffee shop, quoting Kahlil Gibran: *Let the winds of heaven dance between you,* and he had drawn the analogy of two trees standing side by side, tops intertwined, but trunks separate. I remember thinking that the trees' roots, too, would have to be intertwined, and had wondered whether this would be a good thing or not.

'John's got this down already,' I venture.

'Oh, has he,' says Aaron. 'I just hope this guy isn't as loopy as I think he is. One of my girlfriends thought she could trust her landlord. She got raped by him.'

I know this old story and try to reassure Aaron about John. 'John's like a fine piece of classical music,' I tell him, since he relates to pictures so well and to classical music somewhat. 'There's nothing crude about him. He's taking a big risk. He's risking ridicule. He's willing to suffer rather than not say what he feels.'

Aaron seems unmoved when he looks at me.

'This will change things,' he says.

My relationship with Aaron is now challenging him to be all *he* can be — exactly the thing he wanted for me. Becoming all he can be is a task he wants to take on organically. 'Let life teach me,' he says, 'while I do it slowly and don't beat myself up for not doing it faster.'

It seems to me that Aaron's got a lot of growing to do and he mightn't manage it all in one lifetime. He's still so tangled up with his mother, and he's got problems with his father. All his relationship experiences have been coloured by these things.

Aaron is acutely aware of the dysfunctional family he comes from. He used to try to take responsibility for each member of his family, especially his mother and sister. He doesn't do that any more, he says, but still finds it hard.

The other day he found his mother watching television in bed, away from her husband, who was watching the same program, but in the lounge room. The look on her face was heartbreaking, Aaron told me. *Help me! I'm so lonely!* it said. He couldn't say, 'It's your own fault for treating Dad the way you do.' Instead, he felt guilty.

Aaron was once so dominated by his mother, who made him into a pseudo husband. He won't play that game any more, but he still takes all the trouble in the world to make sure his mother has a good computer so she can watch DVDs to her heart's content, to fill in the time she doesn't spend relating to her husband.

Aaron doesn't like to be confronted with my views about his problems. His typical response is to try and turn the tables so it's me and my shortcomings we concentrate on. It's understandable.

I do so want him to resolve all his problems, to find a job and feel good about having money. But I have to be wary not to cross the line and start pushing; or, worse, start taking responsibility for his choices and for what he feels. I have to remind myself that I'm not responsible for Aaron's growth, even if I wish it for him with all my heart. I can get so engrossed in this that I almost stop breathing ...

I take a deep breath and feel like a swimmer coming up to the surface after being swirled and spun by the surf. Good, clean air in my lungs and clarity in my head, although I don't know what all this will mean in the end. What I do know is that, right now, we're good for each other and, right now, I love him and want him.

He's sitting on top of me, delighting me with just very small movements from his hips. I have my arms around the back of my head and start a playful conversation.

'You told me once that you no longer liked me.'

This makes him stop abruptly. With fists suddenly on his hips, he nearly jumps off me. 'What?!'

I laugh and speak slowly. 'You said once that you no longer liked me because you were in love with me.'

'Carla,' he glowers, 'words! When are you going to understand that words are limited and always belong to the moment?'

I'm genuinely amused. He's such an ingenuous, extraordinarily non-political person. Not a single atom in his body wants to rescue him and make the past self who said those words real to me once more.

What you see is what you get is his way. He's always just himself.

And today he *likes* me. I have to be content with that, and I am. At the same time, I feel an inner stream flowing away. I was bathing in this stream once, when it was broad, luxurious and sparkling — the magical waters of in-loveness. The stream is diverging now, slipping away, and I find myself on dry land, beside a colder river, also very clear, clear as crystal, but more ordinary.

'Tell me how you feel loved by me,' he says.

He wants to hear that I understand that he loves me. I like this kind of talk; it allows me to be erotic while I give him compliments and turn myself on at the same time.

'The woman in Carla feels loved by the man in Aaron,' I begin. He smiles. I close my eyes while my litany of praise grows more intense ...

juicy. 'Carla likes feeling Aaron deep inside her; it's always so new, so fresh, so wondrous.' I feel myself enter a warmer current again, once more flowing in the stream. 'And I love your hands on my body ...'

I see one hand approach my face, finger outstretched, heading for a nostril and trying to enter it. It's a gesture that makes me blush.

'I feel ridiculed, Aaron,' I say, eyes closed, enduring the shame.

'No! No!' He's in a hurry to put this right. 'I wasn't ridiculing you. It's difficult for me to comprehend your passion!' He's apologetic all of a sudden. 'I don't know how to take your compliments. I shouldn't hear such things.' And he takes my face in both his hands.

It's so sad. He doesn't realise how much he denigrates himself. He doesn't know how he has just declared himself not my equal.

It's close to midnight and my eyes want to close in sleep. He dresses and sits on the edge of the bed to put on socks and sneakers. I put my arms around his broad back. He's very quiet and thoughtful.

'Things will no longer be simple,' he says. 'Before, there was just you and me. Now there's an extra factor.' He finishes tying his laces. 'It's not easy being Aaron,' he says, and leaves.

In the early morning, my favourite time for reflection, I write my thoughts down on paper.

> *Will I be faced with a choice of either/or? Am I fooling myself, thinking that John and I will stop short of sex, and that I can keep Aaron? If I had to choose, what would I do? Aaron's like a rough diamond, one that might never smooth out. John is like a well-polished moon opal.*

I pull out a tarot card; Death stares at me. *Do not resist sudden change,* it says in the explanation. *The vibratory force around you will provide all the strength needed to accept the new situation.*

A DIFFERENT WORLD

If music be the food of love, play on.
William Shakespeare, *Twelfth Night*

 John's been waiting for an opportunity to take me out. Tonight, he's taking me to the concert hall. I resist wearing my black mini skirt over the new hipster pantyhose I bought recently and opt for a long velvet skirt. 'A pity,' says John.

We hardly talk at all. John takes my hand as we listen and let the music do the talking for us. I love the cultured atmosphere — a different world from Aaron's.

John says he's thinking of buying season tickets. It's an invitation to commit myself to going out with him regularly, but I hesitate. No, there isn't enough in me to want to enthuse about this. So I keep quiet, say nothing.

He takes me home. I invite him in for a drink. Anything might happen now. It's all up to me, how far I want to go.

John takes me in his arms to kiss me. For the first time, I notice how dry and flaky his lips are. Maybe he's nervous, but the kisses go wrong.

'Stand still,' I order. I want to demonstrate to John how to kiss, and approach him with full lips. John, however, is standing so still that he has trouble responding. It's hopeless. He doesn't get that this is an opportunity to learn something new; he believes he's a wonderful kisser already.

I turn to my CD player. It has Emma Shapplin at the ready. The strident music makes my body spontaneously take on a dancer's pose. I'll dance for John! There are no scripted moves for this dance, only a whole bunch of endorphins moving parts of my body into shapes wild, and perhaps grotesque, but mostly graceful. It's for my own enjoyment that I dance. Euphoria builds — I hardly notice John. Until he stands in front of me, takes one of my hands and puts an arm around my waist. He wants to tame this dance!

What's wrong with men that they can't let a woman have her wanton way with music? Like Aaron did a while ago, John unintentionally ends the dance. The euphoria dies, my body comes to a halt. We wiggle our hips together inconsequentially, then sit down again, slightly embarrassed. We talk, and then it's time to say goodnight.

The next time Aaron and I make love, it's after viewing one of David Deida's videos on sexual energy. The trouble with this kind of video is that you start to immediately compare your performance with what he puts forward as the ideal, and then try to enact it.

It wasn't really necessary for Aaron to find out from David that it's a man's job to open the woman 'up to God'. He was already doing that, and he's always been fully present with me. These are the qualities that make him outstanding in the first place. But now he's deliberately upping his masculinity, watching the effect it's having on me. As for me, I become more self-conscious about being a huge 'invitation to be taken'. I decide not to make a big deal out of it: we'll soon forget about the video and come back to our innocence. Cooking up energies, no matter how noble the intent, produces a kind of fakeness that we can do without.

In the video, David Deida asks a man in the audience if he loves his woman enough to let her go and find what she really needs. 'I'm willing to let you discover what it is you really want,' the man says to her.

Aaron had chipped in: 'I want you to do what you have to do, Carla. I want you to be all you can be. That's how much I love you. Sometimes,' he added, 'you don't know what you've got until you lose it. This may be about both of us coming to a deeper appreciation.'

My body feels different tonight. It responds to Aaron's touch, but isn't sharply erotic. Is this the effect of that stupendous orgasm of a couple of days ago? Does it mean I still haven't recovered from it? For the whole day after the event my vagina throbbed non-stop. As from this morning, it's quietly settled. It's taken me two days to come down.

So my body is fairly quiet as I receive Aaron — but, inexplicably, I feel him more deeply. He's sitting on top of me, taking a breather with his hands on his hips, when I look at him and melt. I mouth his name, but no sound comes out: *Aaron*. My eyes are mere slits, lids swollen from the tears that begin to roll down my cheeks. He sees it all, and gets it: this is love as he has never received it before. *He is loved*. He acknowledges it with a movement of his head, a quiet smile. Then he bends down and holds me in his powerful arms so I feel sheltered like a bird in a nest. When I tell him this, his arms tighten around me even more.

We make love until my body can take no more. I'm not sore, just fulfilled and surcharged with love. Tears keep on coming.

'I'm not sad, Aaron.'

'I know.'

And we lie together, until I get chilly. I'm always the first to feel the cold.

And then, that fateful morning . . .

'Aaron, since I woke up today, I know what I have to do.'

'That sounds serious.' His face is all lit up with love. 'You have the face of an angel.'

I fold my face into his chest. 'I don't feel like an angel, Aaron.

You've been hurt by others in the past. It's my prerogative to hurt you today.'

'What do you mean?'

'It's to do with John,' I say, and am surprised that he's taken aback.

'Oh, the John thing ... obviously I've underestimated the guy if he's so important to you. What does he represent to you?'

'I don't know. I have to find out. He represents a mystery.'

Aaron looks suddenly tragic. 'Whatever comes to love Aaron leaves Aaron,' he says, not looking at me any more. 'That's why I've schooled myself about "together and apart". It's never come into its own so much as today. I have only myself and this moment.'

The words go deep into my belly. I, too, have nothing but myself. Absolutely nothing lasts, and absolutely nothing stays with anyone. All we have is ourselves — what we've become through loving and being loved.

'Remember this,' says Aaron. 'What you've done to me today, someone will do to you. Then you'll know what it feels like.' Then, 'You've become like me, that's why you can do this. You've gained a security inside yourself. You've become strong and independent, going after what you want.'

He finds me in tears because, well, this hurts, and I can feel his hurt as well.

'Carla, we've become so comfortable with one another. We love each other so deeply, without doubting the other. You can give yourself unreservedly to me, and I can do the same. This is love, Carla. You've never been better loved. I've never loved anyone more than you.

'Let me have you one last time.'

He stays one more night.

'Aaron, your breathing when you sleep is like a woman who is desperately holding back her tears.'

Snuggled into his chest, I experience spasm after spasm: his chest heaving as he holds his breath as long as he can, then releases a stream of air as if regretfully, then sharply inhales. It's as if he's sobbing non-stop — deep, long, tearless sobs.

'What do you suggest I do about it?'

'Deal with the frozen tears you say this represents.'

'I'll go to Darkan and cry,' he says.

Before he leaves, we have a short discussion.

'I've hurt ever since I felt that my mother rejected me,' he says.

I've never heard him mention this before. 'How did she reject you?'

'She gave me all her attention, then she left me alone. It was as if she trained me to feel dependent on her attention. When I didn't get it any more, the way I craved it, it hurt.'

'And the women in your life have done the same to you,' I say. 'You've attracted versions of your mother time and time again.'

'I've attracted what I needed in my life to become myself,' he says defensively. 'I did therapy three years ago, and shed a lot of tears.'

'But not enough,' I say. 'You didn't finish the process.'

So I've become one of those women who, like his mother, was destined to hurt him.

After he leaves, I tell myself that Aaron can't have me until he becomes more of all he can be. He's opened me to the woman–God energy dormant in me, the force that is now pulling me to be all I can be. Aaron has to find his own way home. In my case, I'm following something positive. In his case, it's a decision to let go of a negative, and that's more difficult. We're friends, good friends, indestructible friends, and our story isn't finished yet.

HEARING THE WIND BLOW

Hear the wind blow, dear,
Hear the wind blow.
'Down in the Valley', traditional American
folksong

 John sends me a text message: *Share your soul with me, love me. Yours, John.*

I try to return a message, but fumble. I've forgotten how to do it, and can't regain the confidence to handle my mobile intelligently just now. Since he's messaged me, it gives me the opportunity to fill John in on what has transpired. I phone him.

'This morning I told Aaron that I'm leaving him,' I say, and hear him gasp.

'What? I didn't expect you to act this fast. I was prepared to wait patiently.'

'I couldn't live with the dichotomy any longer.'

John makes the mistake of thinking this is because of his hold on me.

'No, this isn't entirely about you,' I interrupt. 'It's something I have to do for my own sake.'

'Oh.'

I don't want to flatter John. I don't want to give him the impression that he's made such an impact on me that I find him irresistible and now must break off with Aaron. That's not it.

'Tell me,' says John, because he wants to understand what is going on here, 'does Aaron love you?'

'Oh yes, he does!'

My voice must carry my whole conviction. There's a short silence at the other end.

'I feel for the guy,' John says.

It occurs to me that John's also feeling for himself — his possible future self: *if this woman can do this to her lover, what is she capable of doing to me?*

He's right, of course: Carla, following her heart, can appear ruthless.

'You're doing this entirely honourably,' says Aaron generously. 'You've not used subterfuge or pretence; there have been no lies, no deceit, no negative feelings. You didn't have to hate me to leave me. You love me like no woman has ever loved me. You've healed some deep loneliness inside me, and your love has been a validation of who I am. I've knocked propositions from other women on the head,' he tells me, 'because it's obvious they can't love like you.' He closes his eyes. 'Your love has imprinted itself on me so many times — it's indelible.'

So . . . he's telling me he is more faithful than me.

He reminisces, already looking at the past. 'I've done just about everything on my wish list!' he suddenly observes, almost cheerfully. 'We went to Fremantle together yesterday; we drove down to Darkan; you stayed with me there and made love to me; we saw a movie together, stayed in the car to talk together; we sat by the beach and watched the waves.'

His list is simple. I'm glad it was so well fulfilled.

★ ★ ★

'Are you doing this because I was leaving you to go to Darkan and you wanted to leave me first?' Aaron asks. He's driving my car as we talk.

This has never occurred to me. Obviously I need to explain more clearly why I'm doing this.

'I want to explore what's being offered to me, Aaron. John's an entirely new kind of experience. I told you before that he's like a piece of classical music. You're like some great rock music — Enigma, for instance.'

Aaron's lightly blushing; finesse is definitely not what he's about. I don't want him to feel bad about himself.

'As for John being able to appreciate Enigma or Emma Shapplin, well, I don't know if he can do that.'

Aaron lives in the part of the spectrum that is exciting and alive: the red, infrared and orange. John, on the other hand, lives in the higher and finer reaches: the blues and purples and indigos, with a strong dash of green. What they share is yellow, the will centre where their energies are stored — but such different qualities in both cases. It's yet to be seen how the lower colours will find their way in John's expression. He has big shoes to fill.

'How do you see yourself in the future?' Aaron asks. He's genuinely curious as to how I think I'm going to feel without him. 'By knowing me, you've come into your womanhood, Carla. Other men are getting attracted to you, but when I'm gone, what will they see? Maybe John will get to see who you are without me and not like it.'

It's possible, I agree. If I've depended on Aaron to make me feel fulfilled and sexy, then I may start feeling like a lonely, empty woman. But I really don't feel that's going to happen.

'I feel the future to be exciting and wonderful and full of growth.' Aaron swallows.

After a silence, I add, 'It's like a strong angel energy that's pulling me.'

He looks at me nonplussed. 'An angel? Come again?'

We pull into the driveway.

'Don't underestimate angels,' I say. 'They're powerful beings. I feel one is taking me by the hand.'

'How do you feel now?' he asks later, when we're in the house, because my face is so wet from tears.

'I feel I've done the right thing, Aaron, and that's a good feeling.'

He wants me to repeat it.

'When you've done the right thing, something inside you tells you so, and it's a comfort,' I say.

He watches me patiently.

'Make up your mind and become a single woman again, Carla! You look so sad. Let me massage your shoulders. You're holding responsibility there.'

And it's good to feel his strong hands trying to ease the tension there,

I'm waiting for John, who's phoned to say he wants to meet up with me 'just to say hello'. I see him coming towards me. He's only got a few minutes between work and a doctor's appointment, but we haven't seen each other since last Saturday and he feels he must see me today. He runs and I walk and we meet in each other's arms, there on the footpath outside the Subiaco post office. We exchange a kiss, then he turns to take my hand, leading me back to his car, parked not far away.

'I must be mad,' he says, smiling all the while, 'and I don't care.'

He swings my arm as he walks, but doesn't walk quite straight. Our shoulders keep touching. His mood is infectious. 'Kiss me!' I say mischievously, but the same thought has already entered his mind and my words aren't complete before he grabs my waist and swings me out of the way of slowly moving traffic in the car park.

'My thoughts exactly!' He kisses me, says, 'Damn!' and laughs, then kisses me again, this time more boldly.

He clasps me firmly in his arms. I close my eyes. This is so deliciously strange and wonderful. The conservative John, who swears because he doesn't know this new part of himself, and because he can't help himself, and because it's so foolish of him to love a person so sexually open who *isn't even available* — this man has learnt to live in the moment. And right now, he wants to be with me and hold me and kiss me.

We break and continue to walk slowly. I tell him I want to buy some green tea from the special tea shop over the road.

'OK,' he says. 'I'll walk you there.'

On the footpath, another impulse invades him. He presses me up against a lamp post, pinning me there while he kisses me. He swears again, backs off, comes back because he can't help himself, and says earnestly in my ear, 'I want to fuck you.'

Later, he phones to apologise for being rude to a lady, for using the 'F' word. He stumbles over his words until I interrupt and tell him I'm a woman with a body, not a lady on a pedestal.

'Who are you talking to, John? Am I the virgin Mary?'

He's relieved and laughs.

John's friends are wondering what the hell kind of substance he's on these days. 'I'm on the joy of being alive,' he tells them, and they have a hard time believing him, yet it's true. John seems to have surrendered his desires and just lives in the happiness of loving. Mind you, he's getting lots of admiration in return. This independent, selfless loving is, paradoxically, making a man out of him. A free, sensual and fun-to-be-with man. I can laugh and feel wanted and stay free myself.

I call John on his mobile and discover he's having coffee with my friend Virginia. 'She's a nice woman. I'm getting to know her,' he says. Nothing wrong with that, except it makes me realise what I prefer in a man and in a relationship: utter loyalty — the one-on-one intimacy that I have with Aaron.

This little incident teaches me what it feels like to have your partner's attention wander the way John's does. Aaron leaves me free, but should I choose to wander too far that would change what we have, simple as that. He's an altogether-here-for-you kind of guy, until you don't respect that any more. Then he'll let you go.

'Come to me when you're single again,' were his words. 'I don't do triangles.'

He's not being possessive. He's not condemning me. He's not offended by my entertaining the thought of having sex with John. He's just saying what's real for him, what his values are.

THE TRUTH OF YOU,
THE TRUTH OF ME

Meditation (Truth) is an unexpected earthquake
that shakes our ordered existence
into a thousand directions
. . . and leaves our neat home a total wreck.
Robert Rabbin, 'Truth'

 I can't do this man justice. I want to let John go, although he's offering me what a lot of women dream of. My demands for passion are greater than his gentle, conventional stability. I want to share life with a partner who is my equal in every way; someone who is as strong as I am and demands the deepest loyalty from me.

John wants to 'settle down' for the rest of his life. This would indicate a major change in the way he's been living: loving to flirt with all the women who are open to his appreciative words. John is maturing and aches for stability. What I read into this is perhaps not true, but the feeling is there, nevertheless: that after settling down, everything will have to be hunky-dory for the rest of all time, because we're married, after all. I couldn't try to fit life into a mould like that. I have to let John go.

I may have to let go of Aaron as well. Why? Because of the disparities between us, and because of the long absences. I will have to face these a lot of the time if I'm to have Aaron as my lover.

From my diary:

Beloved, what am I to do?

I love Aaron with heart and soul and body; he's the only one who can draw out this passion I feel.

When I'm with John, dear, gentle John, it's sane, quiet bliss. John, who holds my hand while he watches the tears fall down my cheeks as I tell him about Aaron. No fireworks in our togetherness; just goodness, friendship, the quiet excitement of a deeply flowing, congenial energy. Why do I long for more?

You, Aaron, have taken my heart and set a benchmark in several ways. You know how to surprise me, to make me laugh with your remarks completely out of left field. You knock me off my feet, literally, when you pick me up and take me to bed; your boss nature is something my headstrongness loves to give way to. You take command in little, delightful ways, with your mannerisms as well as your love-making. You guide me, enjoy being the one in charge, even when it comes to undressing me. 'Don't help me, Carla!' You were so disappointed when I did help.

You're so sexy; not in the way you look (very unsexy clothes, Aaron, and not sexy in the way you hobble about, speak nasally and scratch your legs!) but in the way you carry your sexual energy, and you're so full on when you put your attention to it. You know how to take a woman and stay with her for hours. You know how to kiss. You know how to transfer energy and receive it, and send it around in a loop that just keeps on building. When you love, you're exquisite. The extreme tenderness in your face and in your eyes melts me totally. I long to be one with you in these moments.

And then you're gone. Gone for days, long days, gone for a life away from me, to your house in Darkan. Leaving me with my love and my longings. Our energy slowly dissipates from our bellies, gradually disconnecting us. The phone brings us together in a phantom embrace; all we can really say is, 'I love you, I want you, I can't have you, I feel pain.' Then I let your phantom self go, or take your phantom self with me to my bed and my dreams.

There is more that pulls us apart. Maybe it's snobbery, but I want to be with a man who takes responsibility for his financial affairs. You've done so much with your life, being true to yourself as best you could, being willing to suffer anything in the process. At the same time, you left out important areas of your life that needed looking at. *You kept the right to blame others*; this has held you back from success, from peace, even from health. It's made you prone to depression. It has stopped you from feeling worthy of being truly loved. You've led your life as if no one would love you. Now that someone does, you're not prepared, and can't offer a life to share.

You told me about a dream you had recently. You dreamt that I had died and that nobody told you about it. What if you looked at this dream symbolically? What if it means that, at some stage, you realise that Carla has died to you, without you even noticing it? Carla's not the kind of person who takes to relating at a distance. Distance multiplied by absence spells pain, and all organisms will do something to not be in constant pain. Will this love die? Not likely, but the relationship can. Carla may have to say, 'Be with me when we're together, and let me forget about you when we're not. Leave me to lead my own life as if you weren't there, because you're not, except in spirit.'

When a person dies, their spirit is still present, but relating to a spirit is not satisfactory to a person still in their body. On this earth, a man–woman relationship is lived out in the body, or so it seems to Carla, who is a Scorpio.

You say that everyone that loves Aaron leaves Aaron. How can anyone help it if they must live life on Aaron's terms only? What kind of person would want to stick around while being dished out emotional pain all the time? You don't want to hurt anyone. You say, quite rightly, that people only hurt themselves by wanting what they can't have. Well, one solution is to stop wanting what they can't have and go to where they can get it, instead of telling themselves they have to get used to not having it.

High spirituality or bullshit? It doesn't matter; what matters is the truth of what I'm feeling, and I hurt. I hurt and I'm getting tired of hurting. I'm like a widow, or a woman with a man in the army or at sea. I'm not made for this kind of relationship as some women are. That's the truth of me.

Beloved, what am I to do, if I'm to be true to the truth of me?

Life has a way of answering prayers. John's ardour and my good feelings in his company have to come to a point where our sexuality is involved. I just have to find out: what is it like to be touched intimately by John? He seems to think highly of himself as someone who knows how to be with a woman. What will he be like as a lover?

I find out when we come back to my place after a night at the movies. John's hug is particularly ardent; his body is plastered hungrily against mine and only a very obtuse person would not get the message: make love to me or I'll go crazy!

I have a way of coming down to the ordinary, the practical, the prosaic.

'Let's go to the bedroom, John.'

It nevertheless has the taste of an invitation to a ball, to the opening of a mystery, or of Pandora's box, who knows ...

Taking our clothes off is a straightforward thing. I leave my bedside lamp burning, so a soft but clear light shines onto the bed.

And I'm not disappointed; I'm turned on by John's touch. His hands have all the exquisite sensitivity that I noticed when he first clasped my hand in his for the tango lesson. Every nuance of his movements has the quality of music and dance; every touch tells me of the desire that is firing his fingers. I lie on my back, and John lightly massages my legs and feet with the moisturising lotion from my vanity table, moving himself around the bed as he does so. I'm in heaven, receiving his attentions, just relaxing like his massage clients do. John isn't demanding that I respond in kind; he just wants me to receive. My hand travels to stroke his back when it's close enough, just to show him my appreciation.

His hands move to my neck, my chest, my breasts, until they reach my nipples and start a fire there. He notices the effect and closes his mouth over a nipple. A mouth is that much more sensitive than fingers! And John has an experienced tongue; it flicks and loops and licks. He seems to know my body as if it's his own. My other nipple gets the treatment, while the first is gently held so it doesn't feel left out or forgotten. Besides, two nipples excited together exceed the sum of their parts, scientifically speaking. My vulva heaves involuntarily. John brings one hand to it and feels how hot and wet it is. He moves to sit between my legs. He's on his haunches, and from here I notice his hairy chest full of curls, his freckles and his strong and erect penis. John is evidently very proud of his organ: he sits with his hands on his hips and smiles broadly at me.

He moves in closer. The tip of his penis is about to touch me when my energy changes, or I come to my senses, or I'm invisibly hit over the head. Most likely the latter. I suddenly realise I'm about to betray Aaron just out of curiosity! I'm not in love with John. I'm flattered, I'm impressed with his personality and goodness, but I'm not in love.

'John,' I gasp, 'I can't do this! I can't go ahead with this. I'm so sorry.'

John's face registers utter disbelief, but he never for a moment stops being a gentleman. Obviously disappointed, he's even more concerned for the way *I* feel. He soothes me with, 'Never mind, Carla. Whatever you want; it doesn't matter.'

I'm so glad of his generous reaction. He lies down beside me and pulls the bedsheet over us. His face is slightly bemused. Clearly he'd like to know what's happening here.

'I want to belong to Aaron,' I tell him.

That says it all, really. Up until that moment, I'd been wondering whether I wanted to create a threesome. But 'I don't do triangles,' Aaron said, and I realise that's the way I feel as well. *I* don't do triangles. Triangles change things too much.

'John will come in and get the energies I left with you,' Aaron remarked, describing the act as a sort of stealing.

Not that John is consciously aware of that at all. All John sees is a desirable woman, without knowing what has gone into making her desirable. Aaron is right: I do owe some of that to him. He's also right about triangles, how messy they are emotionally. Only when John's penis was within less than a millimetre of my vagina did I realise this.

I explain what I can of this to John, who understands one thing: I've chosen Aaron over him.

He's only slightly awkward as he gets dressed again. He wants me to stay where I am — he'll see himself out.

MUCH ADO

We do what you do until we don't
Byron Katie, healing seminar

 I haven't seen or spoken to Aaron for four days now and I can't stand it any more.

'Aaron, are you there?' I call.

I'm standing outside his subterranean room in the bright sunshine, hesitant to go in. I see him move from his chair near the computer.

'Bloody hell! What're you doing here? You're not supposed to be here!'

He's obviously pleased, though, and motions me to sit down on the edge of his bed. The rest of his room is a shambles: boxes and objects everywhere.

'So how's it going for you?' he asks.

'Not too good,' I sob, and bury my head in his neck. His arm is around me.

'It's not been too good for me either,' he says, 'but I survived. I've been taking the next step: getting ready to leave for Darkan. I want to be in my own space for a while and find myself again.'

But he's so delighted to have me there that he picks me up with one hand on my crutch and circles me around the room, not caring that my legs might knock over a box or two. He lays me on his bed, climbs in and pulls the blankets over us.

We lie looking at each other. Missing one another has created an intensity that shines out of our eyes, draws our lips together again in the sweetest kiss.

'We love each other, kid. You're in me and I'm in you. Nothing can take you from me, not even yourself.' He puts my left arm, the one that lies inert against his body, under his neck. 'There, that's better, isn't it?' It's better for holding his head while I kiss him. He's impetuous; his penis swells against my body.

'Aaron! I'm actually on my way to a meeting and I want to be on time!'

'What about a quickie?'

My belly thrills at the thought of it, but I have an iron will now. 'I want to be on time!' and I wrench myself from him.

He accompanies me to my car. All is suddenly well again.

'You're looking better than when you arrived here,' he says, delighting in being wicked, driving it home to me that it's love that makes me look good, and it's loving him that does it best. His face still shows disbelief as I drive off. I can't believe it myself, but I feel a deep relief at Aaron's genuine pleasure at having me back.

This afternoon he walks in with bags and cases, as if he's moving in, sets them down, walks over to me and without a word picks me up to take me to the bedroom. In moments we're naked and lying close together, not talking, just feeling the joy of having each other close again.

Four days have brought me to my senses.

Four days of thinking he'd have to do without me have made Aaron into a man who knows more than ever what he wants. No hint of a cavalier manner. This time, I don't have to instigate anything.

Making love has an acute edge to it. He seems to take absolutely nothing for granted, and neither do I. He effortlessly flips both of us over from the missionary position. From my vantage point on top of him, his face is as I've never seen it: more rounded, more youthful, intolerably attractive. Seeing him like this, with intense pleasure utterly concentrating his attention, sends me into a paroxysm of desire.

'Oh God! A woman shouldn't want a man this much!'

He chooses this moment to release himself into the vagina of a woman who loves him to excess.

'We've both come over the finishing line,' he says. 'We've been through heaven and hell, and we still love each other. We've managed to be together and apart; we've managed not to hurt each other, or say anything that attacks the other's self-esteem. We've seen the best and the worst of each other, and still love just as deeply. We even know that our future isn't at all secure, and it doesn't stop us from loving in the present. We've made it, kid.'

His eyes laugh with delight and inner knowing. He's a more mature man now, without illusions about himself or me or life. He doesn't have an iota of blame in him. Quite the contrary.

'I'll tell you what you've done for me,' he says. 'You've restored my faith in women. I know now that it's possible for a man like me to have a good relationship with a woman.'

I hear bells pealing in my brain, ringing to celebrate an achievement. This is what I've wanted for Aaron: to heal the awful wounds he's carried from earlier relationships. He's been brought to all women, to trust them and be open to the possibility that they'll respect him.

'And this is what I've done for you.'

I look at his face; I know a whammy is coming when it's not quite convincingly serious.

'You've lost all inhibitions about your body and your sexuality,' he says. 'It's been fucked out of you!'

He grins at the laughter that follows. It encourages him to crack a few jokes bordering on corny. He knows this, but just wants to see me laugh.

'I'm glad to see you've rounded out a bit,' he says. 'When I first met you in your driveway, you looked gaunt.'

'Really?'

I think back to that time. I was thin.

'You were starved for love, and now you've got it and want it forever,' he says. 'You know what you want now, and nothing will stop you from getting it.'

I hadn't been aware of how starved I really was.

'You've been lonely all your life,' he says, as if he's clairvoyant.

Well, I've had my moments, months and years of relating in a satisfying manner, even if it did fall terribly short of what could exist between a man and a woman.

'You're a fulfilled woman now,' he says. 'And I love you. You're in love, but I just love.'

It's good; it wouldn't do for both of us to be moonfaced, both sighing and heaving with desire. I need calm waters in which my passions can take refuge, in which they can be absorbed, appreciated and reciprocated with devotion. My woman's heart lies still in the strong arms of a man who knows how to hold me.

Life is magnificent! *This is how much I love you*, says Life. Life is that ultimate Lover who doesn't desert. Instead, it relentlessly provides all the challenges my soul needs. I knew this Lover during my celibate years in Denmark. My friends used to occasionally swear that I had a man in my life because of the bloom of happiness on my face, and I would say that I was in love with Life. I was filled with gratitude every day for the beauty I was surrounded by: the flowers that grew in my garden, the wild magnificence of Denmark's coastline, its rocks, its skies, its colours. Then this Lover penetrated my vagina with a man's penis; penetrated me right up to my heart, my eyes and the highest energy centres of my body. It blew my mind and took it beyond every concept of what a man and a woman should do or not do when they love each other. Beyond concepts of what our lives should be too.

I look at Aaron and know how blessed I am to know him. Aaron may die before he recognises that his dragons only guard the secret to his emotional freedom. Aaron thinks organically. Change, he says, comes about in its own time, not because it's forced along. It's enough that he does the best he can; that's how my thoughts run tonight.

He'll still leave for Darkan, though, following through with his recent plans. Those cases he brought in with him, they're going south to his house. He says he'll be away for two weeks this time. Neither of us knows what such an absence will provoke.

Aaron returns after nine days, surprising me by arriving back earlier than he said he would. He bowls into my space with a clean-shaven, handsome head. He was sick the day before, but made himself a good meal for the first time in a while and felt better. What I see before me, as he stands there, is a person not exactly gaunt, but drained from all colour, showing the signs of recent, severe stress. A bad diet and being away from me has done something to Aaron.

I kiss him and feel absolutely nothing. I hug him, feel his energy and reciprocate, but there is no shred of passion. I kiss grey lips in a grey face and all my world is grey.

I tell myself to be patient; the world will right itself somehow. He sits down at my table to sip some tea and I wonder at how unlovely he looks. I have never seen him like this. I long for the rose-coloured glasses I used to look through, but for the time being I've lost them. My gaze is ruthless. As I playfully chatter about this and that, I look at his short, grey hair. It sticks out from his head in all directions in an undignified way, on account of him running his hands through it now and again. I see his puffy jowls, and his eyes, so little, too little for his big face.

His breath isn't sweet either, but he says, 'You've got bad breath, too, my oath,' and I laugh and go off to the bathroom. He follows suit, to find his toothbrush, and cleans his teeth alongside me.

'I've been eating a lot of meat lately and haven't been flossing my teeth,' I say to his image in the mirror, grinning shamelessly as I vigorously rectify the situation with open mouth. I am acutely aware that I don't care a hoot what Aaron might be thinking of me.

Aaron is shocked. He knows me as a vegetarian — at least, one that eats only fish and chicken, not red meat.

'It's been doing me a lot of good,' I say, mocking his mild distress.

He tries to reproach me. 'You had no regard for the life of those animals.'

'Sure I did,' I retaliate. 'I thanked those animals for giving their life for me. They were happy to become a part of me.'

For once, Aaron has no immediate response. He's never at a loss for long, though, so it comes a few seconds later. 'I can assure you that all living creatures do not want to die.'

'How do you know that?'

I screw up my face irreverently; he can see that I'm not taking his statement seriously at all.

'What's the matter with you?' Aaron knows something has changed and he's not sure he likes it. 'Have you become independent and don't need anyone any more?'

'That's about it!' I grimace, mouth full of toothpaste. 'Is my breath better now?' I give him a full blast of breath in his face.

Aaron blinks. 'You've lost your vulnerability!' he says, with a rueful edge to his voice but wonder in his face. *What's Carla turning into?* He's nonplussed by my new demeanour.

'Somewhere inside there is still the little girl,' he says, and I don't know whether he's reassuring himself or if he knows something I don't.

The last nine days have seen me change in a way I've only become aware of today — seeing myself through Aaron's eyes just now. For nine days I did without Aaron's physical company. For nine days I went through a withdrawal, much like an addict withdraws when she's deprived of the addictive substance. For a while the longing for a fix is extreme: coarse waves of energy shake the body as brain tentacles reach out for the trigger of a rush of serotonin and a host of painkiller hormones. Then the hungry tentacles shrivel; now there's much less serotonin than normal in an average day and pain is raw and unmitigated. Finally comes a point of balance, a blessed feeling of equilibrium. Then there is freedom, back once more to a point of choice. It took me nine days to come down from the giddy heights of my in-loveness.

The night before he left his home in Darkan to return to Perth, Aaron spoke words of wisdom over the phone, which he may not want to be as true as they are: 'The relationship doesn't own you, Carla; you own the relationship.'

He was probably trying to teach me something, but he only spoke what was already becoming a reality for me. My silence as I ruminated on those words made Aaron ask something quite out of character: 'Do you still love me?'

What a very strange question! How could he doubt it?

'You once said that I was the love of your life,' he went on. 'Is that still the case?'

'I've loved no one the way I've loved you,' I answered.

As I spoke, I realised I was looking in the past for the answer; it didn't tell him how I feel right now. Right now, he represents a benchmark. But that was still created in the past. The truth is, while he was away I didn't know how I would feel when I saw him again. I'd said to John, 'In some way, I wish Aaron wasn't coming back just now. I wish he'd stay away so I can get him out of my system entirely.' How could I say such a thing? I don't know. I'll have to find out.

The question is: if everything that isn't true in this relationship was stripped away, what would be left? I don't know the answer. All I know is two things: one, that pain is a clue to something being not quite true; and two, that more than anything else, more than even the greatest illusion, I want the truth.

I've become a changed person in some fundamental way. And Aaron has spotted it.

He decides to give up on me and his issues, pins me in his arms and walks me backwards out of the bathroom while trying to kiss me. He throws me onto the bed while I giggle and hoot with delight. Aaron's plan is to pull down my slacks, but they are double-buttoned and zipped, so he goes for my bra, lifting it up to expose my breasts. He attacks my nipples with his mouth.

The bold move takes my breath away. Electric charges race down to my clitoris, compelling me to lift my pelvis against his arching body. Then, just as suddenly, he covers me up again. There's no more time for playing around. We are off tonight to attend a lecture in town.

It's nine when we return home, and Aaron makes a beeline for bed. I see him lying awkwardly with his neck on two pillows and ungraciously pull one out from under his head, laughing mercilessly, kissing him without tenderness.

'Are you going to be rough tonight?' he asks. I detect a degree of genuine concern.

'I want to punish you for staying away for so long.'

'Oh,' he says, and watches me as I undress and slide under the cotton sheets to lie next to him. I eye him, checking to see if he looks any different now, in this bedroom light. I light a candle; it softens the lines on his face and his eyes grow bigger and more expressive. It's good to see him like this, almost himself again, I say to myself, all the time aware that *he* hasn't changed, only my way of perceiving him.

It is a full few minutes before he can say that his Carla is back. He can tell from the kisses. I can't tell the difference from one kiss to the next myself, but I've learnt to be astonished at Aaron's perceptiveness. I'm aware of doing just one thing: staying present, not closing my eyes and pretending to be back in some other time with him, just to get myself aroused.

He pulls me to him and the touch of our skin meeting, my chest against his, ignites my pleasure. Aaron surprises me by going down on my nipples. He's figured out that this is the fastest way to get me wet. When he finally hovers his body over me, he waits for me to take the tip of his penis and rub it against my moist clitoris. He then starts thrusting slowly, enveloping his penis little by little, and all the while my vagina gushes out its juices. When his penis finally makes it all the way in, he comes in close, puts his arms around me and takes stock of my face.

I'm home again, says his expression, and I feel that familiar, oh, so comfortable feeling of wholeness, my vagina finally filled again to its sides with what it has been missing for so many days. Fullness. Home. Juices of the mouth. We delight in mingling our juices and the smell of our breath. Satisfaction. No great stirrings in my loins, no lightning bolts, but simple, full pleasure.

As he thrusts, my vagina comes alive again and once more tears are wrung from my eyes in an effort to cope with the exquisiteness. My employers are away, which leaves me free to moan and yell.

He loves looking at me like this, with my head below him. 'Gravity's in your favour when you lie down; you look no more than twenty years old,' he says. Then, 'Hang on, babe.'

I grip him behind his neck and in one firm movement he flips us over, so now I'm on top.

'Have I *aged* twenty years now?' I want to know.

'No way, babe; you're fine,' is his answer, and it's my turn to see gravity do him a wonderful favour: now he's got some colour in his cheeks and the puffiness has disappeared from his face.

In spite of me being on top, he does most of the thrusting, pushing himself up into me, making me gasp and scream, until he finally moans, 'I want you!' and pulls my torso towards him, his head bent sideways, absorbed in his feelings. His great intensity makes me bend over him in a paroxysm of desire as he comes in me. My mouth slobbers all over his neck and face and chest; there's as much saliva in my mouth as there are juices in my vagina, and they both want to be on his skin.

My heaving breath gradually subsides to calmness and I lie on his chest, utterly content. We rest, then Aaron starts philosophising, as he loves to do.

'What they're afraid of in the churches is people having sex, because then the church loses control over them. People would begin to know themselves and not need to be told who they are and what they should be.' He pauses, breathing through a smile, and continues. 'When you have sex, you start off by feeling in control. Then your brain gets flooded with serotonin and hormones, and before long you can't think clearly. And then you blow your mind altogether and for a while you can't think at all. You totally lose control. And you feel satisfied, because now you know who you are without your mind. Look at you! You know yourself as somebody who is mindless, a piece of God. That's sex.'

Aaron, the spokesperson for sex. I think he does it well.

'You were the most woman I've experienced you,' he says later, dressed and sipping a drink before leaving.

I look at him in astonishment, thinking back on past ecstasies. How can he say that? But he isn't speaking of my reactions, my sexual feelings; he's speaking of something more specific to him: Carla as *woman*. He, the man, has experienced me as woman. He has more than a girlfriend in me now: I am *his woman*, that's what he is saying to me. It is a deep compliment, telling me as much of his love as of the changes he's seen in me.

'You were fearless tonight,' he says, and he's right. I lost all fear of not making the right impression, of not doing it right, of how I was seen, of losing him and our relationship. I was without fear, and that meant there was no little girl in there any more, and no blushing, hesitant adolescent either. I became quite shameless.

Aaron's baffled as to what's happened to make me change this much. He doesn't twig it's because I've adjusted to him being away and have become independent of him. I can take or leave this relationship now. He thinks it's to do with the fact that I've recently received a lot of money for my book, *God's Callgirl* — my very first royalty payment; more money than I've ever had in my life.

It's incidental that I should feel freer at the time this happened, but Aaron says, 'Uh-uh, it's all interconnected.'

His body language shows me that he's not quite sure whether he's comfortable with this new Carla. He feels I'm on the cocky side —

in other words, just a bit unbalanced. He also isn't sure whether my new attitude of *I can take this relationship or leave it* quite suits him now that he's revealed his whole heart to me.

'I love you and I want this relationship,' he said tonight, and Aaron would rather walk through fire than say this without meaning it. And then he added, 'I need this relationship; it inspires me to change myself.'

I pricked up my ears: Aaron needing a relationship? However, how I interpret 'need' isn't necessarily the way he does. This need would change if the relationship were taken away from him. Aaron has few ultimate needs. His training in independence is going to be there for him the very moment he needs it again.

IF IT'S A FAMILY YOU WANT

Happy Birthday to you . . .

'What's on your mind?' We're sitting in Aaron's room under the house. We've just shared a meal upstairs that I brought in for everyone. Beryl set the table with all the finery she could find.

Aaron's more aware of my emotional state than I am myself. Since the publication of *God's Callgirl*, only one sister speaks to me at this time; my other siblings — two brothers and two sisters — no longer wish for any contact with me. All they think of is that the family name has been dragged through the mud. They can't see that what I tried to do with my book was provide readers with a first-hand insight into the effects of child sexual abuse. Abused people are often cowed into silence. They often feel totally alone, cut off from the rest of society. My book allowed readers to know that they are not alone, but more than that, to some people my story was an invitation to try and heal from their own experiences. I have been deeply touched by the thousands of emails I've received from readers who identified with my story. There were very few who took any notice of 'the family name'.

I gave my siblings a draft copy of the book to read two years before its publication, but in that time I changed the ending. I doubt that any of my brothers and sisters have read the revised version. My youngest sister mobilised the extended family to try to prevent the book being published. Liesbet, the sister closest to me in age, couldn't take the resulting estrangement any more after six months or so and started communicating with me again.

I feel so sad for my other siblings, and for myself, that they refuse to grant me a worthy motivation for writing the book.

I hadn't quite realised how much my family's cutting me off had affected me. But today's my birthday and I've received no contact at all from them (except Liesbet), much less any cards.

'I'll tell you a secret, Aaron. It's my birthday.'

He looks at me, stunned. 'So that's why you put on a party tonight,' he says. 'You wanted to have your birthday with a family! You should've said something.'

'No! I don't want any fuss, and don't you dare mention anything to your parents.'

'Happy birthday, Carla,' he says softly — the sweetest wish for a birthday in the whole wide world. His face is so full of tenderness; his whole being wants me to know how much he wishes it for me.

'You'll have only one candle tonight,' he says with a wicked grin. I laugh; this 'candle' he's referring to is the only one I want. I'm ready to light it.

'I've never been loved like this before,' he says. 'And I love like I've never loved before. You bring out new feelings in me.'

The sound of these words is unbelievably wonderful. After all, Aaron has loved and been loved a lot in his fifty years of life.

He takes me to his bed. I sit on top of him and insert his eager candle, using it to set myself alight. As we regulate the strokes together, I feel his strong hands around my hips, my waist. Does he have any idea of the energy in his hands?

'Ha ... ppy ... bir ... th ... day ... to ... you ... ou ... ou ...' And then he sings to me, 'Why were you born so beautiful, why were you born at all?'

'I've got a present for you,' he announces.

'So,' I say, 'you want to blow your candle?'

We're taking this symbolism to dizzy heights. We laugh, until the power of his thrusts overcomes us.

'Happy birthday, Carla!'

And as he comes, I really get it: his wish for my happiness, his love, his friendship, his compassion, his admiration. And I get his manliness, in that moment when he releases his potency into me and his face transfigures into ecstasy.

He knows how to give, does Aaron.

We try to sleep together at my place, but it's hopeless. He snores; it's time to let him go home. As he's about to leave, I ask him to get me a glass of water. I rest on my elbow, half asleep, and a few drops of water go down the wrong way, making me cough.

'What were you thinking?' asks Aaron, quick as a flash.

I'm sleepy and can't be bothered with questions. I'm not thinking anything. It's late in the night, for God's sake.

My face probably shows my rebellious thought. Aaron brings his hand up and it hits me. It's involuntary, and he's dismayed. 'Oh, no!' He moves his hand again; this time it turns into a claw and hits me harder. I feel skin come off under his fingernails.

He now has my face between both his hands. 'I'm so sorry!'

My eyes are closed; some part of me is in a dream. There's nothing to say to him. Before he leaves, Aaron fusses with the bedclothes, making everything ship-shape for the remainder of the night.

Dawn breaks and I'm awake in my bed, musing on what happened. When Aaron asked me that question, I think he wanted me to play his game. I didn't show respect for what he considers his 'insightful wisdom' and, almost half asleep himself, his ego was less guarded and lashed out.

What would he come up with himself, if he played his game of *What does this mean?* What would he see if he looked deep enough? Would he be willing to see that his ego was deeply offended? Not just by that one little rebellion last night, but a few similar instances that have been ... well, not so cooperative on my part.

He was pompous with me earlier in the evening, after hooking the video player up to the TV. They'd been sitting disconnectedly next to each other for two weeks, during which time all my efforts to make sense of the leads came to nothing. Then I miraculously discovered how to view the single-digit TV channels via the video. But when it came to double digits, I was once again mystified.

Aaron showed me a button with dots and a dash on it. His explanation was so long and cumbersome that I laughed. He wasn't pleased and said that I must be nervous to laugh like that. I wasn't nervous at all; I was openly derisive of his pontifical attitude. I don't think that sat well with Aaron, though at the time he didn't show it. I kissed him and watched his lips grow full as he pondered whether he would lecture me some more. Then he announced, 'OK, let's go to bed,' and that's what we did.

Aaron's Wise Person is frequently acknowledged by me, but not always, especially when it comes from his head. Well, in this case, the Wise Person felt dishonoured and turned violent. It wanted to deface me, and it did — a little bit, anyway. So, somewhere in Aaron there is a violent ego — the one thing he abhors in others. Isn't it always the case that what we despise in others is the big thing not acknowledged within ourselves? I think of the father of the young man in the film *American Beauty*. His abhorrence of homosexuality came from secretly harbouring those inclinations himself, which he couldn't admit to because of his religious righteousness. Instead, he wrongly suspected his son of being homosexual, and hounded and punished him.

As for myself, why did I allow this to happen to me? It's always so much easier to see another's ego; what about my own? I went to bed with some criticisms about Aaron's pompousness and probably wanted to show him up in some way, and this way was as good as any. He hit me. He would never consciously do that, but he still hit me. Some part of him wanted to.

It's also significant that we spent some time with Isaac Shapiro last night. Isaac travels from Byron Bay to Perth every year to hold *satsang* — a getting-together for the sake of truth. He usually asks penetrating questions, using our own experience to reach the astonishing paradox of the truth of who we are: nothing, it seems, and yet everything. You don't mess with Isaac and hope to remain the same.

Aaron made a point of cornering Isaac after *satsang* finished. He was convinced that Isaac was missing something vital, and that he'd have questions to ask Aaron. Was Aaron determined to show that he, too, was a Wise Person — Isaac's equal? He wouldn't let Isaac go, not even when the organisers started turning the lights off as a hint that it was time to leave. I stood apart from the one-sided conversation, watching as Aaron used both his hands in a throwing gesture toward Isaac's face, literally throwing his ideas at Isaac's head.

Aaron has managed to avoid the obvious kind of egotistical traits — such as greed, possessiveness, status — so he believes he has no ego. But is he identified with being Better and Wiser Than Most, Someone Others Can Learn From? That's what it looks like from where I am. I probably have the same trait, which is why I can recognise it in him. It takes a thief to catch one, they say.

My face hurts, especially my forehead. There are three distinct red spots where skin is missing: between the eyebrows, streaking down the nose, and a place on each cheek under the eyes.

Aha! I suddenly realise what I'm looking at. I'm looking at what sets off Aaron's ego: my stiff-necked resistance to his attempts to change me. He wants me to be interested in computers, electronics, spanners and screwdrivers, to understand how they all work.

'My father used to do that to me,' I told him. 'He was a superbly practical man and he just couldn't accept that I was different from him. I was able to learn about gardening from him, and about animals and insects, but not much else — and he made me feel bad about not understanding.'

Aaron jumped at that. 'You see me as your father!' he yelled. 'You've got to get over that! I'm not your father!'

No, he's not — but like my father, he's trying to change me into what he believes is a better human being — and my neck stiffens up when I refuse. It's one thing to know you're not made for computers, and another to get stiff-necked about being invited to try. I've suffered from a stiff neck for most of my life; all my tension ends up there. It's all about resistance.

Oh, God. It seems we two deserve each other.

I lie down to rest on my bed after this morning's cleaning, and notice that my eyes are wet. Tears hide in the corners, telling me what I'm afraid of. Aaron's going to be hurt, and by me. It's not that I want to hurt him, of course. He's become so vulnerable, so naked.

I've begun to pull back. I enjoy his body, his sex, his energy, his company, but the intensity of it is ebbing slowly away. In-loveness: what a delight, and what a lot of poetic nonsense! I have always known that the honeymoon phase would end; that all-too-human nature would assert itself over projected images. The price of passion is cold reality setting in when you don't want it.

Aaron, I can see, has become attached to me. He can't do without me now. He can't leave without suffering withdrawal symptoms. Worse: he's become attached to our sex, in particular; to the way I respond to his love-making, to be more precise.

'Wowsers!' is his favourite expression of wonder — the exclamation of a teenager, not a mature man. This is the kind of thinking going on in my mind. I know, I tell myself, that all men are boys at heart. You have to take them this way and not expect them to be anything else. It's this boy-quality that makes them so vulnerable. It's the part of them that hasn't grown up and wants women to be nurturing, encouraging, self-affirming, the way their own mothers and fathers were not. In short, a woman is there to serve their self-esteem as well as their pleasure.

Aaron gave me an opening recently when he sensed hesitation in me. 'Is something up?' he asked. His radar is accurate, even though he doesn't quite know what he's picking up. I decided to take the opportunity to be frank.

'I want you to grow up emotionally, Aaron.'

Shocked silence. This wasn't what he expected.

'You're mature in some ways, but not in other ways. You've worked out a world-view that you think works for you, but it's nonsense. Not only that, but you're totally attached to your ideas. You even identify with them!'

I'm referring to his idea of himself as an energy form in a sea of energy in a world that's falling apart because of evil; a universe where UFOs stand by, where the just will make it, and the rest perish.

Aaron took in what I said without seeming overly concerned. But then he wanted to better explain his world-view to me; apparently I hadn't quite got it right. He managed to sound quite convincing; his concepts are uncannily like my own, I realise. With one major difference — the one I believe makes *all* the difference. Aaron talks in terms of information in his head; that's how I see it. He lives in an impersonal universe, even though the creator of it is a He, and He will protect it and intervene when things get too out of hand. But Aaron's never met Him in any believable terms. The closest he's ever come to the embodiment of this Father God was in the person of Fred Robinson, one of the founders of the Eurantia movement, now largely defunct. I rather suspect that Fred was a wonderful father substitute to Aaron, a man who showed him *respect* — that prized commodity he felt he never got from his real father. Also, Aaron's mother is a rescuer type of person: is this where he gets the idea that God will rescue the innocent from the world's evil-doers?

I don't live in a world where God will rescue anybody. I don't have a God who judges anyone, even if I do so myself. Let's face it: I feel disdain for Aaron's world-view, which spills over into his passion for science fiction, especially stories that predict a drastic end of the world as we know it. Robots, aliens, UFOs, *cataclysms*. Cataclysms lead to change, he maintains.

He's right, of course. Cataclysms inevitably lead to major and sometimes radical change. What he misses is that changes can often be made before cataclysms are necessary. Drastic breakdowns can be avoided. Even in his personal life, Aaron misses this, and that's the real point as far as I'm concerned. Instead of paying attention to the things going wrong in his body, for instance, he waits for a disaster.

His right heel has been hurting for months now. He has a chronic sinus problem, and lower legs that are scarred from daily frustrated scratching till they bleed. His car is about to expire due to lack of attention. Aaron dares it to do its worst. He dares his legs and his body to do the same. Where does he think this will end?

I asked him recently, 'What do you think your heel represents, Aaron?'

'Hurt feelings.'

'What kind of feelings?'

'To do with my dad. He's always ignored me. I don't exist for him. I'm his big disappointment.' He looked at the red scars around his ankles. 'This leg will get worse, and then I'll get really angry and create change,' he declared. 'Things have to build up to a certain intensity, then they break and tumble over and a resolution happens.'

'Ah! I get it!' I said. 'You're waiting for life to teach you. If you ignore a message for long enough, it'll get strong enough, and then you won't be able to ignore the message any more.'

Aaron hadn't thought of it in exactly those terms. I felt my anger rising at this great stupidity.

'Waiting for life to teach you is the slowest possible way anyone can learn,' I said. 'Of course life will teach you! But it's only forced to be rude when we don't learn. Look at the millions of people on the planet who are involved in wars, and have lost everything. Their houses have been burnt down. Their children have been murdered. They're wounded, and there's no doctor around. They're hungry and thirsty, and their food has been stolen and destroyed. If enough people suffer like that, consciousness might change because of total hopelessness. It's a hell of a way to learn!'

Aaron started to mumble something.

'Stop avoiding!' I was yelling by then. 'Let's keep this straightforward, shall we?'

Aaron started smiling. 'So, you can get angry!'

The attention was back on me. I hated him doing that. I felt myself blushing and stuttering.

'Sure! I get angry alright, given the right goad!'

I wanted to rescue myself, but I don't know how to stand up to the quiet force that Aaron exudes when he's convinced of what he thinks he knows.

'In your world, everything's white,' he said.

In my world everything's white? Where did he get that idea from?

'My world is NOT always white!' I fumed. 'It contains everything, the lot, light and dark. Only I don't *fight* the darkness. I embrace it, and it transforms.'

I made a gesture with my arms, embracing the air, pulling darkness into myself, but my face was filled with resentment. At that moment, I was oblivious to the fact that what I *wasn't* doing was embracing the 'darkness' I perceived in him; especially his obstinacy. Nor did I recognise that this might also be in myself — my blind spot just then. It's true that I've embraced much in myself that is evil and dark. The power of unconditional self-acceptance collapses negative notions that, until then, seemed unquestionably real. Right then, though, it was more important for me to show Aaron up rather than embrace *his* darkness and let it be.

There's no doubt about it: I'm getting caught up in seeing Aaron's shortcomings. It's not only his emotional immaturity that's been bugging me. It's his manners too.

'You gobble your food, don't you?' I said to him once.

He's aware that other people eat much slower, but he wasn't put out by my impolite observation. Again, in that unflappable way of his, he smiled.

'Eating is like putting petrol in the tank. It's not about tasting. My nose is stuffed up and it interferes with my sense of smell and taste. Plus, my mother's cooking was always very boring, you see.'

My brain seizes on the memory of that conversation: what sort of man doesn't delight in the sense of smell and taste? Might he get fixated on penis pleasure? Is this what's happened with Aaron? My picture of him is becoming bleaker by the minute.

I find myself yearning for a man who doesn't need to defend his self-esteem by subtly putting someone else down. It's a thing he hates to experience himself — he's talked about it so much: the women who put him down with their subtlety. One day we may both realise that the thing we accuse another of is that we most likely do ourselves.

In my imagination, I kiss Aaron. All my judgments disappear when I do that. I'm helpless when I meet who he is. It's so open, so clean, and so precious. As I lie on my bed this morning, I imagine kissing his eyes, his face, his mouth. I'm like a bird that knows where home is and flies to it with unerring instinct, ignoring all weathers.

As I pass the bathroom mirror, I suddenly catch sight of the being who's been in charge of my psyche these last few days: the Mother Superior! The unbending, rigid, judgmental, unsmiling, righteous part of me. I've let her out of the closet, and let her come between Aaron and me. I've seen her once before, in a dream: she's the shadow side of me. She's also the last person a man would feel safe with.

I gape at my reflection, at her and notice that I'm wearing a very straight jacket that has the effect of flattening my chest. Better take it off; it makes me look old. I shudder at what I've become: this unsmiling, judgmental nun. She was there all the time, of course. She came into being over many years of training, first as a scared Catholic girl and then as a young woman in a strict convent. This is the 'serious one' Aaron refers to. 'That one scares me,' he said.

Lynda rings from Bunbury; she's coming up again soon. 'How are things with you and Aaron?' she inquires in that sweet voice of hers. She makes an observation. 'Aaron's the monk among us. He's the best monk there is; he's given up everything to love completely. He's willing to go through hell to accept someone else's choice, namely yours. To accept what is — the only true freedom from pain.'

She listens as I share some of my conversation with Aaron and says, 'Remember to keep it kind.' And with that, she says everything. Suddenly it comes home to me what a stupid person I've been, and how, if I were Aaron, I wouldn't want to come near me again.

After Lynda's call I sit on my couch and read from *The Curious Incident of the Dog in the Night-time* — a book given to me by the president of the Whole Health Institute after I gave a talk there. The story is about an autistic teenager a with peculiar way of viewing the world and no capability to disguise what he feels. He constantly gets into trouble, but is thoroughly likeable on account of his single-mindedness. The reader is privy to all his fears and how he copes with them the best way he can. What can anyone do with a child like that? He isn't teachable. He's like those intractable parts of ourselves that react negatively when someone, including ourselves, wants to argue with them.

I put down the book. It's time for me to come to terms with something, to face the 'shadow' I saw earlier in the bathroom mirror. I decide that the only thing to do is to embrace her. Noticing is the first step. Next is the tedious step of integration. I've accepted so many difficult parts of myself in the past — guilt, shame, fear, despair, the endless failures. Now it's time to accept the side of me that embodies all I've hated about the worst nuns I've known. I see her now. How much damage she's done over the years! My daughters, when they were children, were both at her mercy — lots of times, most likely.

I close my eyes and visualise her clearly as I say the words of acceptance out loud, as if in a ritual. 'Even though this grim, judgmental, unsmiling Mother Superior is part of me, I deeply and profoundly love, accept and embrace her.'

I'll never get rid of her; I can only take away the serious role she's played in my life. I know from experience that acceptance has within it the power of transformation, but maybe I'll have to accept her again and again for the rest of my life. One thing's for sure: if I try to exorcise her — tell her she's not welcome and that she's horrible — she'll grow into a worse monster.

I repeat this unconditional acceptance over and over again, putting my arms around myself in a hug, until I feel totally humble and clean and integrated. My heart breaks to know that it's taken so long to do this. This is definitely one of Aaron's gifts to me: that he's helped me to see myself. I know I won't be as likely to underrate him again. I'll love Aaron, no matter what. Why should I do anything else but enjoy his presence when he's here, for who knows how long?

But he's not here, not tonight, and there's no message.

NEW MOVES

Are you looking for me? Let me come closer then.
Aaron to Carla

 Fate has a way of stepping in and changing our lives. One Saturday in late November I trip and fall on the edge of the swimming pool that belongs to the owners of the house I'm living in. I'm bruised all down my right side and break a couple of ribs. The doctor tells me I need to be off work for six weeks. One moment I'm valued and appreciated by my employers; the next, I'm being asked to leave as I'm no longer useful. I know my rights, but take this as a sign: it *must* be time to leave.

A week later, I move into a house rented by my inventor friend, Kim. I've known Kim for twenty years and have supported several of his inventions. Through pure coincidence, he rang and offered me a room in his house. When he heard about the fall, he was most concerned and told me in his fatherly way that I wasn't to do any housework until I felt better, nor pay any rent.

Kim is divorced from his much-loved wife and was living on his own in the house, which was also his office. Two people come in every day to work in the lounge room that has been turned into a work space: Clinton, the CEO, and Margot, the secretary. Occasionally Chris comes in to look after the accounts.

It soon becomes obvious that Kim needs someone to live with him: his poor eyesight has turned into almost complete blindness. He also had a kidney transplant some time ago, and is now suffering from the long-term side-effects of surviving on only one donated kidney. The plan is that I will become the cleaner of my new home, the cook and occasional driver, as well as the reluctant nurse who manages to inject Kim's insulin.

My bedroom is positioned on the high side of the sloping block, facing the backyard. Windows stretch from one end of the room to the other, capturing a large expanse of sky. To the left, they reveal the top half of an almond tree. On close inspection, the almond tree has a tattered look about it. The cockatoos have stripped it of all its nuts and broken many small branches in the process. I feel an immediate affinity with this tree. I also nurse broken bits, and right now am feeling rather tattered.

When the appointed removalists don't turn up, Aaron and my friend Kate do all the moving for me. They're an A-Team. Aaron knows just how to place the furniture to make the most of the available space. And it's Aaron who spends a whole day fixing my car when I back it out of the garage a few days later without closing the car door. Kim and Clinton watch in fascination as Aaron skilfully and patiently solves the problem of ironing out the crumpled door with the materials he finds to hand: pieces of wood and metal that are lying around, the tools from my car boot, his own strength. It takes him all day. Another man would give up, but giving up isn't in Aaron's make-up. Plus, he just loves being creative in solving problems.

Kim invites him in and asks a few questions. He needs a draughtsman, and because Aaron has been architect-trained and therefore has draughting skills that can be adapted, plus those other much sought-after traits: patience, ingenuity and humility, he is hired on the spot. DeVere Mining Technologies has a draughtsman at last. This is the way things work for Kim, who is a devotee of Sai Baba.

'I could come and live here,' Aaron says on his second day at work. Everyone looks up to hear what Carla's going to say to that.

'Over my dead body!' is my reply, and everybody's head goes down again.

But the idea has been put in our minds, and after everyone has gone home Kim talks to me in his sweet, persuasive way. 'It would be good for us both to have a man around the house, Carla.' Of course, it would be — if only to take care of all the odd jobs that pile up over time. And Kim likes to talk to Aaron; he appreciates their new-found friendship. Besides, Kim is a bit of a romantic and wants to see my and Aaron's relationship bloom.

All the same, I shouldn't be as much of a pushover as I am. In hindsight (such a useful thing when it's too late!) I should be more of a businesswoman and ask Aaron for board money. After all, I'll be doing all the cooking and cleaning! But I only negotiate for food money. And a negotiation it is, with my diet being so different from his. 'I live simply,' he says. Yes; tinned food, junk food and pizzas mainly. Fruit when it's very cheap in bulk. And so we have a discussion about my standards. He has only one choice: to come up to mine, I explain, since I'm not coming down to his. He agrees. Unbeknown to me, a wedge is being put between us already, because Aaron resents being coerced and because he hates to part with money for *food*, of all things. But he wants to be with me, and for that he sacrifices his autonomy in this respect. Later, he will remind me how much of a sacrifice it was for him. Even though it now means he no longer has to drive to work.

So this is how Aaron and I come to live together. It is a big step for me for one reason alone: Aaron will have to sleep with me in my bed every night, not just occasionally, because there is no spare room in the house. This is a leap in our relationship created by circumstance. Or by Sai Baba, if I believe Kim and the way his body shakes when he laughs.

Naturally I'm concerned about how my quality of sleep will be affected. I love having Aaron's body next to mine, but what about his snoring? He tells me to wake him up whenever it disturbs me, but this happens often — and he goes right back to snoring anyway. I decide to buy some earplugs. They work, and the quality of my sleep improves. I start to look better in the mornings.

Aaron doesn't seem to care what I look like in the morning. From the moment he opens his eyes, he's full of compliments. He's charmed out of his mind to be sleeping in my bed.

It's a long time since we both spoke words of not wanting to compromise on being able to be ourselves in our own space; words that seem to be temporarily forgotten in this desire to flow with what life seems to have put in our path. In his own way, Aaron will take care of the house and of Kim, and live rent-free. Would he have wanted to move in if he had to pay rent? It's a moot point.

It's just as well that Aaron has few clothes to bring with him, since my bedroom doesn't have space for them. They have to go in the half-room opposite the hallway, where Aaron erects a clothes rack from odds and ends. He's so proud the day he finds a pretty clothes cupboard with drawers to go into this little room, which doubles as our TV room. 'A gift from God,' he says, because he found it on the roadside. It's white, I discover, when I scrub it down and take off all the labels stuck to it by previous owners.

My couch also lives in this room, only a metre away from the TV, which has been placed on my long, low chest of drawers. It's a cosy place.

THE MANY GUISES OF CONTROL

A molehill is a mountain to those with eyes invested in mountains.
Words of a friend

 I'm in shock; well, seriously unsettled anyway. Aaron's gone shopping early this morning, leaving me to ponder what occurred last night.

I've learnt something and it is this: those who complain about what others do to them are likely to do the very same thing to others. Aaron's great gripe is how others have always wanted to control him. And it seems he needs to make me do as he does — all for my own good, of course.

Aaron likes his computer desktop tightly organised, with icons and files minimised. Last night, when I asked him a question about the organisation of some of my files, he wanted to set them up like his — so tightly packed they seem imploded on one another. I didn't want that; I like seeing the titles of my files at first glance, and feel comfortable with ten or more folders looking at me from the screen. Instead of helping with my immediate problem, Aaron starts teaching me all about folders and storage and retrieval. Worse, he's getting annoyed that I'm apparently not listening to what he's teaching me, because I keep repeating what my immediate objective is. I don't want a lesson about a whole lot of peripherals. He couldn't believe my ingratitude. He couldn't believe what he saw as my inflexibility. I asked for files to stay where they were, and this offended him. I told him what I wanted, but he insisted that I trust him as he renamed things without informing me why. One folder named 'Other' didn't make any sense to me, but when I deleted it he got angry. He dropped his face down — his equivalent of making fists of his hands — and pressed his lips together in a grimace. His face was white and very serious.

'I can't help you any more,' he said, twisted off his chair and left the room. He not only left the room, he left the house. He disappeared onto the verandah, until the mossies started to pester him, forcing him to seek refuge in his car. That's where I found him, keys in hand. I wondered if he was about to leave me, to sort himself out far away from me.

It's happened before that I've been riled by Aaron's attempts to teach me. It's because he reminds me of my father, who also knew how things worked and, like Aaron, always knew how to 'fix' my problem. I'm not nearly so practical, but my father believed it was just a matter of attitude. He threw me into the canal when I was five because he was convinced I'd be able to swim. He had to dive in to save me when I started to drown. Apart from forever disappointing my father, I also made him angry when I knew what I wanted and insisted on telling him.

And now I meet him in Aaron — oh, the irony of it all! My father never saw how his actions were attempts to control me rather than acts of kindness, and Aaron can't see it either. It's his blind spot. Yet he tells me so often about the women in his life who want to control *him*.

Of course, he could be hurt because of my way of speaking to him. I'm not the world's most diplomatic woman; I have no qualms about knowing what I want. It's taken me a long time to come back to myself after my father succeeded in breaking my spirit. I try to be gentle with Aaron, to understand his vulnerable ego. But how can Aaron and I live happily together if I have to walk on eggshells, the way I'd had to with my father when I was very young?

I go to the car to talk to Aaron. He won't speak, but since I don't move away he informs me that he'll go away if I want him to, or stay if that's what I want. I tell him I'd like him to stay, because it's late. He stays.

He's different in the morning: smiling, encouraging me to smile, sexy, wanting me to be sexy too. I want to be near him, to kiss him, but my body is in quiet mode. I'm relieved that he doesn't carry resentment from last night. I don't either, but some part of me is in grief. Tears squeeze themselves from my eyes as he tries to turn me on. My body can't feel the way it usually does. I break away from him. It is then that Aaron decides to go shopping.

Rain is falling on the leaves outside my window — a rare event in Perth's long summer. It won't last; it's just creating a lot of humidity.

What is this grief about?

'Tell me how you feel towards me,' Aaron says, joining me in the kitchen later that morning. He isn't hungry and doesn't even want a cup of tea. We walk to the lounge room, where we sit opposite each other, legs stretched over the coffee table, feet touching. I tell him I'm grieving because of what happened last night, and that this conflict is likely to come up again and again.

'I feel it won't be dealt with, because you can't see past the fact that you want to be helpful,' I say. 'It's your blind spot. Sometimes honesty isn't big enough to see what's going on.'

I remember my own blind spot and how extremely difficult it was for me to see it when I attended an intensive workshop in Holland. My mind knew that if I lost my story of 'my father ruined my life' it would blow apart the structure of beliefs I had built up about being a victim, so I clung to this story for four days. I tell Aaron this story. 'We all formulate a point of view when we're little, in order to cope with life,' I say.

He listens well. He doesn't interrupt.

'I really did get some good results from your efforts,' I tell him. 'My computer folders were all over the place and needed reorganising, and now it's looking good as far as I'm concerned. I also learnt a few things along the way — about selecting a group of files for deletion, for example, and even reselecting one out of a group to be preserved. That was very useful.'

'I admire the way you think and express what you think,' he says with a smile. 'You speak very clearly.'

Really, he's so generous and sweet. He has no problem with me. Will *I* let this go then?

'You're looking serious again,' Aaron remarks.

I am busy at my computer, answering emails. I lean back in my chair and look at him.

'I don't know you when you look like that,' he continues.

He's looking serious himself, but I know what he means. He can be serious without looking grim around the mouth.

'My psychology has become my biology,' I tell him, 'because in the past, I worried too much. I can't change the way I look when I get serious now.'

But Aaron isn't finished with the subject yet. 'It's the "Mother Superior" in you,' he says, 'the one that forgets to have fun.'

I'm defensive now. 'The thing is, I *like* being serious! I'm a serious kind of person! There are people, like you, who have a funny bone. That's not me. So let me be!'

'Okay,' he says, 'but there is a *serious* serious you, and she's *not* funny at all! She doesn't even have a sense of humour!'

I know what he's talking about. I've been familiar with the serious one all my life — well, at least since the age of six, when all of a sudden life took a serious turn. The little girl me followed suit. In time, seriousness became a habit. Right now, though, since the subject's been brought up again, I'm beginning to sense something else about this serious business.

'I know what it is,' I say hesitantly, heading off more comments from Aaron and getting ready to make a confession. 'It's my resistance to the way things are. I even clench my teeth on account of that. At first it was because I resisted oral abuse from my father's penis. I've clenched my teeth so much that it's cost me several molars on the right side of my mouth.' He nods. 'Now I just clench my teeth because of resistance full stop. Resistance happens a thousand times a day!'

Aaron suddenly takes my face in his hands and kisses me.

'For saying that,' he says. 'For owning up that it happens a thousand times a day.'

My confession is hardly a statement of enlightenment! But the magic of Aaron's response is that he helps me to be kind to myself and not make things worse with more self-criticism.

We look at some photos of me sent to us on CD by a journalist who wrote an article about me in a Danish women's magazine. In one of them I'm concentrating while I read a commentary and hey, there's that 'serious' look again. I look like someone who thinks she's doing something more important than feeling happy. That's what Aaron's trying to tell me. It's when I'm concentrating, or lost in thought, that the look comes back.

'It doesn't mean I'm worried, though,' I explain. 'Not any more.'

Aaron has to be content with that. Who knows? Over time, the psychology of happiness may turn up a corner of my mouth. No use worrying about it, though.

'I know why I'm in this relationship,' Aaron says. 'It's because I can be the man I want to be, and everything I do with you lets me be more of the man I want to be.'

Hmm. A telling value.

'When I was with Samantha,' he goes on, 'I thought it was important to do things to keep her happy; I'd bend over backwards. This time, it's about doing what I love to do, to a woman who loves me doing it to her, and who doesn't manipulate me to be anything other than who I am with her. It's such a relief!'

He keeps harking back to the same theme over and over again: this need to be himself; the need to be loved and allowed to be himself. He isn't a conventional guy, keen to fulfil a woman's conventional desires. Paradoxically, he's grown into the kind of man who intuits what I'd like from him when we make love. Perhaps it's because he can feel relaxed instead of under pressure.

I've read articles and books urging women to be more proactive, less passive, to let their partners know what they want. But if you're with an Aaron kind of person, it's best to let him feel you out; he seems to know if you want him to touch your breasts or kiss your nipples. He seems to read every nuance, especially when your enthusiasm no longer matches his. Just a drop of half a degree or so and he notices, enough to inquire later, when you sit beside him to watch TV, whether you did it for him or for yourself. It's so much on his mind, this need for authenticity.

As for me, it fills me with a happy glow to know I have a man whose honesty I can absolutely depend on, and who wants the same from me. Being real, getting honest feedback, him taking the lead when it occurs to him, being invited to relate without any strings attached — all this sits nicely on my soul. We both like our relationship because we both reap the same benefits.

'It's a healing process for me,' Aaron remarks, and looks to me for a rejoinder.

'I thought that from the very first week. It's a healing process for both of us.'

At the beginning, I thought his healing would be by way of preparing him for another relationship. Is it possible that we will stay together after the job, so to speak, is done?

'I don't want to be with anyone else; I can't imagine myself being able to do this with anyone else.' Those are his words now, but they might change. This is a relationship in which Aaron is committed to the truth: not to me, not to the relationship itself, not to the future; only to the truth. It makes for danger, excitement, presence, for the aching, raw reality of now. It's the freedom we long for — and are so afraid of. Aaron is handing it to me. Do I want it as much as he does? Does he really want it as much as he says he does? If so, we'll be a happy twosome, libido built on the knowledge that the only moment we have is now — no thought of the future. The price of this passion for truth is total insecurity.

THE PASSING OF A FRIEND

The rain washes away thoughts of something lacking.
Adapted from untitled poem by Nirmala

 We talk about Kim, who is very poorly now. He can hardly see at all, and his legs are suppurating.

'I'm getting to see the fear that lives in men,' Aaron says.

He's been spending a lot of time with Kim, chatting for hours on the verandah or sitting on the edge of Kim's bed. For one thing, Kim wants to convey to Aaron as much as possible about his visions, so Aaron has the raw materials to work with when he, Kim, dies. Death is something Kim tries to fend off as hard as he can, and he seems convinced that he has quite some time to go. But, Kim reasons to himself, and to us, Sai Baba has sent Aaron to him so he can share his ideas with someone who understands. So Kim scribbles tentative drawings on large sheets of paper, conveying to Aaron his feeling for what he sees more than the actual thing itself. Aaron is just the right person for this type of communication.

'A man gets old and realises he hasn't had a life,' Aaron continues. 'He does the responsibility thing — living for a career or for an idea — and he loses himself. Kim is full of fear, and he isn't quite facing it even now. All he wants is for people to be around him to make him feel better, to give him attention, to distract him from the yawning hole he's teetering above. He doesn't know that he will find *himself* at the bottom of this hole; he's so afraid of his own fear. So he'll go insane, or senile, or pathetic. Men need to feel that they can have a life.'

Kim had great dreams. One of his inventions made him wealthy, before a hostile takeover took it all away again. But Kim's active brain never gave up on ideas. Well ahead of the general community's concerns about water, he realised that water would one day be the new oil. He saw that water evaporation was a major problem and started to design an economical cover for dams and irrigation channels. It never came to a mature enough stage for serious consideration. He once had the grandiose idea that he could persuade governments to adopt his vertical take-off and landing aircraft (VTOL), a wildly clever and futuristic design envisaged to eventually replace cars. The dam cover and the VTOL could have worked, but who would invest the many millions it would take to get them to their various stages of development? All the big projects had to be put on the back-burner in favour of smaller inventions for non-government bodies with money; namely, the mining industry. These projects look promising, but probably won't come to fruition during Kim's lifetime.

What does he know now? That many of his great ideas will come to nothing. His arrogance is melting away in the face of death.

Aaron is thoughtful. 'I'm having a life, Carla. It's caused me a lot of ridicule from people with different values who don't understand how important it is for me to be myself. But I'm willing to sacrifice everything rather than lose myself in some project not of my soul's making.'

Kim and I also have our heart-to-hearts. He is full of kindness towards me. His badly seeing brown eyes take on a sympathetic hue, enhanced by his long, dark eyelashes.

'Don't take Aaron too literally,' he advises me. 'Aaron uses words in his own way, and you misunderstand him sometimes.'

Only seldom does he talk to me about his inner self, the manly, lonely self that is still heartbroken about losing his only love, his wife. It is Aaron who sees more of this side of him than I do; the side that needs attention in the middle of the night. I just notice how illness is humbling Kim, making him more gentle, less assertive, except when he gives me instructions about how to prepare his meals.

From Kim I learn what the best cut of steak is; how to cook it and the chips he loves to perfection. Kim is a gourmet of sorts. He has a love of fine food and doesn't mind spending money on quality. He is supposed to reduce his weight, and does, but somehow never manages to lose his portly image.

Kim suffers from advanced diabetes. He doesn't like imposing on me to take him to the clinic three times a week for his kidney treatment, and in between for emergency attention for the sores on his legs and feet. Although his sight is poor now, as we drive he knows exactly where we are. He has an uncanny memory of the streets and highways.

Gradually, his inclination to tell me how to do everything subsides into trust. Kim is learning to submit to what is happening in his body and life — the strange process of dying. It gives him the opportunity to get close to his son, Nicholas, who comes to visit him more frequently now. His older son, Simon, doesn't drive, so Kim sees him at Simon's mother's place sometimes; these can be times of pain as well as joy since Kim's ex-wife treats him with cool disdain, but he wants his son to know that he loves him.

On Saturday mornings Aaron and I take Kim to meet his very old father and his three brothers at Cottesloe beach for breakfast. It's always a beautiful occasion for sharing, and for enjoying the magnificence of the ocean across the road from the beach café. Aaron and I feel privileged to be part of this gathering, and take the opportunity to go for a walk together and sit and breathe the ocean air.

★ ★ ★

We are sitting peacefully on the veranda in our velvet rocking chairs, watching the doves peck in the garden, when Aaron comes out with one of his great creeds.

'For a man and a woman to stay together, there have to be three ingredients: one, they have to know how to be friends, what it takes to stay in friendship; two, they have to like one another; and three, they have to want the relationship.'

He looks at me with soft eyes.

'You loved me thirty years ago, and kept that experience and protected it, so nothing could spoil it. You kept the innocence of that memory. When you saw me again, you brought this memory out and it was intact, and you loved me the way you did back then. You've never lost that innocence. I love you for that.'

CONFLICT REVISITED

Oh! Brave ones to speak from the heart:
Watch out! The clever mind will trip you up in every way it can.
Carla, in a sober journaling moment

My book is to be published in Holland and I've been asked to go there to promote it. It's two days before I leave. Aaron and I have had a few differences, so he's already a bit strained when I ask him to copy some music I want to take with me onto CDs. He beckons for me to follow him so he can show me how it's done. He tells me to take notes so I won't have to ask him again, and insists I copy him twice after each step. It makes good teaching sense, except I didn't ask for a lesson! I just wanted help with getting a task done in the short time available to me.

Aaron isn't pleased. I can tell from the way he tenses up. I recognise this pattern: it's happened before. Like last time, he leaves the house and goes to sit in his car, which is parked in the driveway. I wait a minute or so before going up to his car and asking to talk.

'Sure, go ahead, talk!'

His body language shows that nothing I can say is likely to make a difference, but I open the car door and sit in the passenger seat. He speaks first. I look into his dull eyes. 'At core, I feel you don't want this relationship, Carla. At core, I feel I don't want this relationship either. This is why I never wanted to have another relationship. This is what I've been trying to avoid.'

'Well,' I say, 'now you can say that Carla was just like all the others. She tried to control you, just like everyone else.'

As I speak, I get an insight. For controlling people, a loss of control over others feels like being controlled themselves. All it takes is for someone to stand their ground and say 'I want this, not that; not what you're trying to foist on me, however well meant.' What is compounding the problem now is that I'm choosing to go far away from Aaron to follow my career, while he stays at home. He had no part in that choice.

We've hit a serious snag here. Or maybe the end. I feel resignation come over me. Instead of trying to talk this out more while he's closed, I decide I need to talk to someone else. I need advice, or help, and I phone Val, whom I've got to know through Kim.

Val is psychic, and a devotee of Sai Baba. She lets me sit in Sai Baba's room, where his picture is adorned with flowers. Val lights a candle and leaves me alone with Sai Baba. I feel so tired that I lie down at his feet, so to speak. I lie down on my side, facing him, and think of nothing, giving my brain a total rest. I lie there in mute supplication, not knowing what to ask for, and drift off into a dozing sleep.

Half an hour later, when I sit down with Val, she notices how my brain has been overstressed. 'You're getting ready to go on an important trip, Carla. You need support at this time.' And then she adds, 'The trouble is that you are a much older soul than Aaron is. He'd do better if he were willing to be guided by you.'

Val doesn't have much of an opinion of Aaron since a conversation she had with him a few weeks ago. Val is still hurting from her past as a nun, and she didn't respond well to Aaron's ideas about what she should do to heal. She actually cried, and she was my visitor! Aaron was remorseful about his callousness. 'I lost it with her. I made a mistake.'

I go home and find him very quiet. Then he asks, 'Did you have a good time with Val?' His question gives me an opportunity to sit down with him.

'Yes, I did. I mostly rested in front of Sai Baba's picture.'

He's silent.

'Aaron, I don't need conflict just when I'm getting ready to go away. I need your support.'

While I've been at Val's, something's changed in Aaron. He reaches out and takes my hands. 'Let's get your CDs sorted out.' This time, he doesn't insist on teaching me, simply goes about creating the copies without a murmur. I sigh with relief.

We look at one another: what has happened?

'Are you going to stay, or will you go away tonight?' I ask him then.

'I'd really like to stay, if that's alright with you.'

He's once more the most tender man alive when we make love, and again when he holds me all night, breathing quietly and normally.

'You slept beautifully last night,' I say the next morning.

He smiles. It is then that it occurs to me that a sort of miracle has happened, and that Sai Baba probably had a lot to do with it.

The next day, Aaron takes me to the airport. From my window seat on the plane, I can see him standing on the observation deck, waiting for take-off. The plane is delayed, but he doesn't budge until it's out of sight and away. As for me, I'm off on a journey that might change us both.

Email from Holland.

> *Aaron,*
> *What if I told you*
> *That I loved no one more than you,*
> *That you have made me feel as no man has?*

Would that give you the sense of richness you deserve?
The kindness of your soul
Healed the criticism of my own carping;
I wasn't good enough in my own eyes until
Your eyes told me differently.
I'm a woman now.
A lover of life, of people, of myself and of you.
Life is my lover; it has me in its arms.
I trust it and have surrendered myself
As a nun surrenders to her God.
I have no God but the truth of my own being.
I have desired you and enjoyed you,
You have loved superbly and healed me;
You and I still love, and respect, and give to each other.
I give you the love of my whole life
You are my friend and I am yours, in tenderness.
Life is taking me away from you, but not all that far.
Be free, dear Aaron, be happy and fly.
Carla

The last time I was in Holland was in 1999, six years ago, and that visit was magical in the way it allowed me to end cycles of sorrow there. I visited all the places that caused me pain as a child, and found only joy because I had ended all blame of my father and myself about what happened to me as a child.

I am welcomed at the airport by an angel in the shape of my promoter: a sturdy woman born and bred in Amsterdam, a superb organiser. Her only flaw is that she smokes whenever she can, which in Holland is just about anywhere. She has my schedule worked out, and in the car we practise my Dutch. It rapidly comes back to me; I have a good head for languages. Her mobile rings: it's the first radio station, checking out how my voice and level of Dutch will come across. And so it continues: interviews for radio, for numerous newspapers, and twice for a TV show.

The highlight is definitely the crowded gathering in the library meeting room on a miserably cold evening in Tilburg, the town of my birth. I have tears in my eyes when I see people who knew my family, and who will remember the war and the way things were exactly as I do. Two cousins introduce themselves to me. I am shocked to recognise their faces and names as those of their mothers', and remember that my comments in the book about my aunts weren't all that flattering. Oh well — it is a heart-warming experience nonetheless.

The next day I am taken by the editor of the local newspaper on a tour of all the sites I missed last time: the cemetery, the mills, which are now a museum, the pilgrimage chapel of Peerke Donders.

More requests for interviews stretch two weeks into a month. During that time, I have limited access to a computer to communicate with Aaron by email. Our exchanges are short, his in staccato poetry:

> there are times when i feel really trapped
> inside my hormones
> caring about everybody around me
> worrying about my other life [his life in Darkan]
>
> the only reason i ever came here was you
> i wanted you
> i am living in a hole without you here
> i will be valid when you are here with me
> to smell you
> see you
> hear you
> sense you
> touch your energy
> lie beside you

It is a difficult time for him, doing without me. I know something's up when he emails me that everyone and his dog is starting to look attractive to him right now. In another email he confesses that he's developed an interest in Margot, Kim's assistant. Margot with her long hair, striking eyes and sweet nature. She's not much of a talker, being conscientious and not wanting to take up work time to chat. Margot is forty something; her big, shiny eyes always tell the truth. She's polite, but not overly so, has a quirky sense of humour and a fine moral sense. The last thing she wants to do is hurt anyone, and it's in this respect that she may get misread by Aaron, who could take her affectionate, smiling return of his attentions for more. Or she may be genuinely interested in him, but would respect his unavailability.

Still, my heart is gripped with fear. I stay with my dear friend Julia one night, and tell her about it and that helps. The next morning, all is well again with me: what will be will be.

Aaron emails me from his house in Darkan one evening:

> Hi babe
>
> In Darkan now.
>
> Just to let you know that my body loves you and my heart agrees with it — have been in agony about having someone to make love to.
>
> Been reading your book [God's Callgirl] to help me identify with you.
>
> Read the draft of The Price of Passion the other night — felt very challenged; scared the living daylights out of myself.
>
> You really are a force of honesty to be reckoned with, so real and honest. I feel honoured to have my dick in you, sacred ground.
>
> The book makes me feel that you are right here with me. You gave your all to so many lovers; you are so brave to bare your feminine soul; you are so real — want you back.
>
> I can have sex with so many women if I wanted to; right now I want to have sex with you. You make me feel that the man in me can talk to you in sex to your soul. Just thought you might like to know that.

And so comes the time for my return, at last, on Easter Sunday of 2005. Aaron comes to pick me up from the airport. I have been looking forward so much to running into his arms that it's so very strange to approach him as he stands there, arms folded, eyes focused as if to read mine. It's good to feel his nearness again — and strange to feel his aloofness.

Once the baggage is in the boot and we're driving home, he explains. 'I wasn't sure you belonged to me any more.'

I can't believe his words.

'You met so many interesting people over there; there must have been at least one person you were attracted to.'

Yes, there had been — two, in fact. What's wrong with feeling an attraction? 'It didn't make any difference to the way I behaved,' I say.

'That's what I saw in you when you came out of customs,' he says. 'You were open and unguarded and I knew all was well.'

I'm intrigued now to know what's been going on in *him*. I ask about his attraction to Margot.

'No, nothing happened, but we became close friends.'

Somehow it takes a while for us to get reacquainted. Strange that. So different from what I'd anticipated. It's as if he doesn't entirely trust me. As if he suspects I'm hiding something from him. I hope the melting of this doubt won't take long.

And then it becomes suddenly, starkly obvious that Aaron has been projecting onto me what's in his own mind. It's Aaron who has become preoccupied with someone else. I notice he touches Margot whenever she comes near — rubs her on the back, squeezes her shoulder, stands so his body is in contact with hers, holds his hand on her.

One evening, as she prepares to leave, he gets up to give her a big hug. Margot is surprised, and seems pleased. She lets him have this closeness with her. I wait near the door; Margot and I are going out to listen to a talk by a movie director. I've already said my casual goodbye to Aaron. It isn't as if we're not coming back later this evening; we've planned to have dinner together, Margot, Aaron and I.

I don't know what I feel as I wait for the hug to finish. Ever since Aaron came to work and live here, I've been aware of the chemistry between him and Margot. While I was away in Europe, my instincts told me it was a close thing as to whether Aaron would take her to bed or not. The fact that he didn't made him grow up in a certain way. He seemed to know more clearly what he wanted. Or else Margot did! But now this.

I could discuss it with Margot as we drive, but the chat is all about movies. I tell myself that I'm being petty and that there's no need to spoil the atmosphere of excited anticipation. Margot's worked as a screenwriter and assistant to movie directors for many years of her life, and she's thrilled to come along to this talk.

Margot's gone home. I run a bath for myself. After my soak, Aaron invites me to sit beside him to watch *Battlestar Galactica* on the TV. 'What is it?' he says. He knows something's going on. He probably knows the cause of it too. Only he isn't admitting anything.

I smile ruefully, not replying, since the only time for talking is in the ad breaks, not long enough for a conversation. Also, I'm ashamed of what I feel. While in the bath, I let my feelings run rampant. I tried to put a name to them. Jealousy? No, not exactly. Insecurity is what I came up with. *Insecurity*! After all we've experienced together! I thought we were so bonded that nothing could destroy what we had. Now I find that there is something: Aaron apparently feels so secure that he thinks he can now play around a bit. Not seriously play around; just have some fun because he loves Margot and he loves women.

Battlestar Galactica finishes and we go to bed. I can't respond to Aaron's touch. The only thing to do is to tell him how I feel — to clear the air so we both know what's going on.

'I've been feeling insecure,' I begin, addressing the semi-darkness of the room.

'I'm aware of that,' he says.

Oh? He's aware of it yet said nothing? I decide to come to the point straightaway. I blurt out the sentence that has been weighing on my heart.

'I want to know, Aaron: do you want to touch Margot, do you want her? Would you want to have your dick in her if you had one to spare? And do you want her to know that?'

My mention of a spare dick is slightly ridiculous, but I'm referring to his oft-repeated words, *I only have one dick, and I choose to give it to you*, an expression of faithfulness decided by physical limitation. He has only one dick, hence he will only have one lover at a time. But what if he had two dicks? Wouldn't that be great?

Aaron isn't pleased with my words and he's not going to answer my question. Instead, he asks me what my problem is. Our conversation goes around and around, gathering darkening clouds, until I ask him to please answer my question. He's forgotten what this is, so I repeat it.

'Tell me if what I think is true!' I insist. 'Tell me if my intuition is right or not.'

He pushes the blanket aside and sits on the bed cross-legged, naked, facing me obliquely. I'm lying down, arms under my head, covered with the blanket, studying his face in the dusk. Aaron's body takes in my request with a slight shudder. Then he straightens his back and is quiet for a moment.

'Yes, your intuition is right,' he says, not sure if he's done the right thing by being truthful. 'And I want you to know that you're the most important person in my life. You know I'm here with you because this is where I want to be.'

When he's finished, I have only a few words: 'Thanks for telling me the truth.'

Aaron's right fist comes down on his crossed thigh. He's furious with my thanks, reading the words to be some version of *Thanks for admitting to your unfaithfulness*.

'This is what I won't put up with any more in a relationship,' he says bitterly. 'I've had a gutful of insecure women! For fourteen weeks I've been bottling up my feelings about Margot because of what you might think, and two days ago I said, "Fuck what Carla thinks! I'm a human being with feelings, and I should be able to express them!" Margot's a lovely woman, and she's lonely. She likes me. I want to show her that I like her too!'

And then he challenges me with a question. 'Tell me what you get out of our relationship; tell me what you get from me!'

He waits in the dark, tense with anger. It's clear that all he can think about is how good a lover he's been, and he wants to stay oblivious to the fact that I have any right to know what's going on inside him that might concern me. He feels outraged by my confessed reaction; feels that my insecurity is unfair, after all the love he's shown me, all the words of reassurance he's poured on me. But I've just been faced with a whole new development: the fact that Aaron's been struggling with his feelings about Margot, and with his fear of my reaction. And that he decided to deal with that by upping the ante, by not confiding in me at all.

I don't have the words to tell him the welter of feelings that come up. For one thing, in spite of what Aaron says to me about my beauty, I don't feel I can compete with Margot. She's so much younger than me. I think of her gorgeous long hair, her expressive eyes, her sweet voice, her sense of fun, her rounded breasts.

'I don't know what to say,' I murmur.

Aaron takes that as a bitter denial of all the good things in our relationship; a deliberate forgetting, an unfair accusation.

'I'll pack up and leave this house,' he says, and gets up and puts on his watch, then, incongruously, his shoes. The rest of him is still naked when I meet him at the foot of our bed and stand in front of him. I reach out to touch him, but quickly pull back my hands from his coldness.

'Well! What do you want to say?'

He feels so badly done by; his love has been so magnificent.

'You've been extremely nice to me lately,' I begin. My words sound like a platitude, a pathetic bribe to make him stay. 'You've been sweet and attentive. I want this relationship!'

He pauses and thinks about how he feels. It's enough to make him stumble, semi-convinced, back onto the bed, toss off his shoes and take off his watch again.

'All I want is for you to be Carla,' he says, lying on the bed with his head supported by his elbowed arm. 'All I want from myself is to be Aaron.' He stares at me in the dark, face stern, determined. *Nobody, but nobody, is going to stop me from being myself.* 'I want to have relationships with everybody! With Margot, with Clinton, with Chris.' And he rattles off the names of more people who come to the house.

'That's fine!' I retort, face close enough for him to see my expression clearly. 'Smiling is fine, enjoying chemistry is nice, putting out friendly vibes and having conversation is nice, but touching and hugging is different. *These are things that lovers do!*'

'I hug Clinton and Chris!' he remonstrates. 'I'm a human being and I hug people! You hug people too, don't you?'

'I don't hug everybody.' He should know this about me by now.

'Margot hugs you,' says Aaron. 'What do you feel when you hug her?'

Aaron's been saying lately that Margot wants to know me better, be my friend.

'I don't feel anything much,' I reply. 'I feel that she wants to hug me because you hug her, and she wants to make it up to me somehow. I feel her discomfort.'

'I feel her loneliness,' he says.

So what? Is he supposed to rescue her?

'If you knew about my insecure feelings, why didn't you talk to me about it?' I ask. 'Why didn't you tell me? Were you scared to discuss it with me? Surely this is the kind of thing that's good to talk about, to prevent problems from developing. Why didn't you talk to me about your feelings?'

It seems a reasonable question. The answer should tell him something about himself. But his answer is one I can't believe.

'I wanted to,' he says, 'but you weren't listening.'

I'm silent. I feel that this is a cop-out; one that's making matters worse.

It's way past midnight and my eyelids want to close in sleep. A riot of thoughts keeps me awake for another hour or so. When morning comes, there will be more thoughts. A decision has to be made. For me to expect Aaron to be different from what he is is to court utter disappointment. I have the choice to accept him as he is, or to say, *Enough. Be yourself somewhere else.*

I could ask Aaron to leave the house, as he threatened to do. That would mean leaving his work as well, for a while, at least. It's not a practical suggestion. I imagine myself in my writing room, feeling miserable and totally uninspired, missing him, wishing our misunderstandings weren't so deep. I'm appalled that in spite of all our bonding, our relationship is still so fragile. That it could be broken so easily.

In the dark, I tell myself that I deserve to be in a relationship with a man I can be totally comfortable with, because the relationship he's in is all he wants. A man whose hormones feel happy with me, and don't want to wander off to eye off all the females they could be playing with. Aaron doesn't have the excuse that his partner is dull and unresponsive to him, not even part of the time. I want a man who is more mature than this eternal Sagittarian . . .

My thoughts run on. Aaron's back is turned to me. I sense an invitation, his longing to have me hug his back. I don't feel like it. I lie quietly, until I, too, turn my back, and we lie apart, and this is the way we go to sleep. Together but apart.

THE PRICE OF PASSION
INCLUDES EVEN THIS

It's only when I'm in your arms
That I realise I'm completely lost.
Simon Gladdish, 'For Rusty'

 I'm always the one who wakes first. My half-asleep brain takes up the monologue of the night before. I don't want to make a decision based on neurosis and insecurity. I want to recognise that men are different from women, and that hormonally healthy men like Aaron will always have their eyes open for feminine beauty and spontaneously fantasise about being with others. I want to admit that Aaron would never be unfaithful to me by having sex with Margot or anyone else. That if I wanted to control him, he'd only get worse. That rather than be controlled, he'd leave me. That he is so tender and close with me. That our love is real. That I want him.

Aaron has also woken, and moves to embrace my back. I hold the arm that encircles me in acknowledgment. No words are spoken in the dawning light. Then he turns. Once more our backs face each other. He sighs when I don't turn to hug him but lie flat on my back instead. His sigh contains a sound of high-pitched distress, very short, almost unnoticeable. But I notice. I find myself turning towards him and hugging his back. It isn't even a decision, just a movement without thought. He turns his face towards me from the pillow and I kiss it with the passion that wells up in the moment.

'My Carla's back. She's left her mind.'

I raise myself up so he can see and hear me clearly. 'I'm happy for you to be Aaron. I want you to be the man you want to be.' It's an exhausted Carla, speaking words she fervently hopes are true.

He hears, and suddenly all seems well again between us. Our bodies once more revel in the sweetness of our blended energies. Our short intercourse confirms that we want each other; then we slip apart again, satisfied for now with this rebonding.

I will have to see how I react in the future. I tell Aaron that it might be good for me to talk to Margot; not to make her feel insecure, but to reassure her that it's fine with me that she's found a good friend in Aaron. I also want to know if she's comfortable with Aaron's approach.

I catch Margot as she passes me on the verandah on the way to her car, and decide to be direct with her.

'Margot, I notice that Aaron seems to be very taken with you. Is there something between you and him?'

Margot is immediately thrown into a terrible spin. 'It's not like that, Carla! I would never . . .' She bends her head, very likely because she is hurt to be seen as untrustworthy, and blurts, 'He seems so needy, Carla! I hate to refuse his attentions because I don't want to hurt his feelings.'

That's good enough for me. I thank Margot sincerely and ask her, please, not to be upset by my questioning of her. Margot leaves as if chastened after a dressing-down. It's not what I'd intended, but I suppose it's inevitable given Margot's humble character.

Aaron's been on tenterhooks all morning. 'What's going to happen to us, babe?'

We're sitting in my writing room. His eyes are baggy. This is stress, not just lack of sleep. I know Aaron well, but will get to know him even better.

For the so-manyth time, he explains how he's always expecting his woman to turn on him. He's never noticed anything in me that tells him I might reject him with the hatred and venom he fears so much, but, he says, he's been surprised by the sweetest of lovers. Total love in the morning; lover gone in the evening. These experiences have carved such a deep wound in him that he's like a warrior in the jungle, always on the alert for trouble.

'It seems to me that we've come across a major incompatibility,' I observe. 'I feel insecure sometimes and need to feel free to tell you about it, and you absolutely can't stand insecurity. You go off your brain when you see it in me.'

I look at him and suddenly sense why he can't handle insecurity in others. He's insecure himself! To see it reflected in me reminds him of his own weakness. Sure, it's a different kind of insecurity — he knows how to be together and apart, to stand in his own energy; he's proud of the fact that he doesn't live off my energy, that he wants nothing from me but my friendship — and yet it's so similar. He's afraid that I will reject him. He's afraid that I will misread his signals, that his love won't be appreciated for what it is. How is that so different from my own fears?

We have the rest of the day to ourselves — two lovers, both ragged at the edges, both in recovery mode from a conflict that has made us breathless because of the raw possibilities it contains.

We talk, and it's so difficult for Aaron to stay with the point. He wants to come back to what, to him, are the important things: he loves me; he loves me a lot. He even says, 'God has put Margot here,' which I know also to be true, but not as an excuse for what has happened.

Finally, I land on the crux of what I'm feeling. 'I feel hurt that you didn't trust me enough to confide in me,' I say. 'I thought that we had something strong enough to weather whatever we are willing to confide about ourselves.'

Somehow this makes sense to him. For the first time, he loses his defensiveness. 'I'm sorry,' he says, and that simplicity conveys everything.

That night, we both go to bed early. It's raining outside. Aaron starts his pillow talk, but I put my finger on his mouth. It's alright. Tonight, let's just go to sleep.

What has transpired doesn't stop Aaron from continuing to flirt with Margot, although there are no more hugs for now. He claims the right to 'be myself' and 'to put my sexual energy wherever it's appreciated'. Margot doesn't know how to be rude to him and say, 'Don't do that'.

'You and I have a great relationship,' he says, facing me cross-legged on a chair in my writing room.

'Then don't throw dirt on it!' I retort.

He closes his eyes, he's so hurt.

After a few moments, he says something that makes me wonder how much he might have been hurt when I was going out with John.

'You were taken with John's energy; there was this chemistry, wasn't there? Plenty of touching, no?'

Oh. The question sits low in my belly. It needs a straight answer.

'Yes, true. At the time, I was convinced that I was feeling something I had to investigate, and yes, I allowed a lot of touching, and I reciprocated willingly. But that was half a year ago, at a time when you and I weren't living together, when you chose to be away for two weeks at a time.'

During Aaron's visits to me in Perth, I didn't go anywhere with John. Aaron had warned me that he wouldn't be part of a threesome, so I had to make up my mind. I did, as soon as I knew John better, and realised this had been a madness of sorts. I'd ended contact with John then.

Aaron didn't want to stand in my way during that time. He'd rather lose me than claim ownership over me or tell me what to do.

Should I accept Aaron's behaviour now, the way he accepted mine then? Even though it's happening right in front of me? I don't know if I can do this, or ought to. Surely it's okay to have boundaries — or compromises, if you want to call them that — as a way of preserving a relationship? If God brought Margot here, it may be so we can both decide what our values are. In that sense, God brought John along too, and I became aware of what I valued most.

No one knows what will happen next. For now, we're lovers. For now, I can't imagine no longer being in Aaron's arms.

FUNERAL OF A DEAR FRIEND

Quiet still sings from the throat of nowhere.
Nirmala, untitled poem

Kim dies. He is so brave at the end. I could never endure what he did with so much surrender. I feel privileged to share his end-time, my good friend of twenty years, before his heart gives out. Kim didn't become senile or insane or pathetic. He learnt to accept his condition as it worsened, in a way that few people could, and so kept his dignity to the very end. I believe he had a life, after all.

The day of Kim's funeral starts with brilliant sunshine. Clinton comes into the office for the morning. He's become the main organiser of the business and its operation now. For years, Kim relied on Clinton's sharp intelligence, his vast knowledge of electronics, his engineering background and his spiritual acuity. Clinton could find a job with better pay anywhere but he's devoted to Kim and what he wanted to achieve.

We get on well, Clinton and I. He's a stocky guy with presence, almost bald in spite of only being forty. He's married to a Chinese woman and they have three delightful children who often keep him from sleeping through the night. Clinton's helped me out of a tight computer spot several times, and enjoys eating the salads I prepare for lunch. I love the way he appreciates a joke, and I trust his opinion on many things.

'Clinton, look at me,' I say. I have on purple pedal-pusher pants and a pink top with an almost plunging neckline. Not the usual funeral attire. 'Do I need to change?'

Clinton's opinion will be executive, considered; that's why I'm asking him.

'Please don't,' he says, smiling.

And I feel that this funeral is, indeed, more of a celebration than a mourning. It's a mild, sunny autumn day. Kim has passed over from this plane of living into another plane, but he's not 'dead', nor ever will be; he's just changed form. For a little while, he'll be in the astral form, observing what goes on. I feel that he gets great pleasure from watching Aaron and me make love. Clinton feels that he gets guidance from Kim, and that for some time he'll help him do what's necessary to get the company on a new track with Kim's younger son, Nick, on board. Nick's only twenty-two, but already shows signs of having the required level head.

Kim's father, three brothers, a sister and dozens of close friends come to bid him farewell. It's a remarkable day, full of marvellous interconnectedness between these people whose paths are crossing each other.

Afterwards, Aaron and I stay on as guardians of the house, as security for the company, which will keep on paying the rent.

Kim's room will stay as it is, until Nick feels it's time to remove his father's belongings.

VISITING DENMARK

Just sit there right now.
Don't do a thing.
Just rest.
Hafiz, 'Just Sit There'

Denmark — so dear to my heart because I spent seventeen years of my life there, and wrote most of *God's Callgirl* there, at a protective distance from the big city, Perth. The unconditional acceptance of my friends proved to be the first real step in my healing process from a difficult past. Those friends are still with me, and one of them, Jill — with whom I've exchanged so many conversations over the years, and who has helped me so many times with her wise insights — has invited Aaron and me to stay in her house for a few days.

We spend most of the first day in my car, travelling south from Perth, for the best part sitting in silence. I've forgotten to bring some music to play on the tape deck. The silence is comfortable; it's just that there's a lot of it. Neither of us wants to chat, to feel obliged to say something for the sake of talking. Aaron remarks on it when we arrive. Was there really nothing to say all that time? Couldn't we have said what we noticed along the way, such as the beauty of the trees that lined the road? Yes, we could have. Yes, we will, in the future.

Jill shows us around her house. It's been renovated and is pristine and Zen-like. I know this place from when she used to live here and I lived five minutes away. It's been empty for a while, but after we leave she will move into it again. The furniture is sparse: a table, two chairs and a divan — the French type with horsehair inside and on castors, stuck in a space all by itself. Aaron tests it briefly. 'It's not as hard as the floor.'

The bedroom has a comfy bed, we discover, after deciding to retire early. I made dinner from what we'd brought with us: eggs and toast and sprouts, followed by tinned apricots. Then Aaron rearranged the chairs in front of the fireplace, which we didn't want to light because it really wasn't that cold. It is the last day of April, overcast and quiet, but still only autumn. We spent an hour or so reading: he from his magazines, me from a book of short stories by Carmel Bird.

Aaron has a shower and comes to join me in bed. I soon discover that he's forgotten to wash under his arms and tell him so, very quietly, not to criticise, just to let him know. 'It's a man thing, I suppose, Aaron.'

He has a solution to that, he says. He goes over to his army duffel bag, where he stores all things manly, and digs out a roll-on deodorant. He smells worse than before, but I haven't the heart to tell him. I appreciate his willingness to please.

He turns to the wall; we're going to sleep. I curl up against his back. Ah, yes, all is well.

My hands are cold from typing this Sunday morning in Denmark. Aaron is lying beside me in Jill's bed, absorbed in his model-making magazines. I duck my left hand under the blanket and onto his warm chest.

'Do you know your hand is cold?' he says, looking up from his magazine.

'Of course I do. I put it there to warm up. You're supposed to love and protect me, remember?'

'Is that so?' he says. 'Where's somebody who'll protect *me*? Hello?'

Oh well, so much for that. But we're friends, better friends than ever, even though he recoils in mock horror when I bend down to kiss him.

I continue to type with a pillow propped behind my back. Aaron stops reading and interrupts me with his affectionate nonsense.

'Ve at headquarters in Berlin haf been obserfing you from our vindows and ve vant to bring you in for questioning.'

'Oh!' I giggle, then say 'How many of you are there?'

'Der is me, Aaron, den der is Fritz, and Helmut, and last of all der is Klutz. Klutz is alvays last, you see.'

At this point Jill knocks at the front door. We invite her in and she's roped into our silliness. It lifts her out of her slightly serious mood.

Aaron and I clamber over the magnificent rocks around Green's Pool and breathe in the vital air. We seem to be alone and Aaron turns romantic. He puts on his Latin lover accent, with a German lisp.

'I vill lie you down on dis hard rock, dis masculine rock, and you vill feel de hardness of my rod inside your softness, and you vill be de bridge between de sky and de earth.'

Matching action to word, he puts his arms around me and lowers me gently to the smooth hardness of the rock beneath us. I can trust the strength of his arms not to drop me, but I think it's in that moment that I lose my digital camera. I don't notice until we arrive back at Jill's house.

Aaron stands against the wall, hands in pockets, one hip jutting out — such a come-on pose, at least so it looks to me. Straight out of a movie. I giggle like a girl.

'Yep, you're a giggly young girl now,' he says. 'That's what you are. You've spent too long being an older woman. A year ago, when I met you again, you doubted who you were and you were sometimes awkward about yourself. Now you're comfortable in your skin and it shows. You are yourself. Sixty-six and bloody beautiful! I'm so proud of you. I'm so happy to be your man.'

THE COLLECTOR

I collect, therefore I am.
Adaptation of Descartes

 Like everyone, Aaron has his quirks, except that he seems to have a double dose. The most peculiar thing about him is his passion for models. It's a world where I can't join him: I can only watch with fascination. He loves to see a whole lot of seemingly dissociated parts gradually take shape: into an aeroplane, a tank, a battleship, a spaceship — every conceivable object to do with war or science fiction. It's a passion that never wanes.

He introduced me to this side of himself rather shyly. He's had a lot of flak, I suppose, from people who think he should grow up — or at least put together a few of his models before he buys more! His collection is already so extensive. He dreams of one day having all these models on shelves lining the walls of his open-plan lounge room. This lounge room is also a dream right now; it exists only on the computer as an architect's three-dimensional drawing. Aaron says it breaks his heart to think of his house. He's collected hundreds of building materials, not to mention mountains of bric-a-brac gathered from God's shop, namely the roadside — things the rich throw out, to be recycled by one of God's more humble servants into a future

268

life. But Aaron can only be in one place at a time, and he's chosen to be with me and the job that promises him a good income when his skills are honed.

In Darkan, where his house is, he feels protected, cocooned and alone — terribly alone. And discouraged, because he is now fifty-one and no nearer to fulfilling his dreams than he was when he built his shed to house all his collected materials, seventeen years ago. The truth is that Aaron can't *not* pick up an item he sees on the road that might provide a future benefit. Old computers, TVs, anything electronic, and items that may be useful for his mother, his sister, his nieces, his friends, me. What he finds is truly miraculous. He has a wish list in his head, and it may take a short time or a long time to find what's on that list, but eventually it appears.

'Even you,' he says. 'I had a picture of you in my mind all this time. It took thirty years for you to come back into my life, but you did!'

When he wanted another Colt to use for parts for his existing car, which was showing serious signs of wear, he manifested not one but two! The first only cost him $150 because it was deemed undriveable and grass had grown up all around. After spending several hours cleaning it up and tinkering with it on the spot, he drove it away. It was in such good condition that he decided to store his original car for parts! The second cost him nothing but an exchange of parts. The owner wanted some parts for his Morris Minor; Aaron had some in his shed.

Today, he comes home from the toyshop with a statue of a flower fairy. She's seated on the stem of a flower, her head resting on her arms, asleep. Her hair flows gracefully around her delicate face; everything about her is delicate, even her hands.

'You're like that,' he says, after he's unwrapped her and put her in my hands for inspection. 'The feel of her is of you. You have her delicacy. Look at her hands: graceful like yours. Those are your arms. You sit like that. That is your body.'

I'm touched by the way he sees me. The statue goes on my dressing table in the bedroom. Later, when we're in bed, he talks about it again.

'You're like a delicate flower,' he says, gazing at the statue. 'You've preserved something I lost: a trust in relationship, a fearlessness, an innocence.'

His fear of relationship has been so profound that I have to be careful what I say to him. If I mention anything that criticises him for the way he relates to me or to others, this may remind him of previous conflicts and immediately escalates his fear into terror — terror that there's going to be a fight. This fear creates a gridlock in our relationship. We need to be honest with one another; but how can we be honest if what we say triggers our sorest emotions? I don't have an answer to that one yet. But I realise that until we find one, our relationship will suffer from a certain lack of depth.

Aaron doesn't think it's necessary to share what goes on inside him. When I talk to him about the importance of communication, he parodies me. 'Do you want me to tell you every little thought that passes through my head? How insecure is that?

'You want me to tell you that I think of nobody but you, don't you! That I will never see another woman as sexually interesting, that I will never feel anything for anyone except you. You want me to censor my thoughts and my imagination, and make sure I talk to others as if they're sexless and I'm sexless. Except you, of course!'

His bitterness is real. He doesn't realise he's insulting me with this exaggeration, and that he's destroying something between us with this attitude. Certainly there's little I can say to defend myself at such moments. The only thing I can do is try to address my own problem — the problem of my remaining insecurity, that is. Even though he exaggerates, it's true that I feel a constriction in my heart when he flirts with the women he meets, lapping up their responses.

It's when I lie down on my bed for a rest this afternoon that the answer comes to me. The feeling is exactly the same as when my father no longer came in the night to molest me. We had moved to sunny Australia, where the house — with thin wooden walls — made his night visits impossible. Also, he'd discovered Melbourne's prostitutes. I felt discarded; no longer his special girl. I was desolate, and climbed up a tree one day and wailed my distress. It wasn't a conscious thing; at the time, the distress was as much a mystery to me as it was to all the people who heard me. The abuse had always happened during the night, when I was asleep.

Now I recognise that feeling again. Oh God! All I can do with it is to accept it, be willing to have such feelings. I apply the tapping sequence of the Emotional Freedom Technique and say aloud, 'Even though I feel this awkward, unreasonable pain in my heart, I deeply and completely forgive and love myself.' The action and the words ease my pain. I realise I can choose to fully accept those feelings, the situation and myself, or suffer.

Aaron comes back from a meeting. It's my turn to go out, so I look for him to say goodbye. He's on the couch in the TV room. Before I can speak, he says, 'I've got a present for you,' and beckons me to sit next to him. I do, and he places the most tender of kisses on my mouth, again and again. In between kisses, I notice his face. It's smooth, with a boyish ecstasy.

'You've got a nice feeling, babe,' he says softly.

How can I destroy this sweetness with my neurosis? I can't say a word that would tarnish the joy of this honest love, not now.

I'm in the lounge room, sipping tea. Aaron sits at one end of the room, Margot at the other. They're both busy and not speaking. Then Aaron pipes up, 'Margot's having a very bad day today.'

'Really? Does she need a hug?'

The words come out before I know what I'm saying, but they do no harm. Aaron gives a short laugh.

Margot says, 'No, it's my tummy that's playing up. I don't even want a cup of tea today. I'll get over it soon.'

The room goes back to silence. I feel in that moment how innocent their whole affair is. Aaron is compassionate towards his friend. She needs his understanding and his attention. They're good mates in this room. I don't have the same natural understanding for Margot that Aaron has. If I did, I'd be closer to her.

One morning she shares with me a dream she had about a letter from her father, saying how proud he was of his beautiful daughter. She is deeply affected by this message from beyond the grave, as she puts it, because her father died when she was fourteen, and in life was never in the habit of telling his children that he loved them. Margot is so keen to tell me about this dream that she comes down the back steps to talk to me while I hang out the washing. It tells me that she's open to me, yet I don't show her the same openness in return. The price of my passion is unkindness.

I feel honoured by her sharing, and pleased for her, and tell her so. We go up the back steps together, Margot in front of me. Her body language tells me how vulnerable she is, and for a moment I feel a gush of unusual warmth. I realise that Margot hasn't a skerrick of bad intention. The last thing on earth she'd want to do is hurt me. I know this as firmly as anyone can know anything. This certainty puts me starkly on notice. It's all *your* stuff, Carla. Aaron may have his problems in other areas, but this is all *yours*!

'I've had so much flak from women about my masculinity,' Aaron muses. 'I'm often terrified that it's not enough.'

Something tears through me as I feel his woundedness. I raise myself up on one elbow and kiss him between words by way of extreme emphasis: 'AARON … YOUR … MASCULINITY … IS … MAGNIFICENT!'

Aaron is stunned. 'I got that,' he says humbly. 'I sure got that! Thank you for showing me myself.' And I feel the glow from his open chest. What a nice thing to teach a bloke: to see and love his own masculinity! Especially when it's so obviously built into a man like Aaron.

'Carla, don't go there,' Aaron says, the moment I begin to say something about my vagina — that maybe it isn't as tight as it should be, or as he's used to feeling in younger women?

'There's nothing flabby about you, take my word for it,' he says. 'And I should know, shouldn't I?'

It's cheeky of him to refer to the number of women he's had in his life, but this time he uses it to drive home a welcome point.

'I want to say this: I like the way your vagina tastes and smells, and the blonde hairs surrounding it. I like the way it sits in your anatomy and the way it gets wet. And I like it because it's yours.'

Well, what else does a woman need to hear to make her feel great about her vagina? I need never have another inferior thought about this subject. Not that Aaron says it to make me feel good. He tells me he wants to express the appreciation he feels, not keep it to himself; he wants to shower his woman with his respect and admiration.

'You make me into a poet,' he says.

He wants me to be more expressive too. I look at him dumbly, stuttering because my brain goes easily to mush and coherent thoughts seem impossibly far away. Then some words tumble out by themselves, uncensored, unmanufactured.

'I open to you like a flower,' they say, 'like a whole field of flowers. And you are the sun, warming all the cell-flowers of my body. The sky is red with the petals of roses, and they are falling down on us, caressing our bodies because that is what they love to do, and then they lie beside us, as lovers, glowing, fragrant and spent.

'I feel like the deep of the ocean, where it's dark and there are no waves, only deep-flowing depths, and then above me I feel slow waves, vast, majestic and broad, and above that, the faster waves of what goes on in the light of the day.'

He puts his hand over my mouth. 'What's this?' he mocks. 'You're becoming a better poet than me! Where did all this come from? Will it ever stop?'

We both laugh. It's a bit of a breakthrough for me, this expression in words.

* * *

'I like your breasts,' he says, unexpectedly. I know he doesn't say anything he doesn't mean, so I ask him, 'What do you like about them?' (My breasts, of all things!)

'I like their petiteness,' he says. (*Petiteness*? How charming!) 'And their extreme sensitivity. They're small, so they haven't sagged; they're like a young girl's breasts. They're cute. And so soft. And they have a trillion nerves in them, that come alive the moment I touch them and make you wet. And I love your nipples; one of them looks almost square when it stands up, you know, and the other's pert and round. They're so big! And they're yours. I like your breasts most of all because they're yours.'

He suddenly holds both my breasts in his hands, and I catch my breath. He holds them quite still; the warmth of his hands courses through their poor flesh, as if he's healing them — or at least my concept of them.

Aaron: 'I had tears coming down just then.'

'Oh?'

'They just came out, no reason at all.'

'Oh.'

'I love you so much it hurts. It makes me sad that I can't love you enough. I try and try, but it's never enough. I never feel satisfied. It's an agony.'

I'm listening to a man in love talking to a woman he's woken up in the middle of the night to tell her how he loves her. I was in a deep sleep. I have a vague memory of being embraced, of his breath close to my face, of the bed wobbling as a heavy body hit it. I woke up slowly to his body pressed against mine from his shoulder to his toes, and his words, *sotto voce*.

'Thank you for last evening. We made such beautiful love, you and I. You're all woman, and I feel all man. It's not just that. I feel your beauty, and it breaks my heart. I try to be like you, and I can't. That's my pain. I can't be like you. I can only love you from the outside. I can only love what's outside of me. It makes me sad that I can't be inside your space; I can't be inside your love; I can't love you enough.'

I recognise this pain. It used to be mine. Only then Aaron kept reminding me that this beauty wasn't outside of me. Aaron's in love now, and not in his right mind. Aaron, the tables have turned. Our previous roles have reversed.

Aaron looks pensive this morning and I ask him what the matter is.

'It's my house,' he explains. 'It wants me to come back to it. It represents my other life that I chose to ignore to be with you. But my house is part of my life too. It's part of who I am.

'It's a bit like being a captain on a ship,' he explains. 'The captain has a wife in town, and he goes away on his boat. She's jealous of him because the ship is like another woman. My house has so much history in it that it empties my soul to ignore it. It's making me feel separate. As much as I try to be here with you, I can't be in two places at once.'

He leaves me to figure out if I'm the ship or the wife. What it means to me is that his house will be a priority at least part of the time.

'What's going to become of us?' Aaron seems fretful. There is never an answer to this repeated question.

'All I know is that we're here now,' is always my answer. There may be endless now-moments, perhaps many of them to be spent together in ways we can't yet imagine.

'I don't want to stand in your way if your life calls you away from me,' he says humbly. 'When you left in that plane to go off to Europe, I stood there until the plane became just a speck in the sky and finally disappeared. In that time, I fully let you go, perhaps never to come back to me. I let you go to your destiny, whatever that was. It was a painful thing to do, but it set me free. Until the moment you came out of customs and met my eyes, I wasn't sure if you'd return to me. It wasn't that I mistrusted you. I knew that your soul could have called you to something different and I wasn't going to stand in your way. That's how much I love you.'

EXCHANGES OF ENERGY

If a mirror ever makes you sad
you should know
that it does
not know
you.
Kabir, 'Where Do the Eyes of Women Fall?'

 We're sitting at the kitchen table. Breakfast for one, me, has just finished. Aaron skips breakfast sometimes. He's not only trying to lose weight (in vain); he explained once that he's trying not to eat beyond his weekly contribution to the food kitty. There's no use telling him that skipping breakfast will only make him hungry later, when he'll fill up on the office biscuits and his own stash of chocolate-coated peanuts.

Lately, I've been waking up feeling tired. That's not usual for me. What's happening? I've become used to Aaron's snoring, but it must still have some effect, the same effect noisy traffic has on people who live close to main roads. Sleeping has been difficult for other reasons as well. I go to bed earlier than Aaron, but don't sleep soundly until he arrives and settles down next to me — often two, three, four hours later. Only then do I allow myself to fall into really deep sleep.

But when Aaron was away at his place in Darkan a few days ago, I was free to go to bed early and get up before six as I used to, which suits my rhythm. My energy was high, and I sat in meditation again — something I've neglected for months as a deliberate exercise. I slept so well that I knew it was a sign that I need more space to myself. I found myself actually excited about Aaron being away. That's not supposed to happen between lovers!

But is this just about sleeping arrangements? Could there be something deeper going on? I desperately need to be honest with myself. I think back to my meditation when Aaron was away. For me, meditating is simply sitting and feeling the sense of my Being. I'd love to do this with Aaron; I feel it would increase our intimacy. We have such good companionship and physical intimacy. Could we have a deeper intimacy, the kind that two souls share when they communicate from Spirit, in silence? Or share their experience of Being? Or share what might stand in the way of that?

It's a slippery path, that. Because I look at Aaron from the outside, I imagine I can see certain things about him more easily than he can. We all have blind spots, don't we? And vice versa: Aaron's also very clear about how he sees me. The trouble is, what we think we see is only our interpretation. It may, in fact, be quite wrong.

Aaron beats me to it by asking if there's anything the matter. Why would he think something's going on with me? Haven't I always been eager to get back in his arms again? Yes. And don't I tell him that I love him? Yes, and I really mean it too. I love him so much. The pain I'm beginning to feel is like the pain of having to leave a loved one behind. I'm moving on, to a far-away country that is no further than my soul and yet may as well be the other side of the world.

Aaron waits patiently for me to get my thoughts together. He's smiling faintly: whatever is in his girl's mind, it's *serious*, and he doesn't easily believe in 'serious'. It usually means exaggeration, illusion, creations of an overworked, fearful imagination. He will listen but won't necessarily hear. *Give her a few days and she'll come to her senses again. She loves me, that's all that matters.*

I take my eyes away from the almond tree in the backyard, it's branches bare now. It looks as though it will never bear fruit again.

'Aaron, I feel that we're so compatible in bed, and we enjoy each other's company, but that's where the continuum breaks off,' I say. 'The compatibility just isn't there in important areas. I'm not judging you for it. It's just me admitting the truth to myself and to you.'

Aaron looks thoughtful but has no reply, so I continue.

'When two eccentrics come together, the points of compatibility decrease as the eccentricity increases. We're both eccentrics. It's a wonder we're as compatible as we are.'

Aaron looks hurt now. He's taken my words about his eccentricity as a form of complaint and is slightly defensive.

'I've never tried to change you, Carla. I've only tried to know you and enjoy you.'

I know this is true. It's always been his intention. Once upon a time he wanted so much to teach me things. He had it firmly entrenched in his brain that a relationship means learning from one another, and he knew exactly what it was I needed to learn. He despaired when I didn't get it, and lost patience, and became insulted when I refused to do as I was told, even though it was for my own good. That was a while ago. Lately, he's been respecting my choices, loving the parts of Carla he likes. And the other parts? Well, he's decided they're my business, not his.

'When you want to change me, I feel violated,' he says now. 'That's why I don't come from my head. Mind is destructive.'

I think of how I may have wanted to change him lately. There are some clear examples. Last week I begged him to please, *please*, leave the cups and glasses on the draining rack after washing them so their rims could dry, and to please, *please*, put the cutlery in the receptacle provided so it could dry as well.

He'd ignored me at first. 'Calm down, Carla, let me do it my way.' *I'm doing the dishes, isn't that wonderful enough?*

But I'd explained the reasons for my request — 'If you understand the logic of what I'm saying, why don't you want to follow it?' — and he'd promised to do as requested. However, it just didn't happen. A few days later I asked whether he was deliberately refusing, or just kept forgetting. Aaron was apologetic: yes, he'd forgotten.

I realised that if it's so difficult for him to change a simple habit, how much more difficult is it for him to make deeper changes; changes, for instance, on an emotional level.

I have no right to expect Aaron to change. But it's time for me to realise that in spite of his good intentions, he *isn't* going to change. It's time for me to work out what I'm prepared to live with and what I'm not, and to let him know.

Lately, the amount of stuff he keeps bringing into the house has really piled up. Some of it — his music CDs, two large boxes of them — have ended up on top of the filing cabinet in my writing room. They don't look bad there, but he didn't ask me if it was okay to put them into the special space that is my writing room.

His other stuff has piled up in the small room opposite the bedroom, which serves as our clothes room as well as a TV room. There is another room available — the room that was Kim's — but Aaron doesn't seem to like the idea of putting his things in there, or sometimes sleeping there to give me a break from his snoring. He doesn't feel comfortable about infringing on what was Kim's space. I find this difficult to understand when it's been almost two months since Kim's death. It seems my space doesn't matter, but Kim's space does, because he's dead. That's Aaron's eccentricity; nothing I can do about that. What I can do is move in there myself, but that doesn't seem fair. I like my own bed, having my dresser near, and the light that floods my room in the morning.

Aaron says he'd rather sleep on the old leather couch in the lounge room. And he does. For three nights this week, he's worked on his computer in there till very late at night, then flopped onto the couch.

This doesn't resolve the problem of his things cluttering the small TV room. The pile gets so big that the door can't be shut any more. I notice this just before leaving the house for an appointment, and ask Aaron to rearrange his things so visitors on their way to the toilet won't see the mess. There's to be a board meeting in the office that morning, which means more people passing the room than usual. He promises to see to it straightaway, but when I return it's obvious that he's forgotten. Nothing has been moved and the door has been left open, yet again. Mess doesn't matter to him; why should it matter to me?

When we have the house to ourselves, I tell him about my misgivings.

'Aaron, you came into my space, so you should honour my boundaries. You have them in your place, remember? I was told about your rules. When I'm in your space, I have to fit in with your boundaries. You need to respect mine.'

Aaron sees the point, and apologises, but there's another incident a few days later. He's casually dipping used teacups into the dishwater in the sink, supposedly washing them up as he sits at the lunch table. I interrupt my conversation with Clinton and Margaret to throw a comment at him. 'Aaron! Cups don't get clean like that!' Everyone is stunned by the tone of my voice.

Aaron slaps his hand as if he's a naughty child and says mockingly, 'Bad hand! Not supposed to do that! Don't do it again!'

It's a relief that he treats the episode humorously, but I can't stand finding cups on the shelves with lipstick stains on them or tea or coffee stains inside. Aaron couldn't care less, believes it contributes to a healthy immune system. I have no idea why cleaning up is such a big turn-off for him, until he tells me.

'You make me feel like a little boy again,' he says, 'being picked on by my mother.'

It makes sense now. No wonder he often 'forgets' the things I ask him to do, like closing the TV room door or taking the rubbish bins out to the kerb. Forgetting is his form of rebellion against his mother. It's easier to cope with his untidiness and forgetfulness when I understand, but I still find myself wishing for a man who has broken free of all that.

Aaron sees my wish for him to change as an insult to love. 'I'm here with you for what we have in common,' he says. 'I don't concentrate on differences.'

It sounds heroic to me. Can two people do this together, or will it only work when one person does it? Or will it not work at all, because differences have a way of asserting themselves whether you want to concentrate on them or not?

I feel upset, but realise there's no use giving in to that. Aaron is just this way; I can choose to take him as he is or decide that I don't want to live with him. Aaron calls my upsetness 'ego', but if wanting things my way is 'ego', then that's what it is, and it's up to Aaron to decide whether he likes that or not. I'm weary of trying to live beyond my evolution, trying to accept something when I don't feel like it.

'There are other exchanges of energy,' I say. 'For example, when one person does all the cleaning in the house and the other does none, that's not a fair exchange of energy.'

His face becomes serious. 'If you don't want to do things for me, then don't.'

'How would your life be if I stopped acting like your mother? Would you be able to look after yourself?'

'I'd live a different lifestyle from yours, but I'd survive.'

It would never work for us to live as separate people in this house, each only looking after ourselves. Aaron would never clean, because he's not used to that. His house in Darkan is one big dust bowl.

'I'm grateful to recognise what's under the dust when I wipe it away,' he said once, and that just about sums up his interest in keeping things clean. He says this will change when his house is finished. Well, why not practise doing it here?

'I don't want to go there just now, Carla.'

Aaron doesn't envisage anyone sharing his future house, it seems. If anyone did, it would simply be on his terms. Is wanting to live in a clean house a sign of insecurity? He says it is. I don't agree. Does it matter? Right now, he lives in *this* house with *me*, and apart from the washing up after lunch and dinner (and he usually skips the stove), I do all the cleaning. And I don't like that arrangement.

And so it happens that a small incident becomes the trigger for a deeper upset.

One small incident can be a symbol for what is unresolved in a person's wounded psyche — and the catalyst for change or an ending. When such an incident happens, a person like Aaron is faced with a choice. Do I want this relationship? Because if I do, I *will have to change*. Or do I feel sorry for myself and my pain and get angry and say, *No way! I will not have drama in my life, never again!*

Well, life with Aaron has come to this. It's the incident of the door to the small room being left open again. I confront Aaron about having to close the door at least four times that one day. He stands there in total disbelief: how can leaving a door open mean anything to anybody? His immediate reaction is to make a beeline for the office where Margot and Clinton are packing up to go home.

'Hey, guys, does it matter to you that the door to the small room in the passage is left open?' he asks, his tone of voice and body language saying, *Back me up, guys, back me up!*

Margot's instant reaction is to smile and laugh. 'Of course it doesn't matter!'

But Clinton is more thoughtful. He looks straight at Aaron and nods. Yes, it does matter to him. Like me, Clinton is probably thinking of the company image.

'You bastard!' is Aaron's reaction.

'He just did that to support you!' he says later, when both Clinton and Margot have gone home. 'He couldn't have meant it. He didn't want to upset you.'

Aaron's not around when dinner is ready. He's gone outside, to mull things over by himself. This is looking serious. I let him stay outside, leave him to get his own dinner when he's ready.

That night, he has a dream; a nightmare, rather. It occurs three times. In the dream, he is trying to protect a fluffy little dog from a huge mastiff, which is mauling the little dog in its teeth. The only thing he can do to get the mastiff off the dog is to poke his fingers into its eyes. His hands get damaged trying to get the smaller dog out of the mastiff's jaws.

To Aaron, the dream is about how he protects relationships: the innocent, fluffy little dog. *I will not have drama in my relationships!* is Aaron's mantra. To me, the parts of the dream represent parts of Aaron's psyche. He will poke his own eyes out rather than see that this is all his own doing: it is he who's setting the scene for the drama. When I insist on boundaries, does that create drama? Or is it his reaction to my insistence that creates drama?

It's hard to believe that he can't — won't — see what I so patiently describe when he asks for my interpretation of his dream.

WHEN IT STARTS TO MATTER

The only sin which people never forgive in each other is a difference in opinion.
Ralph Waldo Emerson

 I'm sitting in one of the easy chairs next to the sofa Aaron's been sleeping on. It's past eight o'clock in the morning, and I've made us some tea. I return to his dream.

'The dream shows me that when you're asked to change your behaviour to suit someone else, you feel attacked at your core,' I say. 'You feel you can no longer be yourself. No wonder you must resist by "forgetting" all the time! And I'm the terrible mastiff, the baddie! If I'm the mastiff, I create the drama that you don't want in your life, but for some uncanny reason it inevitably turns up. Again and again and again.'

'When someone tells me how to live, I want to get out of there. You just want things your way,' he says. 'You're completely unable to compromise.'

'Not true!' I retort. 'I've been willing to put up with the mess, provided that you keep the door shut on it. That's a compromise, isn't it?'

I don't get a reply. For Aaron, to be proved wrong is a wrong in itself.

'I just feel into the relationship,' he says eventually. 'Feelings are what matter to me, not bloody reasons.' There's another pause. Then: 'I've had this dream many times.'

'I rest my case,' is my reply.

It may be years, if ever, before this conversation makes real sense to Aaron. It may take the breakdown of several more relationships. He may never understand it. Somehow, it's all too difficult for him. What is curious is the thought that he is totally devoted to the preservation of his drama-creating values.

We continue our conversation in the kitchen, where I prepare breakfast for myself. Aaron's dream has given us both the opportunity we need to say some things clearly.

'I feel that I was badly treated as a child.' Aaron looks at me, hoping for compassion, and of course there's plenty of that in me.

'I understand that it's your woundedness that makes you overreact the way you do,' I say. 'Small incidents can trigger the dreadful feelings of unresolved events in your life. So far, all you've wanted to do is find compensation instead of examining and learning from them.'

'Yes, alright.'

His reply comes too fast on the heels of my words for me to believe he's taken them in. But he does own up to the reality of the bloody welts now disfiguring his legs.

'I scratch my legs because of the pain of that,' he says.

But I have no mercy. 'Here's something for you then. While you scratch your legs, you'll never have a relationship that lasts.'

'Hmm.'

It's the end of our talk. Clinton has come into the office early.

There's a lot of banter and good feeling among Clinton, Margot and Aaron during the day. It's good to have the others there — to give Aaron a break from me, for starters.

Margot and I have cleared up the awkwardness between us. Margot, as it turned out, was never interested in Aaron in a sexual way at all. She didn't want him to feel rejected, which was why she allowed him the hugs and touching. That's changed. Margot has firmly drawn the line now.

When the day is over, and Margot and Clinton have gone home, Aaron returns to our conversation. 'You talk about acceptance: doesn't that mean accepting me as I am?'

I've thought long and hard about this one, and I've come to some conclusions. Yes, it does mean accepting him as he is, but it also means accepting *all* the facts of the situation, not just him; accepting the *whole* truth. That truth includes how I feel about things.

I make some tea and invite him to sit down at the kitchen table.

'It surely doesn't mean I should be walked over, Aaron. I have standards. They're higher than yours. You can't ask me to come down to yours. You only have the choice to come up to mine.'

He looks astonished at what could be interpreted as my brashness. It is bold: lovers have split up over less. Aaron is silent, nods ever so slightly as he takes this in.

'I live here rent-free,' I say, 'but I work for it by keeping the house clean. You don't do any cleaning; you don't even take the rubbish out. I've been letting you get away with it. You don't do any of the food shopping, so you don't even know the price of food. It takes time and petrol to do the shopping.'

'How much money do you want, Carla?'

Aaron agrees to pay the amount I suggest, but what is he going to do to equal the *energy* output from my side? Isn't a relationship an exchange of energies? In all areas, not just in emotional terms?

Our differences don't end there. There's the huge question of how we are growing apart because I attend gatherings and weekends on spiritual awareness, and have weekly sessions in bodywork. Aaron thinks he doesn't have the money for this kind of thing, nor for any other therapy that may be useful.

'You're treading water standing still, Aaron. You know an awful lot about *why* it is you scratch your legs, for example, and why you have a chronic sinus problem since forever and why you snore, but you don't do anything about it!'

'I *am* doing something,' he says. 'I'm reducing my things!'

It's true that he is sorting through the huge collection of data, and numerous backups of data, on the various hard drives of his computers. This has kept him busy for three weeks already, till deep in the night, every night.

'After that, I'll start going through all my clothes and getting rid of really old things, and as soon as I get to Darkan again I'm going to go through my junk and get rid of all the things I know I'll never be able to use. You've shown me how good it is to live simply.'

That would be a major change. Yet when I accompanied him the other day to get something he needed for the office, he couldn't resist buying a whole lot of things just because they were cheap, and always in multiples of at least three. He can't help accumulating things when they're going cheap. It's an addiction.

'As soon as you have enough money, you'll buy more models,' I say. 'You already have hundreds of them, all still in their boxes, because it would be impossible in one lifetime to put them all together!'

Models enable him to enter a world of make-believe, the one safe place he had as a child, and he wants to endlessly recreate this safe feeling of childhood by buying more models. I understand this, but there's a certain edge to my tone as I make my observations. Aaron notices. His extremely tolerant nature doesn't want to interfere with what I'm expressing, but he does want to make it clear to me that what I'm thinking and feeling about him isn't necessarily his own reality. Despite that, Aaron has no bitterness towards me whatsoever, not an iota of desire to harm me or get back at me. It's disconcerting, because it brings my indignation into sharp relief. I have the grace to tell him that I appreciate his softness, that I recognise my critical attitude.

This night I go to sleep feeling remorse and tenderness for this man with many faults but such humility. I decide to have a little bit of humility myself.

Aaron comes to bed for a late cuddle and falls asleep curled around my body. At some very early hour in the morning his sniffles and sneezes develop and he decides to continue his sleep on the lounge room floor.

'I want to make love to you before I leave for Darkan,' he says as I pass him at seven in the morning. He's planning to go to his house and reorganise his things there, as he said he would.

'Join me for a cup of tea then,' I say.

When the tea is made, he drags his sleepy body into my bedroom, just as my daughter Caroline phones from Melbourne. He gratefully sinks onto the mattress. My daughter and I have a leisurely conversation while one of my legs is wrapped around Aaron's torso. I sip several cups of tea. She finally hangs up.

'Wake up, Romeo!' I snuggle up to his back.

He stirs immediately. 'It's so good, this wrap-around feeling, Carla. Your femininity against my back, your all-female body along the whole of my body.'

He turns his face towards me. His breath smells, so I don't attempt to kiss him on his mouth. I caress as much of his body as my right hand can reach, from his face to his testicles, and he comes alive, moaning. I decide I'm the more awake one and make a move to sit on him. His face, with its round, wide-open eyes, is below me, expressing his surprised delight and appreciation.

After our crescendo, I lie beside him as he pants, allowing my vagina to subside from its deep excitement.

'You're a beautiful lover, Carla. You're so in your body, so focused. Your intensity fires mine. You're fearless. You surrender to what is happening in your body; you're so in the now when you love me.'

Aaron loves to say something sweet to mark the moment. I listen intently and look at myself through his eyes. If only I could transfer this kind of fearless surrender and focus into the rest of life!

'How did you feel when you made love to me?' he asks.

'I felt surprise. It's always new. I never know what's going to happen.'

'It's the only security — the security of never knowing what's going to happen next. The security of insecurity. You relax into insecurity when you make love.'

Where does he get all those words? Yes, I do 'relax into insecurity' when I make love. The challenge is to go for this all the time, without the help of hormones. I sense the freedom of this, again and again; yet again and again my mind asserts itself and tells me I should worry about getting something out of life that isn't there. When will I finally wise up to my head enough to not listen to it?

BUCKETS TO CRY

The storm, the shifter of shapes,
drives on across the woods and across time
Rainer Maria Rilke, 'The Man Watching'

 'If you want me, you'll have to come and get me. You'll
have to take responsibility, Carla.' Aaron's preparing to go to
Darkan. He says he might be away for weeks this time.

'I'm glad you'll be there for me when you come back,' I say.

'I mightn't be.'

'Oh?'

'Three things could happen. One, the relationship could dry up in
me; two, it might be that I want to keep to myself, be in my own
space and not have it disturbed; and three, someone else could come
into my life.'

Well, that's telling me.

'We don't know what life will bring us, do we?' I reply.

'Don't get me wrong: I won't be looking for someone to replace
you. I want to find myself again without you around, find out who I
am when I integrate all that's happened between us. But I do want to
love and be loved.'

Meaning, *if you leave me, Carla, I won't want to be alone.*

Since he isn't in a hurry to pack and leave, we keep on talking.

'I'm just grateful that we can sit here and talk about this,' he says. 'I'm so used to girlfriends going berserk on me and spitting the dummy. I'm used to tears and begging.'

I ask him again why he scratches his legs.

'I scratch when I feel your judgmental attitude, your "headiness"; when you talk about my options about what I could do, how you want me to be, what you see wrong with me. All that makes me feel very nervous and freaky, and it makes me scratch.'

'But you scratched way before you knew me. When did you start?'

'It started when I was with Veronica.'

'You were in your twenties then.'

'Yes. It started with the stress of that relationship. I used to get severe cramps in my right leg as well. I haven't had them since I've been with you!' Aaron seems pleased by this improvement. 'This relationship has its downsides, but the upside is the positive warmth you've given me. I used not to be able to feel my leg, but I lie in bed now and I can feel it. I have a shower and the skin softens, then I lie in bed and feel it dry and stretch and hurt, and I let it. When I've dealt with everything, the scratching will finish and I'll be able to feel my legs completely.'

Aaron leaves for Darkan around noon. There's no pain in the parting. I know that he'll love the feeling of being in his own house, and he'll get absorbed in his tasks. He so badly needs a break from his computer work and from me. And I'm already feeling the wicked joy of not having to take anyone into consideration for a while.

I have time to think things over while he's away. We all have our obsessions, I tell myself. The more wonderfully eccentric we are, the more of them we have; and the more we haven't faced our issues, the more eccentricities we'll have. It's just how it is. But what has happened to the exquisite pleasure I felt when I decided to take everything about Aaron in my stride and not get offended by anything?

There's a conflict going on in me. I do a lot of thinking about unconditional love. It seems to be a must for the complete happiness of my heart. I wither when I judge and am judged. Yet there's a 'but' that follows, and I don't want to ignore it. I believe the 'but' belongs to love as well, because, above all, I need to be honest with myself. It's no use imposing unconditional love rules on myself when a) I'm not ready for sainthood, and b) this means ignoring taking care of myself.

Maybe it's only a partial truth, an incomplete and painful lesson, but I feel relief at the relative clarity I've gained. This relationship is over. I feel it, even while my brain doesn't want to recognise it.

Slowly, I consider the facts of the matter. We're so good together in bed, we enjoy each other's energy immensely; it's comforting, so comforting. I curl up to Aaron the way a cat curls up in someone's lap. The tendency is like the cat's too: to go to sleep like this, or go to sleep and never wake up

Who wants to wake up to the reality that this is it? I don't. My head's been in a fog because I've denied it. Today, I lay down because my whole body was feeling heavy. I lay down and snoozed, and awoke to tears in my eyes and the knowledge that I wanted to cry buckets because this relationship is over. We just don't have enough in common.

Part of me is saying, *I can do better than this, so I'll leave Aaron.*

In my mind, Aaron says, *You'll be sorry. It's the energy that matters, nothing else, and you won't find this energy again. You'll find out how your mind has tricked you and you'll be sorry.*

In spite of his words, Aaron is back again after four days. It's hardly been long enough to miss him.

We spend the night together. Aaron, exhausted, falls asleep in the middle of making love, and I follow seconds later. We both sleep deeply and well and wake up together at around seven o'clock, when the sun begins to play over the bed sheets.

Aaron's happy. 'I had such a good sleep. Did you?'

Yes, I did.

'Do you want to kiss this rosebud?' And he offers his lips. 'Be careful of the bristles.'

I do, and he moves to put his arms around me, but I get up, returning after a while with a tray of tea for two.

Aaron's cheerful. He's worked out what's been going on, he says, and lets me know his thoughts.

'You always sort yourself out before long,' he says. 'You've changed; you've really learnt about together and apart. You don't need the attachment any more and you're much more confident in yourself. I'm sick and tired of rescuing little girls who want a free ride on my dick. They forget that having sex doesn't mean you still lead two lives and you still die alone. I feel safe with you.'

It never ceases to amaze me how he always compares this relationship with his past experiences, and how he's always grateful that this time there is no impossible price to pay for having sex. 'Thank God, thank God!' I've heard him whisper to himself. 'It *does* exist. It *is* possible. Thank God!'

'I always test things out; that's what I do,' I say softly, almost to myself.

'I want to take up where I left off,' he says, pulling me towards him under the blankets.

Is he assuming that I want what he wants? I don't struggle to avoid him, and discover that this morning I've metamorphosed into a different kind of woman. I succumb to making love because I enjoy my lover's pleasure, knowing that at some stage I will enjoy it intensely myself. It always happens: the moment when tears come to my eyes because of the overflowing pleasure.

He ejaculates, even though this wasn't his intention, and I hear him say, 'Oh God! Oh God!' as he shuts his eyes and waits for things to subside. Later, I ask him what he meant: did he mean *Oh God, how good this is,* or *Oh God, how tired this is making me*? It could easily have been the latter, judging from the rings under his eyes, but he laughs at the very suggestion. Oh no, to him this was soooo good!

He's so light, I have to believe him. But I believe my own perception as well: I think it's a big bit of both.

Aaron continues with his observations.

'You put yourself first now. This relationship has become expendable to you because you're following the call of your life. You've grown up and I'm pleased for you! As for me, I'm here to know you and love you, and for the love I get from you. You still like me and enjoy me, and you still want the relationship. Am I right?'

He waits for my answer.

'Yes, you're right, but this relationship needs redefining, Aaron.'

Aaron's done some thinking about my 'you can't change' assertion and comes up with a typically Aaron answer.

'I came to Perth thinking I'd become a teacher. Then I met you, and as a result I abandoned my studies. I was introduced to a lot of lovely people, I got a job, and I started to live with you in this house. Those were massive changes in my life. My house in Darkan was my focal point, but when you came into my life, my priority changed to living with you. Don't you think those are phenomenal changes?'

I have to give it to him: I never considered these events to be changes that he'd made; rather, they seemed like changes that happened to him. But they did involve his choosing, and he chose a complete turn-around of his usual life.

'Three years ago, I was a depressive person,' he goes on. 'That's changed. I've come to myself in a lot of ways; I know more about who I am. I'm different from the person I was two years ago. I've changed even more in the last year, and so have you!'

It's all true. Full marks to Aaron.

Our conversation isn't over.

'I'm the kind of man every woman wants to be with and no one can live with,' he quips, plumping a pillow as he laughs and looks at me.

The devil! He knows he's attractive, that women love him as a lover and for the energy he has. Yet, so far, no woman has been able to stay with him. I'm just one more lover about to call it quits, but I want to understand my motivations exactly before I do.

'Why do you think no woman wants to stay with you?'

'Because of their insecurity.'

'Their insecurity? What might be the reason if I left then, since I'm not insecure?'

'Ah, but you are,' he says. 'I can see your insecurity . . . I can see how vulnerable you are when you love me. I will never want to hurt that. I want you to be the Carla you can be — so happy with yourself that you're unbreakable in your sense of self. You always had beauty, but you couldn't see it. Now it's coming back to you that you can be yourself again, and have it all. You're waking up to yourself, and I'm here to make that happen for you.'

He waits for all of this to sink in, then continues. 'When you made love to me thirty years ago I learnt your energy. I let you go, thinking I'd find it somewhere else. But I never did. The Cogs worked their ways and now we're together again. I'm aware every day of the energy that you are, and that keeps attracting me to be where I am instead of somewhere else.'

OK. That's beautifully put. He does love and appreciate me.

'Will it make a difference if I say that I love you?' he says, smiling at me. I think I can read the rest of it — what he doesn't say. *How can you be so obtuse? Why are the things in your head more important than this simple feeling between us?*

Later that day I go into the lounge room to find Aaron sitting on the floor surrounded by computer parts, concentrating hard on putting them all together. He's making a new computer for his mother; the project has taken him hours already. And I suddenly remember how much time he's spent on my computer, installing software, installing quantities of music, helping me produce a bookmark and stationery. In fact, he's done as much as he can regarding my computer to make my life easier. He copies CDs for me when I ask him, and shopped with me to buy a decent CD and DVD burner, then showed me how to use them.

And I shouldn't forget all the work he did on my car when I had my little Honda. Since I bought the computerised Camry, he's been unable to do any mechanical work for me. I've taken this particular way of contributing out of his hands.

Aaron would never defend himself by reminding me of any of the above. When I go to thank him, he says, 'I just love you, Carla.'

How can you leave a man like that?

RISKING IT ALL

Give me your deepest fears ...
what use have they ever been to you?
Nirmala, untitled poem

 It's my birthday. I'm booked for a telephone seminar from the United States, starting at 7 a.m., which goes on for more than an hour. In the meantime, Aaron has to go out to a job that will take him away for hours. The office staff come in at around nine with happy wishes, and it's not until after midday that Aaron bursts through the door. I happen to enter the office from the kitchen at that moment and see him rush over to Margot and haul her up from her chair to give her a big hug and a kiss. Margot squeals in surprise. I'm stunned.

Aaron takes me out for lunch — the first time ever and a big deal for him, so I don't want to spoil the event. He notices that something's not quite right with me, but drops his concern when I get genuinely enthusiastic about the menu.

My belly's in turmoil all afternoon. I back my car out of the garage and finally do what I've avoided for so long: I collide with Aaron's white Colt parked in the driveway. Luckily there isn't much damage, but I see the incident as symbolic. It's time to talk before we do more damage, but I want to leave it until tonight, after the others have left. I remember Aaron's reaction the last time I brought up the subject of Margot, and don't savour the prospect of him going into another angry defence.

We're sitting on the lounge in the TV room when I describe to Aaron what I witnessed in the office.

'I can't remember that,' he says.

Not a good start, but I guess it's hard for him to immediately come to terms with what I'm bringing up.

'You think that I would have a relationship with Margot if you left me, don't you?' he counters. 'I just want to be a sexual man. I love to flirt and be nice to the girls. I love feeling appreciated for the man I am. Margot often comes in on a cloud of hormones. She's lonely. I want to take the edge off for her. It doesn't mean I'm going to have sex with her. I have that with you. You're all I want.'

This is beginning to sound like the conversation we had several months ago. 'You can be the man you want to be,' I had said at that time.

Now I say, 'Since then, Aaron, you said that you no longer wanted to hug women.'

'That was then, Carla! You know that things change all the time. You're not always available to me. You stick yourself in your writing room and I don't see you for hours at a time. Is it any wonder that I turn to an attractive woman in the office who likes me?'

It's late in the evening and this conversation is making me really tired. I decide to go to bed and leave Aaron to finish watching his TV show. It's been a hell of a birthday. Aaron won't apologise; instead, he claims his right to be the way he is. As for me, it's not so much that I want to criticise him for flirting as that I want a man who doesn't need to do that. A fierce feeling of wanting utter loyalty from a man rises up in me. It's too fierce, ignoring the fact that Aaron is actually totally loyal in his own way; but for now it serves to tell me what I really want. The pain in my belly continues. There's an equally strong pain in my heart. I feel the need to pray.

I surrender to grace, my soul moans when I go to bed. *I surrender this predicament to grace*. The pain eases somewhat and I'm able to walk through the unseen tears as if through a soaking rain.

I keep feeling sad because Aaron doesn't seem to respect me or our relationship enough to keep his sexual energy within boundaries. I believe that he should value what we have so much that he's willing to grow up from his sexual immaturity and offer me his whole self. He doesn't have anything else to offer: no financial security, no possessions to speak of that he can share. He only has his whole self, and he chooses to give only part of that. He wants to be sexual with anyone who appreciates his sexuality. He calls that his freedom. To me, it's the choice of an immature soul, and I feel so sad.

If I am to stay with Aaron, I'll have to be content with his love as it is. I know that he won't go so far as to have sex with anyone else, no matter how much he might be attracted to them. I know that when Aaron makes love, his attention is with me one hundred per cent, that his love is genuine and deep. That his sex is as strong as it is because he loves so much.

This demand for loyalty that I feel inside me is a scorching flame. It's the Scorpio's unreasonable demand! I can feel that now. It's time to tame this down and recognise that Aaron gives more than many a faithful man gives to his wife, much more. It's not easy to face one's pride. It isn't easy to override the ego and tell it to be quiet, that it's making too much bloody noise.

Aaron shouldn't be asked to do what he isn't capable of doing. Aaron's just himself, and he's innocent.

I give a huge sigh. It's so hard for me to not be right all the time. I love being right, and to suffer for it.

And then, as I walk through the doorway, he stands there, dumb, forlorn, but with his arms half-stretched out.

I take nothing for granted. 'What do you want, Aaron?'

'A hug?' he says, without knowing what sort of reply he'll get. We've been following a no-hug pact for two days now. There's been no touching at all.

I don't hesitate to walk into his arms, to hold him and be held. He feels so vulnerable. It's good to exchange close, friendly vibes again. He allows himself a chaste kiss. If only he could kiss other women like that!

Still, the hug has broken the tension between us. That evening, we sit beside each other on the couch and I take his proffered hand. He's tired, very tired.

'I'm done with being the seducer,' he says. 'I'm tired of trying. I'm withdrawing from you, Carla. When I come out of my space, you will see a different side of me. I won't be there for you any more. You will no longer be able to depend on my warmth.'

A coldness runs past my heart; a sudden doubt enters. I may be making a huge mistake and could lose him for nothing! But I'm also aware of a sort of light inside me — a small voice. I listen to it the way a shipwrecked sailor listens for sounds of rescue amid the turmoil of the waves.

'I'm willing to risk losing your warmth,' I say. 'I'm taking a risk all round. I don't really know what I'm doing. Don't think that I'm judging or rejecting you, Aaron.'

I have a dream that night. I come to Aaron in my astral body, wrap it around him, breathe his sweet flesh.

I feel love for him like a white heat coming straight from my heart.

And then I wake up in my own bed and feel pain in my belly. It's sore, excruciating. The instinct of my half-dreaming self is to cut the cords tying me to Aaron. That definitely makes my belly feel better.

When I awake fully, I'm afraid I've made a mistake by cutting those cords. I'm afraid that my deceptive ego is making a demand that will ruin what we have.

'You came to me in my dream last night,' Aaron says, the next time we're alone.

Well, yes, I know I did. I remember that myself. I decide to take him off the hook.

'You didn't hurt me, Aaron.'

He relaxes visibly. 'I needed you to tell me that. I feel so guilty about not being able to give you what you want.'

He's torn now between what he calls being himself and what he now wants to be: the man who gives his woman what she wants, but doubts that he can.

I want to fall into Aaron's waiting arms, but don't. Something tells me, *Don't do it, Carla*! It doesn't seem to be my stubborn voice. It feels, instead, like a voice from a wiser part of myself, whispering urgently. I decide to trust it.

'I want to wait this out, Aaron, to see what's on the other side. If I'm making a mistake, I'll wear it.'

Aaron doesn't exactly like this. He wants to warn me.

'It might be too late by the time you change your mind, Carla. I can be very thorough when I want to get someone out of my system.'

I know what he's talking about. If he truly loves, though, he won't want to get me out of his system. And, if he succeeds, he didn't really love. And so I test his mettle — although I only become aware of this later, when I look back.

'I'm prepared to make a mistake,' I say.

I wake up and know I'm over the hump. Last night, the sexual urge and the clamp in my belly was at its worst. Normally, I'd call this sort of thing a need to punish myself, or denial of my real need to love. And *still* I feel that inner voice urging me on; not ruthless, not revengeful, but quietly persistent. It's not a question of not loving Aaron. It's a question of becoming free of the need to belong to him. I need to belong to myself again.

Today I know the triumph of following this smallest voice, this little bit of sanity. I'm energised with a new vision: I see myself doing my work with the public, and I'm not alone. I have a partner who supports me in my work. The future is full of light, pulling me. I know that all is well.

I can also see that Aaron needs someone other than me to make him happy the way he wants to be. He's made so many sacrifices to be part of my world in the city.

'You need someone who can enter your world in Darkan,' I say later, 'and your world of models and sci-fi and computers.'

He quits his computer and sits down on the couch near me. 'I think that when we've both learnt what we need to learn, we'll part. We're discovering how much we're alone,' he goes on. 'We try to keep ourselves harmless. We keep respecting each other. We're prepared to undress and be raw emotionally. We won't eat each other alive.'

'I feel OK with you and without you.'

Aaron's incorrigible. 'So when are you getting your ass over here?'

Aaron has finally claimed Kim's old room. Without telling me, he's moved all his stuff into it. The small room looks so neat now that it will be fine to leave the door open.

From the outside, it looks as if all we've done is stopped having sex (except for the occasional aberration). But what I feel is much more than that. The distance of only another two days of celibacy has given me more clarity. I can see with clear eyes that being tied to Aaron also means tossing my future in with him. But our paths are so different, and our core values just as much. I've been holding myself back, experimenting with his way of seeing things. It feels as if I'm being dragged down by him. I won't let this happen.

He was so proud of himself when he was offered a pay rise at work and knocked it back in favour of shares in the company. Not a bad move really, since in a couple of years those shares will be worth quite a bit. But that's not what Aaron was thinking about. He was thinking about saving the company some cash that it could use for other things! He wants to keep living on the minimum he can manage, even though it means he can't afford to see an optometrist, something he desperately needs to do. He can't buy parts for his car either. It's all so lopsided to me, but valid for Aaron.

Now that we have separate rooms, I feel I should make something clear.

'When the door of my room is properly closed, that means it's private. It means I really want to be left alone in there.'

He nods, smirks a bit, because it really marks a change.

I make this new rule because he's come in twice now, without invitation and without knocking. Twice I said, 'Invading my privacy!' and once was genuinely embarrassed. It means nothing to Aaron. After all, *he* doesn't need to shield himself from *me*. The door is always open with him, in every way.

'When my door is open, it means you're welcome,' he says. 'And if it's off its hinges, it means the same thing.'

He goes on his way, laughing, but from now on he will respect the new rule that's come between us, a symbol of our apartness.

'You're forcing me to fall out of love with you,' he says.

In the morning, I sit on his bed and ask how he's slept. I love this man, and am still my affectionate self with him, so I kiss him and stroke his face. Does he mistake my intentions?

'I'm not playing games with you,' I say.

'I know that.'

It's very important for me that he understands this. I am in a position of power here, with perfect choice. Aaron is dependent on my decisions, making absolutely no secret of the fact that he wants me, all the time.

'Do you know how beautiful you are? How good a feeling you are?' He smiles.

'I have some clues because I can feel the good feelings you are to me!'

'Good answer!' he says.

Aaron's humble love is a mirror for me to see more clearly who I am. The contrast is sometimes so sharp it's painful. I am a judgmental bitch compared to his softness. Aaron's been consistently kind, refusing to make a list of the things he doesn't like about me when I ask.

'I just let them be. They're not important to me, the things I don't like about you. I remember the feelings we have together; that's what matters to me.'

That evening, I kiss him a quick goodnight; it's so late, close to midnight. Once my head is on the pillow I seem to go to sleep, but wake up disturbed. Where is Aaron? Did I hear him go outside? Why would he go outside just now? The questions aren't clear in my mind, but I find myself getting out of bed.

'Are you there, Aaron?'

I address my question to the house, and get no answer. Aaron's bedroom door is slightly ajar, and when I push it open carefully, so as not to disturb him should he be asleep after all, he suddenly sits up and throws the blankets open.

'Come in!'

I wander over as if in a dream. 'What were you doing? I was wondering where you were?' I'm under the covers now.

'You just committed suicide by coming in here,' he says, embracing me firmly. 'Suicide of the ego,' he explains later. 'Suicide of the part of you that's in denial of what you really want.'

Oh! He's so ardent just now. He can't conceal his utter delight in having me there, and ducks under the blankets to delight my fanny with his tongue. I hold the blankets up to the night air so he can breathe. Up he comes in a few moments, ready to insert his phallus. How could he be ready that quickly? I don't think I even touched him!

Aaron stops midway as he enters me, breathing, looking at me, waiting for me to catch up with what's happening, waiting for me to be with him totally before he proceeds. He sinks himself into me and we both just feel this moment.

I'm so warm, he says, and so wet, but after a while, he goes in search of the lubricant in my room. He gives the tube to me as he steps up on the bed and places his hands on the wall. His legs taut, he stands away from the wall, his torso above me. I apply the lubricant to his stallion penis, in awe of its size and straightness, in awe of his powerful and fearless stance. 'Wow!' I whisper, 'Wow!' And stroke his organ up and down, straight and strong as a rod. He lowers himself down on me, parting my legs with his.

He's in no hurry, bringing me to a point of ecstasy over and over again, and coming back from the brink over and over, finally pulling me on top of him. I roll off him before long, both of us panting.

'Let's relax.'

We wriggle back under the warm blankets. I enjoy the delicious feel of his hands stroking me, attaching themselves to my breasts.

'Your breasts are big tonight,' he says.

'They ache to be touched.'

My nipples are raw with desire.

'Touched they shall be,' he says. 'All you have to do, any time, is ask. How we love each other!' he breathes. 'Do you realise how much we love each other?'

I'm a bit shocked. This desire to be with one another, this enjoyment of each other, this delight in the energies we create together: is that love?

'Do most people love like this?' I wonder out loud.

'No,' Aaron says, 'because of needing. People want to add something to their lives. They don't see how it's all about expressing what's already in them. They just need to find a person to do it with, not a person to have and possess. Look around you — there's so much loneliness, and it all begins with SEX! We're all sexual beings; this is how God made us. We can be mirrors for each other, for the God in each of us. Misery comes from not understanding that. Men and women are meant to fuck each other.'

Aaron's energy is full on tonight, and his breath is sweet. The moment of his orgasm was huge. It was as if he were a god from another world, not the simple Aaron I know in the daytime. 'Don't underestimate me,' he's said a few times in the past. No — better not to underestimate Aaron.

'You're something else, Aaron.' What else can I say to express my respect for the love and potency this man can exude? 'You're awesome.'

'So are you, babe. You're such a beautiful woman.'

I drift off to sleep as he watches me, hand under his head. This man has had the most enormous orgasm and *he* isn't falling asleep, *I* am! I open my eyes now and again; his radiant face is still there. Finally he laughs as I peep yet again, and lets his head fall on the pillow.

Perhaps he knew that I would leave as soon as his sleeping breath became an inevitable snore; perhaps he was putting off this moment as long as possible. I get up, look in vain for my nightie, and leave naked for the peace of my own bed.

If I love this man so much, why would I plan to go somewhere far away from him so all this will be destroyed? There isn't a good answer for that. The best answer is that we both sense that the Cogs are working away in the ether and we shall obey them. I feel fear, but know that I won't hesitate when the moment of leaping into the future arrives. For now, it seems we're being given some indelible memories to take with us, like some special sustaining food before we set out. Maybe we'll need this along our individual journeys of probable aloneness, to revitalise us when our energies run cold and low.

A NEW FACE

This lover never shows the same face
always a new disguise
keeping mind in suspense
and senses alert.
Nirmala, untitled poem

 A whole week goes by amicably, with my sexuality having a bumpy ride of on and off, and Aaron patiently watching what's going on in me.

'When we first started this relationship, you kept saying that it was new every time. Now we've gone everywhere we can and the relationship has died down.' That's his way of putting it.

Since the possibility of me leaving this relationship has come up, I feel free to discuss any aspect of it. I've nothing to lose by speaking up, and along come words that are closer and closer to the mark.

'Perhaps this relationship has achieved its purpose, Aaron.'

We're sitting in the lounge room with a hot drink, and he looks up from reading the newspaper as I continue.

'I think it has healed certain things in both of us. You know now that you can have a good relationship with a woman. Even if it ends, it doesn't have to end with a lot of bad feeling. This is a major change for you. You know that you can be good for a woman, and that you don't have to live alone any more. You feel much better about yourself as a sexual being. As for me, I've come to myself as a woman. My sexuality has come into its own. I feel good about myself too.'

Aaron smiles a huge smile. 'For you to say those things about me means they are true for yourself too, Carla.' His pleasure is genuine and undisguised. The biggest compliment anyone can give Aaron is to be a happier person for having known him.

Life is arranging our immediate future. Aaron's late nights and long days at the computer are wearing him down, so it's plain he has to go away to Darkan more regularly for a break. The plan is for him to disappear to Darkan for a whole week as from next Tuesday. I'm looking forward to this.

Aaron's a bit hurt. 'Why are you looking forward to it?'

'Because absence makes the heart grow fonder — I do believe that's true. And because you need a break, and because your house needs you, and because you'll enjoy being away looking after your house and projects.'

'Hmm.'

My pleasure sounds less heartless put that way. Still, we will have to wait and see what a longer period of being apart will do for both of us.

I don't know what Aaron's up to. He won't come to bed tonight, he says. 'Why not be cuddly in bed?' I ask.

'Not tonight. I'll burn myself out tonight.'

I don't like the sound of that. Is he intending to burn away all his desire for connection, to make himself unapproachable? Is he doing a telephone job on me, the way he did when Rachel spurned him all those years ago and he watched a telephone — the symbol of their communication — slowly disintegrate in the fire?

I know there's something going on in him. He showed me his legs this morning: he's started to scratch again and his flesh is scored and bleeding. Maybe tonight he'll think about what it is.

Despite my concern, I luxuriate in being able to stretch out and have the whole bed to myself. Another part of me misses Aaron and wonders what's going on in him. I have three hot-water bottles to compensate for his absence and still I feel cold around my knees. I fall asleep but wake up at intervals through the night. The light in the lounge room never goes out.

The next morning, Aaron looks under the weather. He spent a couple of hours on the couch, fully dressed. Every time he stirred and woke, he got up and worked on his computer.

'I thought that maybe you wanted to cut yourself off from me,' I say.

Aaron looks shocked. 'No, Carla, that's what *you're* doing.'

'You wanted to burn out, you said.'

'Yes, I wanted to burn out all the *crap*. I've had to come to terms with the fact that we won't be together any more.'

'We're still here now.'

He smiles. 'I'm looking at the *feelings* that are here,' he says. 'You're running away with the future. There isn't room for me in your pictures of the future.'

It's evening now, after a day of tension for both of us. It's as if he's taken the lead now in pulling us apart. I still don't understand exactly what he burnt last night.

He finds me in my writing room, where it's dark except for the light filtering in from the street. I'm close to tears with grief. I sit There for no more than three minutes before Aaron senses what's afoot and finds me. It's real, his ability to tune in to someone else. He sits facing me, earnest, kind, hoping to be of some use to my crumpled emotions.

'When I said last night that I'd burn out, my intention was to burn away all the negative ideas that wanted to come into my brain about you and about what you're doing and what it means about myself,' he explains to me. 'I wanted to burn away my ego.' He pauses. 'I don't want you to implode on yourself.' And then he says, 'You're not losing me.'

He's quiet, watching the effect his words have on me.

'I never lose a relationship,' he says softly. 'I'll never lose you. You're part of me forever. I love you, and your love for me has changed me. The only thing I want to take with me is the good feeling of how you love me and what you've given me. This grieving over what no longer is and what you can't have — I've done a lot of that in my life, but I left it behind a long time ago.'

Again he waits. His attitude is so sweet that it makes my tears bigger. He's intolerably good! I envy him his ability to be himself, no matter what others may do around him, what they may give or take away; his ability to be content with himself.

'I envy you,' I say aloud.

He's intrigued and waits for more.

'I envy you for what you have achieved in yourself.'

Aaron didn't expect that. He straightens up, lost for words, curious and pleased.

'That is the nicest thing you've said to me.' He smiles. 'Thank you for saying that. You've seen something in me that you value. You want to make that your own. I'm so pleased.'

There's nothing in me that wants to cook dinner tonight, so we go to the Chinese restaurant to pick up takeaway. Once there, we decide to stay, and we sit in the same spot as twelve months ago, when Aaron first came to live with me. This is significant to both of us. The food is always very good here, and our appetites are fully revived by the excellent honey and satay chicken.

Aaron has changed. He seems to have indeed burnt away a lot last night. His defensiveness has vanished completely. However, my resolve to move away from him is strong.

Tonight, he'll sleep in his own room, but he'll come into my room for a cuddle first, he says. We go to bed at the same time. This happens so rarely these days that it's a remarkable coincidence in itself. We're also both semi-naked, wanting this to be an intimate closeness. Neither of us expects to be carried away, not after all the effort we've put ourselves through to be separate.

Aaron pulls me to him by tucking his right arm under me and rolling my back towards his front. This way he can run his hand over my torso even if it's encased in a cotton nightie. He loves the curve of my hips; he loves the softness of my breasts. His energy's alive; his body's soon on fire. What am I to do? I turn around and face him. He takes the opportunity to clasp me close, then suddenly lifts himself up to enter me. To my astonishment, I don't resist.

When we make love like this, it seems nothing can ever stand between us. Why shouldn't such a thing be an absolute priority in the scale of values? What on earth do I want, if this isn't enough? But I push thought aside for now. Let's just enjoy each other; let life take us where it will later.

Reality sets in when Aaron starts snoring. It's time to nudge him, ask him to leave my bed. Then I turn over and have the soundest sleep ever.

Aaron shows me his plans for revamping the bedroom in his house at Darkan and the studio next door to it. He'll not be short of things to do when he gets there. There's not a single bad feeling between us, a good way to part.

The days pass peacefully when he's gone. I find my thoughts wandering to him in every unguarded moment. I imagine him in his work gear: the torn stretchy shorts he will never throw away; or, if it's cold, the grey over-sized prison overalls he got for a song from the op shop, with arms and legs too long even for him. And a beanie on his head. I daren't think of how he eats, when he eats: these are unknowns to himself till the last minute, and that might be very late in the day. I imagine him taking delight in using his power tools and moving things about in space the way he can't on a computer. After a long day of work, he'll soak in a deep, hot bath. He won't have time to miss me.

I don't ring, and he doesn't either. After three days, a letter comes for him — an excuse for me to phone.

'I was about to phone *you*!' he laughs. 'I was thinking about it and you rang!'

A few days later, when the same thing happens, it doesn't sound so convincing. I think he just doesn't want to use his phone to contact me because he reckons I can afford it more. He wants to save money. It's a small example of the one thing I find irksome between us: his lack of money and how it makes him think and act. I may be wrong, of course. After all, it's *me* that's moving away from *him*, even if he's gone to Darkan for a while. If I'm not content with his silence, then it's up to me to tell him.

I'm in my writing room when he comes back. Writing is a healing experience for me. Putting words to my feelings clarifies them. My feelings aren't taken for granted; they don't happen without my noticing them. Writing is a way of becoming more aware of what is happening inside me as well as outside me: I become a witness to my own life. When Aaron is away, there is more time to write and reflect.

It's been a whole week and he's just come into the office. I can hear welcoming sounds from Clinton and Margot, and happy banter. I stay where I am until I feel the excitement has died down a bit. I don't want to do the happy couple thing, where we run into each other's arms. Aaron doesn't make a move to find me either.

When I enter the room, he acknowledges me briefly. He's giving an interesting account of some experience to his friends and doesn't want to be interrupted. I walk past him to the kitchen to put the kettle on for all of us. Then, I sit and watch him.

He's dishevelled, even feral. His flannel work shirt is hanging partly out of his pants and so is the T-shirt under it. His T-shirt looks as if he's been sleeping in it too. There's blood on his pants; he's been scratching his legs until they've bled. His face is dusty and stubbly. The strange thing is, none of it matters to me any more. Once upon a time I'd have been mortified that my man looked like this. But Aaron's his own man now, and how he looks and what he does is his affair.

In one week, we've drifted apart significantly. I've so enjoyed being by myself that I almost resent his presence. At times, I was even greedy about having my own space! On the other hand, it's been tough coping with hormones that are trying to find their way to pleasure only to get a rude refusal from my stubbornness. One occasion of masturbation brought relief, but this was no answer to the army of hormones relentlessly cloning themselves in spite of me. I have watched my face tense up, become long. The challenge to change back to simply being with my inner Beloved is not as easy as I'd imagined. And yet I'm determined to continue my celibacy. It has been hard for a full week, but I feel I've gained ground in my attempt to be separate. I can't ruin all that now.

He looks at me intently, reads my energy and smiles wryly.

'What are you looking at?' I say.

'I'm trying to find Carla,' he replies. There is obvious pain in his heart.

That evening he takes a long shower and appears at the door of my writing room to say goodnight. It's around nine o'clock. I'm reading a terrible novel, a detective story with so many inconsistencies that I wonder what the dickens the editor must have been thinking. And the book cost me $32.95! I'm disgusted, but the storyline is set in a convent so I can't put it down.

It's a reversal of roles, the irony of which doesn't escape us. *He's* going to bed before me, and I'll follow when I'm ready. I decide not to be ready for quite a while. Hopefully he'll be asleep when I make it to my bed and find him there. He didn't ask if he could be in my bed, did he? He just assumed it would be okay if I didn't say anything.

One thing I'm sure about: I'm not going to have sex with Aaron, even if it's difficult for both of us. Even if he sleeps in the same bed with me after being away for seven days.

I won't have sex with Aaron, although I burn. I lie on the edge of my side of the bed, avoiding the slightest touch. His foot wanders over to my side and I stick mine out of the blankets. I'm a Scorpio. I know what I want and I'm resolute.

A CELIBACY OF SORTS

Even when the truth shatters your dreams
even when the truth leaves you emptied out . . .
there is no other possibility than happily ever after
Nirmala, untitled poem

We feel strange in this frail space, with the winter sun streaming into the lounge room. The noisy reverse-cycle machine in the window is pumping heat into the air. I look into Aaron's eyes. Unlike me, he's not slept well, and they're red.

I start the conversation on a positive note. 'We've learnt a lot from each other.'

'Oh, the real learning begins when we've lost each other.' Aaron's telling it how it will be, talking from experience. He stops for a moment. 'You will miss me — once the energy's gone and you don't have it any more. I'm coming to terms with the idea of not having you in my life. I'm grieving. Now I know what Kim felt like when he lost his wife.'

I look inside myself and finally come up with something that is unquestionably real. 'Aaron, my feelings are pulling me into my future; they're doing the same for you.'

Margot comes in, bringing the sun with her, then Clinton arrives. The day in the office has begun.

I'm having bodywork with my therapist, Bernice. It's day number eight of no sex. Bernice is a good therapist because she can read what's happening in a body and work accordingly. I lie on her massage table, and she's holding my head when she asks what's going in my life that's making my brain behave in a way not usual for me. I tell her I'm moving away from Aaron. Bernice asks whether I'd like to do a cutting of the cords that hold Aaron and me together. I remember my dream about cutting the cords tying me to him and the relief I felt then. I agree. It's a scary decision, a feeling of no return.

Bernice asks me to visualise Aaron's face and surround him with a shape and a colour. My shape is oval and its colour is pink. Now I'm to think of all the negatives about Aaron and tell him them out loud. I prefer to do this silently, and Bernice easily agrees. 'Just let me know when you've finished.'

So I tell Aaron about how his self harm distresses me; how I don't like the way he's not dealing with his problems, not even his eyesight. That I can't wait for him to change, since it'll take him all of his life, if not longer.

You have no money and you're scared of having significant money. You can't even afford to look after yourself properly. You live on dreams; the way you're going, you'll never build your house. You live as if you've made a vow of poverty.

I don't like how your belly protrudes and how your breath is foul in the morning, and that you don't seem to care enough to get up and do something about it before you hug me and breathe on me.

It's a pity that your feet are so sore and unwell that you can't go for walks with me.

Your love of science fiction leaves hardly any room for movies with any human content.

You don't like my kind of movies and my kind of music.

You don't know how to dance.

You don't know how to dress up.

You wear the same clothes you sleep in.

You're a slob in the bathroom. You leave puddles of water instead of using the bathmat.

I don't like your attitude to the so-called assholes of the world. I don't like the way you keep being sore about the past. I don't like the childish way you expect God to step in to fix up the mess on this planet.

Phew! The list is certainly long enough. Bernice now asks me to let this image of Aaron recede. In my mind's eye, Aaron's face becomes dimmer and smaller; it sinks into the darkness, into oblivion. I swallow hard.

My next step is to visualise Aaron's face again. This time his face is in a round, green shape, and I'm to tell him all I appreciate about him. Again I speak to him in the silence of the room while Bernice holds my head. I sense my face going pink with the enthusiasm I feel while I silently 'speak' my list.

Aaron, I love you for your generosity and your honesty.

You have no nastiness in you, none whatsoever.

You genuinely love and respect me; you don't want to stand in my way or try to force me to do or not do anything I don't want to do.

You practise what you preach: you stand apart even while you are so magnificent when we are together.

I like the way you make me feel calm. It's nice to feel your energy in the house. It's nice to hold your hand and feel its warmth. It's good to lean against you and feel your sweetness.

I love your masculinity, your hormonal self, your male power and the strength in your arms.

I love the way you're total when we make love.

You're so articulate. And you keep telling me that you love me.

I love your kisses, and above all I love the way you feel.

Is that it? No, there's something else.

Your constancy. I love your constancy. You never stopped loving me, whether I wanted to be with you or leave you. It made no difference.

I'm asked to put this Aaron somewhere in my body, and it goes straight to the middle of my chest.

The session comes to an end.

I go home. Aaron's face looks unusual, so I ask him what's going on. He leans back on his computer chair and swivels a little as he speaks.

'I feel the connection between us breaking up,' he says. 'It's making me feel a bit bad in the tummy.'

'The umbilical cord being severed, eh?' I stroke his face as I pass, amazed that Aaron should be so consciously connected to what's happening.

An hour or so later, it's my turn to feel queasy. Aaron notices. 'What's up, babe?'

'I feel sick. I think it's the coffee and cake I had this afternoon.'

Aaron gets up immediately to hold me in his arms.

'Babe, it's the cords disintegrating between us. It's alright. We'll be alright.'

That evening we both attend one of Peter and Pearl's *satsang* evenings, a gathering of friends interested in spiritual truth. Pearl, whose exquisite heart is always wide open, gives me the most loving of hugs. I confide in her that I'm moving away from Aaron, but that we're still very good friends.

'That's beautiful!' she says, her blind eyes shining and her pink cheeks glowing. 'What fierce grace! Consciousness is arising in both of you.' She puts her face next to mine as she speaks. 'You're doing what's right for you without blaming him or hating him. Good on you, love.' I can feel her joy seeping through to my belly as she holds me tight, then plants a humungous kiss on my cheek. It gives me a warm glow. I have the right kind of friends.

'Is Aaron here?' And she goes searching for him.

The evening begins. After a time of sitting in silence, we watch a video, followed by a period of discussion. There is time for meeting and chatting, so I catch up with Maureen and Peggy. The conversation touches on my book, *God's Callgirl* — am I still giving talks? This time the question has significance because these two women are in contact with people who organise big-time circuits.

'Are you ready for the big time,' they ask, 'to earn some really good money?'

'I'm free to travel anywhere in the world!' I can say that honestly now.

'How would you like to be on a cruise ship, giving talks and workshops? Would that be your scene?'

A cruise ship? Would I have to be an entertainer? I'm entertaining sometimes, but mostly my topics are deep stuff. 'I don't know.'

'Most of the passengers are older people who'd love you,' says Maureen. 'Send me your CV via email.'

I look around and see Aaron sitting on a couch by himself. Just then he's joined by Peter and they start a lively conversation. Aaron tells me later how alienated he felt while I was connecting with people so easily, and how no one had wanted to talk to him while he was feeling like that. He'd worked on that feeling, and as soon as he'd integrated it, Peter had entered his space.

'Cry and you cry alone,' he says, as we drive back home. 'It's only when you're happy that others want to know you.'

We arrive home. It's late, but he wants to do something on his computer. 'Goodnight.' From his chair, he pulls me down to kiss me.

I feel a surge of passion, a sweetness in my mouth. He pulls me onto his lap to kiss me some more, since I seem to be willing, then gets up with me in his arms and staggers across the room into the corridor. He makes as if he's going towards his bedroom, before suddenly turning and going towards mine. Then he drops me onto my bed.

'That scared you, didn't it?' he laughs, poking my belly button and leaving the room.

I lie there, astonished. My God! If he'd stayed, I'd have allowed myself to be seduced! I am lying there quite still, thinking, when he comes into my room again in a playful mood. He jumps up on the bed and straddles me, bouncing our bodies up and down.

'What're you doing?' I ask.

'Playing. Better to play than lie in my bed thinking about you.' And he nudges my breasts, then lowers his body to bite my fanny through my jeans.

'Aaron!!' I'm indignant, but he laughs and sits over me, taking all the stances of making love in quick succession.

'You're seducing me!'

Aaron stops, turns serious. 'Remember, it's you who makes all the decisions. I only want you to be yourself, a woman who knows what she wants.'

He gets ready to leave. 'Just know that whenever you want to wrap yourself around my dick, I'm there for you.'

It's too much. I want this selfless Aaron and I get off my bed. I've been so hard on myself these last few days. It's been eight days of aloneness. Eight days for Aaron as well, who hasn't lost his sense of humour, his interest in me or his love for me. I move to undress myself.

Aaron's eyes boggle. He really didn't expect me to break my resolve, but he's not in the mood to analyse or hesitate. He takes my arm and pulls me towards his bedroom. 'That is *your* place of singularity now,' he says, referring to my room. 'I'm taking you to my bed.'

Undressing is a matter of seconds for him, since he never wears anything more than pants, shirt and undies. Already in bed, he watches me take off jeans, socks worn over pantyhose, pantyhose, jumper, shirt, bra, underpants, all in conscious, deliberate moves. I could change my mind at every new item of clothing and head back to my own room, but the undressing proceeds without hesitation. I'm soon under the covers and next to his warm skin.

Aaron isn't all that sexed up. He holds me close: it's this closeness he loves. It's our kisses that turn us on towards each other. Aaron can't believe this is happening. He'd never expected to do this again. Maybe I'm perverse, but this very fact is a turn-on.

My own eagerness takes me by surprise. Aaron is fully awake to it and matches it beautifully. It's as if we're in a dance that knows no choreography except its own exquisite sinuousness. It has its fast paces and its many pauses on a fine point. Aaron makes no demands. He varies his position on top of me, and I direct him with my hands, pressing on his shoulders, on his head sometimes, keeping in rhythm with him, thrusting myself up towards him. I feel his hands on my head as he gently thrusts and kisses.

'Don't wear me out; I want you to come in me now!'

'I don't want to come. I just want to enjoy you.'

'Okay.'

But he starts to exert a tremendous energy now. It's like a gallop to the finish as his penis engorges to a fullness that drowns the shape of my vagina, until the surge of energy engulfs both of us in bliss. We subside into an embrace.

'What can I do for you?' he asks, not doing what I expect him to do, which is fall asleep.

'A lot, if you're up to it.'

'Give me a few minutes while I recover.'

I stroke his head, his back, his arms. We lie still for a while. Then Aaron wants to tell me what he experienced.

'You were different! You were so strong and focused — doing exactly what you wanted ... I wish I could really say what I felt.' Pause. 'I was holding my hands over your head and I was fucking an angel in a Gothic window.' Another pause. '*We* made that moment. It's unrepeatable. No one else could make that moment. It's what we're both made of. We're good at what we do!'

He closes his eyes again. 'I feel a new life in me, a new discovery. You have my undying love for that! You're a beautiful woman, Carla.'

'And you're a sweet lover. *You* are beautiful, Aaron.'

'I love being a lover,' he says. 'It's all I ever wanted to do, to love a woman. I could never understand it when this beautiful thing developed into the woman wanting me to be someone I wasn't, having to relate in a way that made no sense to me.' I've heard this several times before, but he really gets my attention when he says, 'You've done me a great favour by ending our relationship.' He looks at me because he knows there'll be a question coming.

'How so?'

'I've felt a burden leaving me. I no longer feel pressured to become something for you, and I don't feel judged any more.'

I blush. I hate being lumped in with his previous demanding partners. Have I really been like that? Well, yes. I have to admit that I've wanted him to dress up when he's gone out with me, and that I've criticised him for scratching his legs, but, more seriously, that I expected him to do what could be loosely described as 'something to fulfil his potential'. There's probably nothing more deadly than that. Until this moment, I didn't clearly know that this is what I particularly loved in Aaron: his potential!

It's true that since I've said this relationship is over, it hasn't bothered me to see him all messed up, like when he returned from Darkan. He's gone back to looking feral and I haven't cared. I've taken the pressure off myself as well.

It feels like it's past midnight. Has he forgotten what he said about wanting to do something for me? Even as I think this, he leaps into action. He knows me so well, what I like, what turns my body on. His hands and mouth pour attention on me; he loves feeling the crescendo build, and to hold me as the waves of bliss run through me. They keep on coming, longer than ever. I gratefully subside into peacefulness beside him. His eyes never leave me as he keeps holding me. Finally, sleep beckons.

'I want to sleep in my own bed,' I say.

'Of course. Do you want me to carry you there?'

'Hmm, no thanks.' I imagine that in his half-awake state he might drop me.

Any doubts about whether I did the right thing or not are taken away when Aaron comes into my room at around eight in the morning.

We've both slept till this late? He jumps on my bed and sits cross-legged on what used to be his side of the bed.

'I can't tell you how I felt last night. I'm lost for words.' He hangs his head for a few moments, then looks up. 'It was like two hungers coming together!'

'It doesn't happen every day, Aaron.'

He looks puzzled.

'I mean, if you're sated all the time, you can't be hungry. We were that way last night because we'd been away from each other for so long.'

'I'm OK with either,' is Aaron's rejoinder. 'I just like sticking my dick in you. You're a good feeling.

'This bed was about our love' he says, looking around. 'My bed was just about hormones. You wanted me for yourself, and you decided to take your clothes off and be with me. I didn't expect you to do that, but you made a woman's choice to be with a man. I was shocked by your passion, but just as much by my own.' He laughs.

'What's funny?'

'You were once doing a song and dance about me and other girlfriends, and now you don't need me.' He waits before he says, 'I know what's going on with you. It's your mind getting in the way.'

I'm disappointed that he's hanging onto this explanation. Isn't it possible that in this lifetime, I'm ending cycles: cycles with my parents, daughters, ex husbands, and with Aaron. But it's true that my mind played a part.

I'm often disgusted by his habits. Even this morning, he put on the T-shirt that he'd worn for three days and slept in for just as many. His trousers have a bloodstain from his scratching, and he wears them nevertheless. I walk into the bathroom and my brain spasms when my bare feet land in a puddle of cold water — he hasn't bothered to use the shower curtain properly. He sometimes cleans his mouth in the morning, and most times doesn't, and doesn't care that it disgusts me. All these things have had an impact.

Aaron says he's going to make some tea.

'I'd love one of those ginger and lemon ones,' I say.

'Who said I was going to make one for you?' he teases.

It's how it is between us now: the relationship that isn't but is. We're not together, we're apart, and the odd and unexpected thing is that we are happier than we've ever been.

I feel so well in my body today! It's the best indicator yet that it sometimes does me no good to impose my will on my body for the sake of a decision. Besides, it's clear to both of us that our coming together last night wasn't a change in my resolve to move on. I chose to make love to Aaron, and let myself be remarkably loved.

'It was a fitting closure,' Aaron says, when he comes in again with a tray and two cups of herbal tea. 'I felt that something was left hanging in the air. Even though you'd given me lots of warning, it was still so sudden. But understand this, Carla: I never owned you. I'm happy to be myself. Relationship is a bonus to me, not something I require for my happiness. And I want you to know this too: I'm happy to be with you. I don't want anyone else. While we're psychically connected I won't have sex with another person, because I know that hurts. I won't be looking for another relationship, not even when this one's finished. I'll want to be on my own for a bit. I know you're moving on, because you're choosing your life, and I don't want to stand in your way. I'm proud of the woman you've become. After all, I put a lot of my energy into your growing up.'

At last I realise that it's our apartness that is creating the quality of our togetherness. It challenged Aaron's need for emotional security to let me go without any strings when I said I wanted to end our relationship. He thought he was losing me. It challenged mine as well, as I thought I was losing him. Nothing has really changed between us except that now, for the first time, I've truly let him go to be his own man and let myself be me. Our very apartness allows us to be together now that we've both outgrown our puppy ways and our attempts to show only our good sides to each other. There's nothing now that we don't know about the other.

I'm not doing anything to 'sell' myself to Aaron, and that is wildly attractive to him.

I'm only with Aaron when all of me wants to be there. And that's exactly what he enjoys about me.

I suddenly notice that the almond tree has blossoms on it, and cry out with surprise and delight. The tree has no leaves at all, but on the very bottom branches the most delicate pale pink blossoms have appeared overnight.

SOME KIND OF DIVORCE

I think that we have come here
A thousand times before,
You and I
Barbara Barton, 'We Have Been Here Before'

 Something's changed this afternoon, I can sense it. Aaron's upset about us moving apart, contrary to this morning when he'd agreed that we couldn't grow without parting. 'We both have to live out what we've learnt,' he said then.

For a brief while — as if a star burns brightest just before it dies — our togetherness has had a special tenderness. We've had such a keen appreciation of each other's qualities. We so much enjoy just lying together and basking in the energies we create between us. Our language is simple.

'I love you, babe. I love telling you.'

'I love you, too, Aaron.'

'I'm glad.'

I hear him whisper, 'It's hard to believe. This is the beginning of the end of us.'

★ ★ ★

'Kim warned me about you,' he says some time later.

'Oh? How so?'

He doesn't enlarge on this except to say that Kim said I was a 'wilful kind of woman'.

I think back to Kim's philosophy about relationships. It was his main reason for wanting to write his memoirs, to disseminate his ideas. Kim cottoned on to the idea that the male and female sexual energies are present in a person in different degrees and people could be categorised accordingly. For instance, Kim described himself as a male–male, meaning that he was exclusively expressing masculine sexual energy. I recognised that: Kim wasn't macho, but he was what he described himself to be. His ex-wife he described as female–female, and that therefore they were a very good match for each other. As for me, he pointed out that I was a female with quite a bit of male energy, and so he called me a male–female.

Kim also had theories about the various combinations of energies. The all-male and all-female lovers are interested in lifelong partnerships. People like me, according to this theory, are more inclined to be serial monogamists. We get bored. We don't know how to be faithful to one person because we're always looking for different experiences.

Well, Kim may be right. It's been the case so far. I managed to be in a relationship with Hal for many years, but only five consecutively. Maybe I should warn anyone who wants to be my lover in the future: *I'll only be there until I won't. I won't force myself to stay when the energy goes.* To be like me isn't a bad thing; it's just how it is and needs to be taken into account.

I have more thoughts on this. What would have happened if Aaron and I had rationed our sexual togetherness more? If we had deliberately not spent so much time together and slept more in our own beds? Would my passion have survived in better shape? Possibly. I wanted more space between our love-making, in order to keep the edge of newness intact. It didn't make sense to Aaron, who never lost his ardour. And all the time a slow erosion was taking place. And then the energy failed on my part. And here we are. The price of my prolonged passion is the emptiness of now.

Even if all this is true, there's something even truer. This relationship is over because it has done what it was meant to. It has made me flower in ways I could not imagine before I met Aaron. In fifteen months I've grown up emotionally and have become fearless. I'm willing to make mistakes. If this decision turns out to be a mistake and I desperately want Aaron back in my life when he's no longer available, well, I'm willing to take that risk. If my emptiness is the price of passion, then I'm willing to be in it for as long as life dictates. Was my life ever entirely in my hands? 'Of all things, love is the greatest mystery', writes Roger Housden in *Ten Poems to Open Your Heart*. 'Better, then, not to hold fast to certainties about where it came from or where it might lead.'

Then what about my certainty that this is over? Love is more than a relationship to a person; it is altogether mysterious, I can't fully explain to myself what I'm doing. But there is that voice in me: *Carla, stand apart for now.*

'It's not until the person goes away that you notice what you're missing. Then you really feel the emptiness. Then it's time to integrate all you've learnt, or lose it.' It's Aaron, trying to warn me.

Is he trying to tell me it's better to hold on to him because it's easy to underestimate what I stand to lose? If so, I resist this subtle ploy. Fear of losing his energy has made me avoid making a final decision for almost a month. It has stifled me. Yes, his energy will be withdrawn. Yes, I will miss him. No, I won't miss him so much that I will lose my own warmth. And I *am* integrating what I've gained — and becoming myself in a new way.

'Emptiness is frightening, Aaron. People will do anything to avoid that emptiness, no?'

★ ★ ★

'I told Margot.' Aaron is washing up, talking to me with his back to me. The way he half-swallows his words tells me this is a confession.

'You told her what?'

'That we're going our separate ways. I told her how good you've been for me. She seemed pleased.'

'I guess she is sympathetic.'

'It's tiring for me to keep trying,' he says. 'I have to give up chasing you; I'm too old for that.'

My heart pinches when I hear him say this, but it's fair enough.

Aaron keeps talking to me when he gets a moment off work here and there, visits me in my work room, keeps me in the loop.

'I'm feeling sweet grief, not bitter grief. It's sweet because I allow what's happening to happen; I'm not resisting it. It's a discipline for me, but really I have no choice because I know what the alternative is: just a lot of the wrong kind of pain. I'm careful to watch my thoughts, and when criticism comes up I ignore it and concentrate on appreciating you. That's how I protect my heart.'

It's awesome for me to watch Aaron's choices. I'm proud of him, for always growing past his ego.

'I admire you, Aaron.'

I swallow, looking at the man I'm giving away, who is growing more and more attractive by the minute. He's healing himself from his mother and from all his past relationships. He's getting himself ready to fall in love again with a woman who will suit him, because he will be an emotionally strong man and she won't be demanding and won't be a drama queen and will know how to appreciate a rare character like him. The thing for me to do is to stand back and let all this happen.

I bring Aaron a cup of herbal tea while he's still under his blankets. He stirs, invites me to sit on the edge of his bed.

'I've had a dream. I woke up with a pain in my heart,' he says. From the look of his white face, the pain is every bit as physical as emotional. 'The pain comes from this heavy weight right here' — and he indicates the middle of his chest. 'It's a black, cylindrical weight, like a piston, which is bearing down on my heart and squeezing it. My heart's murmuring right now with the weight of it.' He shapes his hand as if it's holding this piston, and winces with the pain of it. 'When I die, it'll probably be of a heart attack. God! I don't want to die that way!'

Aaron's dream was about a memory of himself when he was a very little boy — only about six — and felt very lonely and unwanted. His memory of his father was that he was often angry at him and impatient, and his mother often tried to get him off her hands by leading him to his toys. 'Here, play with these blocks,' she said in the dream, and Aaron's little heart broke. He felt so sad that he lay down on the lounge room floor beside his toys and prayed to God. 'God, nobody wants me. When can I leave this planet?' And the answer came: 'You can leave when you're fifty-four.' The child Aaron worked it out: that wasn't until 2008. It seemed an awfully long time away. But now that time is approaching, and Aaron, fifty-two, says he doesn't want to die.

He lies with his eyes closed, left hand over his chest. All I can do is watch and feel for him. He's longed so much to be wanted in his life. He's been disappointed so much, as well. This wound has recreated the feeling of 'nobody wants me' time and time again, each time his lovers left him.

'*You* don't want me either,' says Aaron, eyes open now, not accusing me, just talking to himself and to me. 'You don't want to share my life.'

I sit there knowing it's true. Aaron has created a singular life for himself, not easy for anyone to share.

'There's more to this,' he now reckons. 'You have the same wound, Carla. You weren't wanted either, and your greatest desire is to be seen for who you are so you can be loved. We can't help each other because we have the same wound.'

He looks at me. I've been silent all this while. 'What are you feeling now?' he asks.

'I feel your feelings, and I feel that I don't know how to help you.'

He strokes my face. 'Thanks for being honest,' he says. 'Here, come under the blankets for a cuddle.'

I obey and lie there quietly, facing him.

'The feel of you, always present in the background throughout all my relationships; you've been with me all those years.' He lifts himself up on an elbow. 'Look at those deep eyes, looking at me and loving me. Ancient eyes, showing the wisdom of countless lifetimes.'

He sinks back onto his pillow.

'I never felt truly wanted by my parents,' he says. 'Because a child needs its parents, the parents feel wanted themselves. I grew up always wanting more affection, especially from my mother. I was dependent on her emotionally for a long time. I looked really sexy in my twenties, and she loved it when I lavished attention on her. But even then, the affection she gave me still wasn't the same as being wanted for myself.'

I'm gobsmacked by Aaron's perspicacity. It also occurs to me that his father might have noticed this special relationship between his wife and his son. His usual strategy was to ignore Aaron when he wanted something from him, especially fatherly attention.

'Your father might have developed an aversion for you because you stole all the limelight,' I say.

'That could be true. He made me feel desperate. The one thing I couldn't bear feeling was not being wanted. I felt lost when nobody wanted me. Now *you* don't want me. The big difference this time is that you still love me, and so my wanting is standing out in stark relief. If you hated me, I wouldn't have noticed my own wanting.'

'You're really doing it this time,' I say. 'You're not scared any more to get to the bottom of your problem and face it completely.'

Aaron is growing at a rate of knots. Not that he's consistent. He sometimes crumbles, and then I notice the office biscuits disappearing before lunchtime. His stomach is growing during this attempt to find peace from his biting thoughts. He takes one step back and two steps forward, like most people going through this kind of process.

'I refuse to implode the way I've done in the past,' he says. 'I'm concentrating on making moments out of the time we still have together. I'm not concentrating on your feelings, otherwise I'll become reactive. The least painful way to go through this is to allow the grief and the wanting. When you let go a great love, there's grief; you can't escape it. I haven't lost any relationships because I still love my partners. I will always appreciate the way they loved me. The rest I don't care about.'

'I still love you, Aaron, and I enjoy your company. Don't we hold hands as we watch TV together?'

Aaron's relieved to hear this. 'I'm aware of how a woman's judgments might want me out of the way,' he says. 'At least you still enjoy having me around.'

He puts his hand out, I place mine in his, and the energy runs between us like a sunny, healing stream.

He tells me what's happening to his body. Lately, he's been seeing a doctor for his knees, and his hips have been hurting too.

'All the pains are coming back into my body; I feel raw again. Everything's sharp instead of soft. I need sex. My body needs sex to feel good. I need to be in a relationship.'

I know that whatever words Aaron says to me, he also hears himself and checks them out sooner or later. When he says he needs sex and to be in a relationship, that's true for him in the moment he says it. Once the words are out of his system, they have a chance to mutate into greater wisdom. Just now, he's concentrating on expressing the feelings. He pauses and breathes deeply.

'I'm scared. I might lose you soon to another bloke, or to life, or the Cogs might send me another girlfriend and then you'll be out of my system.'

I have nothing to say. I wait for whatever else comes out of his mind.

'It's no use me trying to find a replacement for you. I wait on the Cogs. The way to judge any situation is by the feeling it produces. If it's right, there'll be warmth.

'I'll miss you because you're not me. You're you, with your own energies. I've tried as much as I can to make them my own, so I won't miss you as much as a romantic would. I'm way past romancing anyone, with the terrible grief when that someone leaves. I'm convinced that the happiest I'll ever be is now. Grief is about looking back and hoping for the future. I'm going to be happy — with or without you.'

Aaron looks up at me with clear eyes. He's not asking for approval or ratification. He's getting stronger, learning the lessons he once taught me, at a deeper level. It's losing a grand love that gives a person the opportunity to learn great lessons well.

I wake with a start from a nightmare. My heart thumps so much that Aaron seems to feel it and turns over from the side he's been sleeping on. I was curled into his back. He came into my bed very early in the morning and we both kept on sleeping.

He wants to know what my dream was about. He is an intuitive interpreter of dreams. 'Each image represents a type of energy,' he says.

'In the dream, I'm in a room with a woman called Michele and a man,' I say. 'I'm suspicious of the way he leers and smacks his lips. All of a sudden I realise what he's done: he's eaten Michele! I can't see her anywhere, but there's a telltale bit of her dress clinging to his mouth. I rush to the room next door where there are a lot of women to tell them and warn them, but I don't know what to say: they simply won't believe me if I say that the man in the room next door has eaten Michele! I don't have time; the man follows me into the room and looks at me menacingly. He doesn't want me to say anything, and grabs my left arm to pull me towards him and pokes a finger into a spot under my other arm in order to make me lose consciousness. That's when I wake up.'

'Can I offer an interpretation?'

'Of course.'

'You're afraid that in a relationship with a man you'll be swallowed up, eaten alive, and that you'll lose control over your life.'

What a stunning thought. Dreams don't lie. I think this over, and Aaron continues.

'It's probably because your father overwhelmed you when you were a kid, and ever since then you've had a fear of being overwhelmed by a man. It's prevented you from being able to surrender completely in a relationship.'

A feeling starts to emerge from my subconscious. Aaron has put a finger on something.

'My father managed to break me and I lost my sense of myself,' I say. 'That's it! When I chose my partners, I chose kind and gentle people — James and Hal — the opposite of my father, guys who couldn't control me. They couldn't hold me either.'

'You still carry a fear of being dominated and of not being able to be yourself in a relationship, of being controlled by the relationship if not by the guy,' Aaron adds.

Is this what my desperate attempt at disentanglement has been about? About protecting my sense of freedom? To ensure a sense of being able to be myself? If so, then what I've been doing has nothing to do with not loving Aaron any more. It has nothing to do with taking account of his shortcomings. It has to do with my own neurosis.

Since we have had our own bedrooms and our relationship has been declared non-existent, I feel as if a noose has been removed from my neck — the neck that has suffered from chronic stiffness since my father tried to strangle me as a child. My father's hands around my throat! I'm stunned by these revelations coming to light as a result of my dream.

'It's scary,' I say.

'Tell me about it.'

'I know myself so poorly. I wasn't aware of my motivations.'

The phone rings. It's my grandson, Damien; he wants his Oma to take him and his sister to the playground. While they play, I sit and breathe easily. It's good to get to know something about yourself. I feel relaxed, relieved, grateful. Deep, easy breaths. I've got something to work on now: it won't do to let Aaron go because of a neurosis. I already know, however, that if this is part of my reason for leaving Aaron, then it isn't all of it. It isn't the darkness but the light that is calling me.

★ ★ ★

Aaron wants to show me something he's excited and proud about. It's the leg that he's been scratching so relentlessly; it's beginning to heal because he hasn't touched it for a while. The reason? The pressure's off, he says. He feels he's single again, responsible for himself only, and free from the thought that he has to change himself to fit into my life.

'I've been in a twist because I felt I couldn't be good enough for you in lots of ways; and that's what I've suffered from since I was a little boy.'

I'm glad for him, but can't quite share his enthusiasm. 'So it's the little boy in you that's off the hook. He's no longer getting challenged. His buttons aren't being pressed any more. Is that why you need to be so apart in a relationship — to protect your little boy? Wouldn't it be better to grow him up instead of protecting him and basing your life on his neurosis?'

'Do you hear your tone of voice when you say things like that to me?'

I take this as a way for Aaron to deflect what I've said to him.

'So what? Who cares how I say it? Just listen for a change!'

'I have a vulnerable little boy in me, and you have an authoritative person in you,' he maintains. 'You grew up with an authoritative dad and mum, and lots of other people, and you adopted their strategy. My little boy; that authoritative part of you — one needs the other to be triggered.'

He has more to say.

'I'm healing because I wasn't even aware of this pattern before I met you again. Awareness is the first step. I've been very honest with myself and haven't tried to hide my awful scratching habit from myself or from anyone. I knew it would freak people out to see me scratch; I knew they'd be horrified and appalled; and I didn't want to hide it from them when I needed to scratch. That to me is a healing in itself — not wanting to hide it.'

I have to agree that he has been gruesomely honest — a first step in his healing, as he says. But will it ever go further than that? I don't get it. He scratches as a result of feeling rejected, yet his scratching produces rejection, if only of the silent, appalled kind. But this kind of rejection he can understand; he has deliberately caused it himself, and deliberately uses it to not reject himself in spite of that. Aaron's a complex character. I sometimes wonder if he has made a contract somewhere in space and time in which growing up is associated with blood-letting.

'You've done me a great service by splitting up from me,' he says, smiling. 'You're loved even more for that. You might have thought that you were giving something up, but you've lost nothing. I love you even more.'

This morning, Aaron lies in his bed and wishes for love. He doesn't feel free to invite me any more. He's just lying there, wishing for someone to love him, when I pop into his room. He opens his blankets in welcome, and in moments I'm snuggling next to him.

The feeling between us has changed. For me, there's no longer the passion that used to make me open to him. There's a friendship here, plus a present desire on my part for sex. Not a violent need, but why forgo a pleasure waiting for me here, in Aaron's bed, with a man I can trust to not misunderstand my intentions?

It's different when he enters me. Again, there's no immediate thrill, just a welcoming. It's when he continues his thrusting from a half-sitting position that my body wakes up and tears are again wrung from my eyes. We climax at the same time, and I can tell how good we both feel. Our hormones have found a way, as well as our friendship.

'You're so much like me,' says Aaron. What he means is, I find sex when I need it and someone who likes me is near. I'm not attached, have no demands, have no expectations, have no promises. That's his world. I can enter his world now as a visitor while I'm still moving into my own world.

'I know what good love is now,' he says. 'I'll settle for nothing less.' And he adds, 'You're a woman now, in control of your destiny. You're no longer a little girl. You don't need anyone now you have yourself. I know that you'll find what you want.'

I woke that morning with a new, steady feeling of freedom. I was free to choose, and in that moment I wanted Aaron.

'We have a deep affection for each other and we like to give sexual pleasure to and receive it from one another,' is Aaron's observation. Then he talks about how passion naturally wanes for a couple over time, and friendship becomes more important.

That's where I disagree. Passion in my next relationship, I assert, will be maintained by the ... I search for the word and realise it's *husbanding* ... by the husbanding of energies within the circle of the relationship. A fierce appreciation of the relationship, and a natural desire to guard it from corruption of all kinds, such as comes from dishonesty about sharing feelings, lack of communication and putting sexual energy outside of the circle. This kind of commitment would allow me to be free to be passionate in all of life, because its particular, deepest expression would be channelled in one direction only.

GETTING DOWN TO IT

There is no end to pain
nor an end to joy
within the soul of freedom
Nirmala, untitled poem

 Again, our relationship changes. I blame it on a three-week intensive course in Theta Healing. My eyes see differently afterwards. I clearly see what I want from a partner, and what Aaron's not offering.

We're sitting on the deck of the *Duyfken*, the little wooden replica of a ship that bravely left Holland in the sixteenth century and traversed the oceans to reach Australia. We enjoy the balmy, fresh air that wafts over the Swan River where the *Duyfken* is docked in front of the Swan Brewery buildings and the expanse of water before us. On the far shore, traffic moves along lit highways and freeways.

'I want to be with someone who can share my space with me.'

It's Aaron, finally voicing the words of ultimate truth. I hear them, and know that it marks the point of no return. He's given up on me being interested in living in his house in Darkan. He's also given up on me understanding his stories. I no longer believe them the way I used to, and that has become an unbearable insult to a tender part of his nature. I may still be a child–woman, as he says, but I'm not naïve and gullible any more. So I feel relieved at what he's said. I know what I want: I want a gentleman kind of guy.

'You want someone who can look after you financially too,' he says.

Well, not quite. I want someone who is my financial equal, that's all. But I can't say this to him. To me, Aaron's a bit too proud of his ability to get by on a minimum.

I pay for the parking and drive us home again in my car. We head for our respective bedrooms. Tomorrow is Saturday and there'll be enough time for talking then.

I spend that Saturday with a total alien. Aaron has completely disconnected from me. I've never seen him like this before: a seeming lump of humourless moroseness. There is no light in his eyes.

I know to leave him alone when he's like this. Once, it took him a week to go through his personal hell; another time he shortened it to just an hour. I know he'll come out of it and be a better man for having resolved something inside him.

When he does want to talk, his face is paler than I've ever seen it before. His lips aren't quite in control as he speaks.

'Are you sure you don't want our "us-ness" any more?' He'll go and burn our relationship away unless I say something *now*. This is crunch time. 'I really love you, Carla, but if you don't want me, I won't stand in your way.'

I look at him. I've never been loved so steadily and so unconditionally before. Am I deliberately destroying something precious? Why would I do that? People do that sort of thing because they don't feel worthy of being truly loved. They believe it can't last. Is it because I'm older than Aaron, and feel the age difference between us will become too much, and I want to be the first to leave? Is it that I wouldn't be able to bear *him* leaving *me*?

These are all serious questions, because, once upon a time, that's exactly what I did. I tested my partners by being rude and crass: *Now, do you still love me?* Usually it was too much for them, and I thought it was a good thing to discover they didn't love me unconditionally after all. I was like a child testing its parents.

But there is a steadiness in the midst of my sorrow now. All day, tears surprise me, coming out of nowhere. I can feel Aaron's pain. I can feel the beauty of what we once had, and how it is still beautiful for me now that it's over and I have to move on. It's not as if I've fallen for someone else; there's no other lover on the horizon.

'I'm obeying what you call the Cogs, Aaron. I'm following an unknown call, the same way I've done a few times in my life — like when I left my home in Denmark to come to Perth.' I had no idea why I had to make that break, but the call was unmistakable. 'It's an unknown future that's pulling me. I'm not leaving this relationship because I judge you. We're good friends, but we aren't partners.'

'You know what you forgot?' says Aaron, with a hint of bitterness. 'You forgot to *ask*.'

What does he mean? To ask him to change into partner material for me?

'I don't want to ask you to change, Aaron!'

He looks away. He knows it's hopeless. Carla's going places he's not *interested* in. Aaron's saying, 'No one wants to walk with me. Everyone loves how I feel to them, but no one wants to walk with me.' But Aaron himself doesn't really want to walk with me. He wants me to walk with him, that's all.

'All I want is a friend to hang out with.' As he says this, he knows that he's just described the main difference between us. I want more than to 'hang out' with someone.

'It's not enough for me, Aaron.'

He nods. He knows. He's so sore.

'It's unbelievable, the way my chest hurts,' he says.

The pain will end when Aaron finally lets go.

Aaron's fist comes down heavily on the kitchen table when I refuse to let him have the last word. The cup in front of him spills its contents over the table and onto the floor, but doesn't fall to the ground itself.

'Enough!' he shouts. 'That's enough! Not another word!'

His fury has the desired effect: it shuts me up. There is silence in the room. Aaron stands on the other side of the table, then sits down again. My gaze is down, eyes welling with tears. Tears always melt Aaron. He pulls a chair over to sit opposite me and takes my hands in his. 'Tell me what the tears are about.'

When the words don't come fast enough, he lets go of my hands. I'm too silent now. Too wordy before, too silent now.

I grope for words that don't amount to a negative reaction, which would infuriate him even more. 'I don't know!' I whimper, not able to put my finger on my grief yet.

'You're so dry, Carla. I never get any juice from you.'

But the truth does come.

'My father used to silence me like that.'

Aaron sits back on his chair. This isn't what he expected, or wanted, to hear. I continue.

'You're not violent like him, but he couldn't bear me challenging his opinions. He would use his fist and his voice to silence me.'

'Do you feel safe with me?' Aaron wants to know.

'Yes. I feel safe with you.'

'I would never hurt you.'

'I know.'

Anger like this is rare with Aaron. What it tells me (once again) is that the barriers between us aren't going to be breached by talking. What's more, the closure we're seeking will stop short of us completely understanding one another. There are too many buttons that get pressed on both sides. Neither of us has the maturity or the skills to navigate the rocks we know lie hidden under the water but don't want to see.

After this incident, Aarons wants to build a bridge between us again. He asks me to sort a huge pile of nails with him that he has recently found. He sits himself down on the steps in front of the house with the nails in a bucket of water and invites me to sit next to him. I am aware of the pleasure he gets from my cooperation. I feel him smiling inside: we are healing our friendship again.

'I've always loved sorting things,' he says. 'When I was a little boy I found comfort in it. It was something simple to do that created order. It gave me a sense that my life was more in order.'

Yes, I believe that. This wonderfully creative person, this recycler and mender of broken goods, developed his skills from a desire to create order out of emotional chaos. I admire this in him; if he were free of the compulsion, it would still give him pleasure. It gives him great pleasure to provide for others — to give someone a computer built from scratch from salvaged parts, for example; to provide me with the best office chair yet from three disparate parts creatively put together. And now he is the company's valued problem-solver and designer. He can be justly proud of Clinton's appreciation of his contribution.

Aaron is leaving for Darkan this morning. I cut one of the first roses of spring and put it on his dashboard. He'll be away for as long as he likes — the company is grateful to him for what he has achieved by making a magnificent model and solving an important problem with a principal design. As he drives off and our hands part, I know it will be a different Aaron who comes back.

It's the end of our relationship. It feels complete, if raw. Rawness is perhaps necessary for a couple to be able to part. They have to face the negatives and incompatibilities; feel them in order to break away from each other.

It had to happen. Aaron had to get thoroughly disillusioned with me. When he's away in Darkan, I forget to record *Dr Who* for him. This is an important request from Aaron, who has religiously collected every episode of the series — up to now. When he returns from Darkan, he's shocked at my failure; tries hard not to read betrayal in it.

Just the next morning after this disappointment, I compound the problem of his struggling emotions. On my way down the corridor,

I hear the video tape recorder in distress — it's whirring and banging. Has the machine been left on all night and now it's reacting? Not knowing that Aaron put a tape in only minutes earlier, I push every available button to stop the fracas. Out pops a video.

'And it was broken,' he tells me later, with lead in his voice. 'That's never happened to me in all my life.'

Aaron thinks in symbols, and this extraordinary event must mean an extraordinary lack of something on my part. That night, he goes to bed and closes his door without saying goodnight. I notice, and inquire from outside the closed door how he's feeling.

'Just quiet,' he says.

'Quiet, not depressed?'

'No, just quiet. I know you weren't being malicious when you stopped that VCR, Carla.'

Okay, but some permanent damage has been done to his image of me. I'm witnessing the disassembling of a relationship. Part of me is glad it's happening. I want Aaron to start looking in another direction.

It's time to say it all now and see if we can still stay friends. We're sitting on the couch in the little TV room. I'm tired, having watched *When Worlds Collide* with Aaron. Now it's late. Watching that movie fulfilled a dream for Aaron, who saw it on television way back in the fifties, when the quality of picture was poor. It doesn't hold the same interest for me. This is one of Aaron's sadnesses — that I am downright unappreciative of the clichés film-makers indulged in back then. He knows they're clichés, but it doesn't matter to him.

When he asks how I enjoyed the movie, I tell him straight. He's aghast. 'There's your complaining self again,' he says.

'I know I complain, Aaron. You keep your complaints inside, but they're still there! Then you say *I'm* the one who always complains! Probably the things you don't like about me have mostly to do with you feeling judged by me. I should be able to ask you to please do this or that and not the other without you going into a crisis of feeling judged.'

'You're *so* critical, Carla! I wither when you open your mouth and tell me how I should be. It's your voice. I can hear it in your *voice*, your condemnation. It's horrible! You never take responsibility for that! You say it's all to do with *me* and nothing to do with *you*.'

We sit there a while in silence, before he goes on.

'You don't care about joining me in my space. You *hate* my space! You come to my house like a tourist, and want to get away from it as soon as possible because it's not like your space. You can't see what I've achieved on my block in Darkan. It's all meaningless to you. You don't know how much that hurts me — that I choose to be in your space and you never choose to be in mine.'

'How could I have chosen to be in your space, Aaron? Honestly? Could I really have come to live in Darkan? Or moved into your parents' house? I invited you to share a house with me but you said you could never afford that — that was out completely.'

Aaron doesn't want to concede this. He's talking more about my willingness and ability to share his space *emotionally*. For instance, he would have liked me to yearn to live in Darkan, even though that was impossible. He would have liked me to want to go to places like the video shop, the toy shops and the recycling shops just to be in his company. His space, his values. I know what he means. I am worse than half-hearted about these things. His (to me) strange obsessions were something I put up with and didn't let stand in the way of loving him. In the end, my indifference hurt him.

Aaron has more to say.

'You go off to your meetings and talks and leave me alone in the house. You don't think twice about that, and I'm the last one to stand in your way. But it doesn't matter to you that you do so many things without me.'

I feel very tired but don't want to walk out on him and this conversation.

Aaron installed an air conditioner in my bedroom yesterday. He has comments about that too. 'You've now got a bedroom where you can control the temperature the way you want it. All is exactly as *you* wish. In my room, it's close to natural — just what the fan can do to give me a little cool. Your room isn't mine any more. I won't go in there any more. I've made the effort to install your air conditioner and that's it. How do you like that analogy?'

'I think it's a bit unfair, Aaron, because my room gets much hotter than yours. It's too uncomfortable to be in it without cooling.'

'I'm saying things to you today that I've been holding in for a long time, and now that I've said them I have to accept them as real and deal with them. I'm alone and have to find my own space again. I have to find out who I am without you in my life. How does that sound to you?'

'I feel sad, but I know it's inevitable.'

I feel Aaron's need for companionship and for sex. Not that he won't be able to adjust; he will. But withdrawal makes him heavy and broody. He doesn't feel he's the man he wants to be when he's on his own.

'We're walking on different sides of the river now.' That's how he puts it since he's come back from Darkan. 'We're each determined to walk alone on our side. Sometimes we make a bridge and get together. Then, *poof!* The bridge evaporates and we find ourselves walking alone again, attentive to each other all the same. We build fewer and fewer bridges, just parts of bridges now, that get broken before they meet in the middle.'

It's an evocative picture, quite accurate. He's convinced it's the way my mind is working: I'm thinking too much, I'm judging him too much, and that's why my interest in him is waning. He's right to a degree: I get appalled by some of his habits. The bad habits seem to get worse in company, when he might be a bit nervous about what others think about him. Then he seems not to notice that he scratches his legs and picks at them, and speaks with his mouth full. It gets worse when he takes off his sandals and puts his feet onto the coffee table, often the more easily to scratch his legs. I've asked him before to take the offensive-smelling sandals away, and he has thrown them across the floor and out of the way. But he forgets. The list goes on.

These things don't matter to those in love, or to those who can love unconditionally, or to those who can stop listening to what their minds are yacking on about. After all, a person has redeeming qualities. A man, in particular, needs to be taken with a grain of salt, especially if a woman wants the genuine, not-too-polished article. It's no use, though: my insides revolt, and that's that.

I ask my friend Lynda how she sees Aaron and me as I drive her in my car to the train station after her visit. It's always good to get an outside point of view, and I know she loves us both. Lynda is careful to put things in general terms; she doesn't want anything to sound like a criticism of either of us.

'When two older people choose to be in relationship, it's for reasons other than raising children,' she says, relaxing back in her seat to face me side on while I drive. 'It's for reasons such as companionship, mutual support for a chosen goal, enjoyment of what you have in common. There will always be areas that create irritation, because that's human nature. The older you get, the worse that sort of thing can get.'

She's right. I've noticed this about both of us: how we like to have our own way about things.

'You and Aaron love each other, that's obvious. There's a strong bond between you.'

'And we can't help loving each other; we enjoy each other's company and touch. There's so much good feeling.'

'Then unconditional love has to take care of all the differences,' she remarks, neatly hitting that most important nail on the head, and echoing Aaron's attitude: *I love; that should be enough.*

'Love has no price and is of inestimable value,' she says, 'and yet it costs everything! What it costs is the death of the ego. The person has to decide: is this enough? If it is, the ego dies.'

I carefully consider Lynda's words. She's really clarifying things for me.

'You know what, Lynda? I can't do it! I haven't got it in me to love that much. It just isn't enough for me. I want more compatibility in the everyday areas of life!'

I'm finally able to say it as it is.

'Well, that's honest enough,' says Lynda. 'Love-making shows us what we're made of: all the truth and all the baggage.'

Now that I have this final clarity, I need to tell Aaron. As soon as I'm home again, I ask for his attention.

'You know how to love unconditionally, Aaron. I can't. It's too hard for me.' I look at him hopelessly.

Aaron suddenly lunges forward and takes my hands, unexpectedly grateful for my honesty.

'I have a confession to make myself, Carla. You treat relationships like a shopping list. You don't know how to appreciate me! You shit on my love. To you, relationship is about making your partner suit you. If I take my love away from you, you'll fall off a cliff. There'll be such a big hole.'

I should despair, but I don't. Somehow, I welcome this: he's given himself the voice of grief at last. He's aggrieved just now, and a bit sour, but I remember that he's been through worse and come out of it loving even more.

He moves himself along the couch, further away from me. 'You treat me like a commodity,' he says dully.

And yet, when he's done, he thanks me for listening and we get on with the day.

THE BYWAYS OF LOVE

Love is a thing of twoness.
But underneath any twoness, man is alone.
DH Lawrence, 'Deeper Than Love'

 We sit on the verandah before the day gets hot. This is how we talk now, gradually coming to terms with our own thoughts and feelings.

'I woke up with a terrifying thought this morning,' says Aaron.

I wait, but he won't say anything more until I prompt him. 'And what was that?'

'I have to go find another girlfriend,' he says and sighs wickedly.

Our conversations are becoming clearer about what we've decided to do.

'Lots of people wouldn't mind having what we have, and would compromise themselves all the way to hell to keep it,' says Aaron. 'They'd decide to compromise and stay together because they appreciate the good parts. That's fair enough.'

'Well, they might put moral obligations on themselves, such as "I have to accept this person for the rest of my life because I promised",' I rejoin. 'That usually goes together with "I *should* love this person in spite of what I don't like about him. I *should* be able to overcome my dislikes and maybe other, more violent reactions and I *should* take on this challenge for my growth and the glory of God," or something similar.'

'Yep,' says Aaron, 'and then there's genuine unconditional love. The other is loved and enjoyed and simply forgiven for his or her foibles. That's really the only way a relationship can flourish. It's what you and I did, until we didn't; at least, you didn't, and lately I haven't either.'

'At those times, we came up against something more than a foible, Aaron. We hit some basic incompatibilities, which is more serious. That kind of thing shouldn't be ignored. Then you can't go around saying, "I'm here for what we have in common", when what we have in common is on top of some deep stuff we *don't* have in common. That's where I see us now. We've arrived at that point. I'm just the first one to see it clearly, so it's more painful for you.'

His women, Aaron says, used to come up to him with a banner in front of their face with the words, *Change! Be the person I want you to be!* 'And I have a banner that says, *I want to be Aaron! Take me or leave me!* That crude demand for change is brutal. It's more than disrespectful. It's —'

'Are you sure that's what it said on those women's banners?' I interrupt. 'That's what you might have interpreted it to mean, but you have a terrible propensity for feeling judged. Could it be that they were asking for something valid?'

He can't answer that. His memories are only of being attacked and discounted.

I try to put it into words for both of us. 'It's as if God is telling us, "Hey, this doesn't work, therefore it isn't what I have in mind for you. Quit this. It's had its time. It's fulfilled its purpose. Don't be attached to memories and don't force it to be what it isn't. There isn't a need for you to compromise. Have faith and move on. There's Life; life that can provide exactly what's right for you."'

Aaron nods, but I know he's only half-convinced. *Love conquers all* is what he believes, and wants to make true for himself, at least.

'From my side, Aaron, what comforts me is knowing that this break-up is meant to happen. That strong intuition I had at the beginning of the relationship is a comfort to me now, because I was given a hint of what to expect.'

'Maybe you made it true because you believed in that vision,' he says. 'You declared it true, and as a result it happened.'

A self-fulfilling prophecy, in other words. He's implying that I could have rejected that vision and chosen to change it. Only it wasn't like that. It was as if, back then, I already knew at some level that this relationship was only for a time. That it had a built-in ending.

'I've had a vision too, Carla. Ever since I was a boy, I've known that I'll die at the age of fifty-four. Now my knees are packing up and my body is full of pain.' And then he adds, 'I want to change that vision. I don't want to die.'

I listen to his inner sorrow. His strong body is still remarkably strong. He has an amazing constitution. And yet it's breaking down in important ways. His eyes, for instance. He often complains about the strain in his eyes, but hasn't been near an optometrist because they cost money.

'You've got a huge challenge, Aaron. God won't blame you if you decide to put it off for another lifetime.'

I know he knows it himself already — that he really won't change. I can bring it out into the open so he doesn't have to fool himself about it and hurt himself by continually failing.

'For instance, you say that you want to heal your knees. If that were true, the first thing you'd do is reduce your weight, because your knees are stressed carrying that load all the time.'

Aaron nods, slightly embarrassed.

'You know you won't do anything to lose weight, Aaron.'

But he's off the hook as far as my expectations are concerned, and that's what brings a smile to his face. Then he asks, 'Do you have any challenges?'

'Sure,' I answer. 'Sometimes I still feel some sort of existential terror come up through my body. It lives in the cells of my body, and I haven't managed to shake it out and live in complete faith and comfort. I also feel fierce criticism at times — towards myself and towards other people. I'm intolerant, as you know! I have my challenges, alright.'

He needs to hear that, to know it's not all his fault that this relationship has ended.

'Yes,' he agrees, 'that intolerance. It's the one reason why this relationship has to end, as far as I'm concerned. 'Your love was total and pure, Carla. It gave me back my innocence. That's a great gift. You enabled me to be the man I've always known I could be: someone who loves without reserve, loyal, attentive and gentle, forgiving. There's a lot I don't like about you, but I never said anything because I'm not here for those things. I'm here for the energy. I just love the feeling of you; that's it.'

In the end, it's no one's fault. We've both come to clearly face issues that we will eventually deal with. That, in itself, is quite something.

Tomorrow, he'll go to his house again and stay there for the weekend. In spite of all that's transpired between us this evening, he takes my hand and leads me down the corridor to his room. And so we lie on his bed. Even though my body is sleepy and not interested in sex, his touch and desire might arouse me. I want this to be a goodbye present for him. He perks up so much after sex that it's a joy to think of giving him this. As for Aaron, he reckons it's his gift to me. 'You'll feel better after this,' he says, as if he's following the dictum: *Complaining women just need to be laid*. Well, I'll let him have that.

This time, though, my body won't play its part the way it has in the past. Pleasure surfaces, but soon dies again. Aaron's thrusting awakens my sexuality in an ungentle way that has nothing to do with him; it's just my body that no longer responds to him the way it used to. In spite of the help of lubrication, my fanny burns at the edges before he's finished. He comes uncontrollably, releasing the tension built up over the past few days of celibacy.

Aaron stays alert, his head on his elbow, watching me until I stir to get up because I want to sleep in my own bed.

The next morning, I notice how happy he is as he packs. His mind is completely clear. When he sees me, there isn't a hint or gesture that speaks of anything but the task in hand. Sex has miraculously restored his balance, as it does for so many men. Maybe that's why women allow their men to have sex with them even when they don't feel like it. They have the satisfaction of seeing their man in a happy mood. A happy man is a cooperative man, a man who does things around the house. It was after we had sex that Aaron decided to install my air conditioner! It wasn't my intention — far from it — but it's just occurred to me that this is what happened. No wonder sex can become a political tool in a woman's hands! No wonder that a man, because of his need, can become extremely cautious about being used by women.

Back from Darkan, Aaron's approach is guided by the love he feels we still share and by his hormones. I'm having an afternoon lie-down on my bed when he knocks and enters.

'Aaron, I don't feel seducible!'

'You still feel lovable.'

'I feel languid.'

'That's alright; be as languid as you like.'

By now, he's hovering above me, legs straddled on either side of my supine body. He's ever so attentive, ever so careful to not go where he isn't wanted. His caution reminds me of the dance of the male spider as he approaches the much bigger female, even if she seems unsuspecting and friendly. As he gets closer — all the while waving the legs containing his treasure, his sperm — he constantly tests the taste of her feet, to judge if she's turned on by him. Even when she spreads her eight legs in a gesture of invitation, he can't be sure of his ultimate welcome. She can still make a meal of him, and she often does.

I like the fact that Aaron expects no more of me than to not reject his efforts. His hands run over my body with tenderness, respect, longing. He peels off my skirt and panties so he can caress the parts that are exposed. He licks my clitoris into awakening, and my vagina spurts out its juices in spite of my languor. He inserts himself ever so carefully. Every movement is so gentle, so measured and considerate.

He lunges forward and pulls my top and bra over my head. This makes my arms go up, and I grip a vertical slat at the back of the bed. My breasts are still so insignificant compared to some, but he loves them and lowers himself onto them. His mouth finds my nipples as he gently keeps thrusting. I open my eyes now and again and see the intensity of pleasure on his face.

He wants me to come to a point of excitement before he releases, so he suddenly adopts a posture that allows his penis to go deeper. My body is compelled to respond, and as it climaxes so does he.

I lie back in total satisfaction, eyes closed, as he sits back and comes down from his feelings, his penis still inside me. When eventually he lies next to me, I open my eyes to see him regard me with tenderness.

'Your friend is still here,' he says.

Afterwards, I wonder how he can do that. And how he could be so willing to take the lead all the way and not have any expectations. Our roles have been reversed so much since I first met him.

Aaron comes in one morning (after knocking politely on my closed door and waiting till he hears my 'come in!') and commands me to lie down. He wants to hold me. So I rearrange the pillows and stretch out. Aaron holds me close in his powerful arms. I breathe quietly into his chest and ask him what he's doing.

'Diffusing the tension between us,' he says.

It's a tension only he is aware of. He just can't believe that I am OK. I hold his body, naked except for a brief pair of red jocks, and am careful not to give him the impression that I want to turn him on with my touch.

His hands pass over my back with firm strokes. I relax and enjoy his touch, until his hand passes over my front, strokes a nipple and makes a move to remove my dressing gown. I stop him.

'I'm not sexually interested.'

He snorts. 'That's entirely your affair,' he says, 'that's got nothing to do with me. I'm just here, inviting you, and you can do with that what you want.'

I'm silent as we lie there. He takes up the silence between us. 'I need affection,' he reiterates softly for the so-manyth time. He tries something else. 'It used to be fun between us. Now there is so much tension. I want us to go back to the way we were. I know you. You're a sexual woman. What's happened to your spontaneity?'

He almost has me there. No one wants to be called unspontaneous! But my mind is firing rapidly, even though it's early in the morning. There is a place for self-control in sexuality; indulgence of a superficial desire isn't the same as spontaneity.

'When I had sex with you, I was a radiant woman, Aaron. Since I stopped making love with you, I've noticed myself getting dull. But I don't want to be dependent on sexual intercourse for my radiance. I want to enjoy whatever I'm doing in the moment and make that the reason for being happy.'

'Been there, done that!' he says gruffly.

'Are you talking about yourself?' I'm incredulous that he would dismiss what I've just said with such cynicism and disrespect.

'Yes. I've been there and done that. I'm Aaron and it's not my way. I'm happy when I'm being me.'

He's implying, of course, that I'm not being me, and that I'm fooling myself if I think I'm going to succeed in being happy while not having sex.

He no longer holds me as tightly. His breath is above my head, but I can still detect the sourness of early morning on it.

'Where is the intimacy we used to have? And the affection?' He's plaintive. 'We were so happy once.'

I can't tell him again that it's no longer appropriate for me to be intimate with him. I tried only a minute ago, by sharing something truly important to me, only to see how bored he is with what he can't imagine as part of his own life.

The front doorbell rings. It's Pete the vegie man, delivering his organic goods. I break away from our embrace and answer the door. Pete is used to seeing me in my dressing gown.

After Pete leaves, it's time for my morning Pilates exercises. I promised myself to be regular, and being true to my promise is paying off. I notice how the life force is flowing strongly in me as I swing my arms above my head and down again and as I include my knees and pelvis in the movement. *'Feel!'* sings the woman on my CD. *'Feel the return to yourself!'*

The music and exercise is intoxicating. My stomach and vaginal muscles tighten with pleasure and good health. I AM being me! I'm enjoying feeling sexual and intensely alive and still content to have no sexual partner for now.

'I was shocked by your selfishness last night,' Aaron says from his chair on the verandah. It's early in the morning. The birds notice us and come flying in the hope of some seed thrown on the ground. 'I could never do what you did last night,' he elaborates.

Last night, when Aaron once more bared his soul to me — his need for affection, his desire to be a sexual man again. And I said — as emphatically as I could this time and probably without the softness that the occasion warranted — that it was time for me to create distance between us, not intimacy. Affection from me would be interpreted as a sexual invitation, a sexual interest, and create new hope.

'I have never met anyone who could just put a person outside like you did,' he says. 'You can pick a person up and drop him just like that. You are incredibly selfish.'

It's true that in a similar situation, Aaron would have made love to me; his compassionate heart wouldn't have hesitated to love away the hurt and need.

'It's the way I am, Aaron.'

'Yes, I can see that now. It's made me think I could do with a bit of that myself. I like the idea of being selfish for a change.'

He sounds bitter as he says this, and I know he doesn't quite appreciate that my so-called selfishness is my ability to do the right thing once I know it. I've learnt to follow an inner directive with trepidation, but also with courage. The judgmental streak in me confuses the purity of this ability, hence the doubts that come up when this is pointed out to me. And Aaron, above all people, will point this out to me, because the child in him begins to panic and break its heart anew whenever it thinks it is going to be rejected again. Aaron the man is there to protect that child by firmly never ever going to the depths of that pain. This is his no-go zone. His wounded heart is surrounded by barbed wire. When his little child is challenged by me, Aaron's eyes become steely and his manner takes on a soldier's stance: *Go no further!*

Aaron encloses me in his arms.

'Do you want to be the woman who tastes the love I have to give?' he asks. 'I know you. You love being loved. You don't have to do a thing: I will pleasure you. Do you want me to love you?'

I listen to my body as he holds me closer. I so appreciate his energy. I haven't had sex for weeks now. And I don't want to make love to Aaron.

'It's just not coming up for me, Aaron. My body is just staying very still and there isn't anything in me that wants to make love to you.'

'It's a case of an under-inflated tyre with a fully inflated one,' he observes. 'It just doesn't work, does it? It's under-inflated and will never be fully inflated again.'

COMING HOME TO OURSELVES

Do you imagine that the future
is predictable — even by God?
Neale Donald Walsch,
Conversations With God Book 2

Aaron takes a trailer-load of building materials down to his house in Darkan on Thursday and isn't expected to return until Monday morning. I double-lock the front door each night when I go to bed.

It's past midnight on Sunday when I half-wake from very deep sleep to the racket of Aaron breaking awkwardly into the house. My brain isn't awake enough to function when he places his chilly body next to mine and puts his arm around me. He's overflowing with love and warmth. 'I love your beauty, Carla!' And then he says, 'I'm not afraid of not being loved.'

My sleepy self just manages to put an arm around his big torso. I fall asleep again the moment he leaves my bed.

In the morning, though, I remember his words. While he was away, he seems to have overcome his tendency to dwell on my rejection of him. He's not even afraid of me not loving him; he's just going to love anyway. But he's different when I see him get up. He's morose.

'Yes,' he says, in answer to my questioning look, 'I'm angry. I'm angry at myself for always falling back to my illusions about you. That's got to change, and it changes from this moment.'

I can see that he's close to tears, and his skin is grey.

'I want affection,' he says. 'I want us to be emotionally alive. I love being a lover, and I love being affectionate. That's who I am.'

I listen to and feel his pain. I should break down now and rescue him — that's the message — but I decide not to take responsibility for him. He may call it cruelty, I'm aware of that, and still I don't want to step over what I genuinely feel.

His face is grim; this is a challenge coming hard on the heels of his loving overture of last night. He thought I would do the same: rise above what he calls my negative ego, as he's done. And so, in spite of his previous insights, Aaron spirals down another level.

'You can't see me any further than you can see yourself. You don't know me, Carla!'

I want to tell him about an insight I had last night. It's always awkward saying something that I know isn't going to be quite understood.

'Well, what is it?'

'You know how you've always said that love should be enough, and I always said that it isn't? Last night, I realised that love of the truth is more important than love of the person.'

Aaron looks nonplussed, but he doesn't seem to be offended, so I continue.

'When two people don't share the same love of the truth all the way, then the one who wants more honesty is still lonely. My heart is committed to the truth the way a nun is to God.'

It's a huge statement, and it doesn't sit entirely right. I have my pride; I have a tendency to think of myself as better than him, and so it's easy for me to say things like this and fool myself again. Even so, in spite of the danger of failing to live my truth consistently, it's still my biggest passion.

'I'll sacrifice everything for this, Aaron. It means that eventually no part of my ego will be safe from the searchlight. I feel that's where you won't join me.'

Poor Aaron has to hear this from the woman he loves beyond reason. It's not that Aaron isn't a lover of the truth himself. He tells me now, with unusual shyness, how he's been dealing with the pain of his recent terrible loneliness.

'You pressed buttons in me and started a process I just had to finish if I wasn't to die,' he says.

He looks at me and smiles, because he knows how much what he's going to say next will astound me, showing me how much he can, indeed, change.

'I looked down that corridor to your bedroom so many times and felt so terribly lonely, wanting you.'

Yes, I had a fair idea about that. I used to listen to his occasional dry cough, indicating his discomfort and his tortured brain.

'You know what I did, Carla? I comforted the little boy in me that had those same feelings so many years ago. I felt so little and helpless and alone. I held him close and healed his little heart. I did this day after day, and now I think I've grown up.' He pauses, a little shyly. 'I'm a man now, Carla.'

I can feel his confident, clean energy. Yes, he's a man now, owning his own energy. It's phenomenal. Aaron is coming to himself again. That irresistible beauty once more begins to shine from his face. His sexuality is once more asserting itself as innocent, expectant and now free of attachment to me. I am so immensely pleased for him.

'My love,' he asserts, 'is mine. I can't *find* love; I can only generate it myself and find reflections of it outside of myself. When I love different women, it feels the same, no matter who I'm with, because the love feelings are mine, not theirs. God is one, and so love is the same everywhere.'

These aren't words he could have spoken a month ago. He must be changing, because, according to his own laws, change brings accidents, and he has gashed both his right thumb and his left big toe in two incidents only three days apart. Both times, my heart almost stood still as he dealt with the pain with every expression open to a man. Theatrical, but not acted. 'I do pain well,' was his comment to my white face as he finally relaxed again and bandaged his wounds the way he likes it: simple, effective, no fuss.

Although I don't expect Aaron to be free of all his defences, he's fast becoming the person I wanted all along; the boy in him becoming a man now that I've let him go, and now that it may be too late.

Still, I know that Aaron hasn't faced his last and most awful demon: the core of his greatest pain. He dealt with his lonely child because he was forced to make himself feel better. He's not ready yet to let the truth burn away the supposed ideal of feeling better.

Burning away fear has been a big part of the story of my life; it's been the one thing that frees me of dark inner secrets. Once the passion for inner truthfulness gets hold of a person, nothing less will do, even faithful, delighted, affectionate and devoted love like Aaron's. I would have to sell my soul to stay with Aaron, and give up my eyes and ears for the sake of safety and security, for this in-love attentiveness, this chrysalis cocoon. Without the creative courage to shed the old skin and metamorphose into a glorious butterfly, the chrysalis dies anyway. At least, in this way our love for each other is being preserved, allowing us to evolve, albeit in our separate ways.

'I've learnt from this relationship and from all my relationships,' says Aaron, sitting across the coffee table from me after Clinton and Margot have gone home. 'A total relationship is a myth. From my relationship with you I've learnt to stay in my own centre while relationships come and go. I don't control what other people want to do. They decide to leave; it's their affair. I'll be open for what comes next.'

I feel the new strength that Aaron has found, mixed with his defiance.

'Did you ever find out why your women left you?' I ask cautiously, trying not to awaken his suspicion that I'm about to say something that feels like an attack.

'They leave, and that's their business, not mine,' he says.

'So you never found out why they left? And I'm leaving, and you won't know why I left either?'

He looks at me with flat eyes. I know what he says to friends who inquire why we're splitting up. *I've reached my use-by date. Carla has a vision of where she's going in her life, and there isn't any room for me there.*

'It's not the whole story, Aaron.'

'I don't need to know any more,' he says. 'And you're making me feel uncomfortable now.'

'The discomfort comes up rather easily, doesn't it.'

This comment is filled with a great deal of sadness, and isn't a question. This is the brink from which he could jump into the feeling and find out what is really inside it and beyond it, but he habitually retreats. For him to understand why I am leaving him, he would have to face this innermost reality, and it's just too unbearable.

We sit in silence while he looks at me with a straight face that I can't read.

'What are you thinking now?' I ask.

'I'm admiring your beauty,' he says. 'You're so young.' A slight smile returns to his face. 'You were young and innocent when you introduced me to love all those years ago. You're still like that. I have that same innocence inside me because of your example.'

He has changed the tone of the conversation, and it's good this way. I also have a compliment for him.

'You are a warm and generous lover, Aaron. You know how to make a woman feel good.'

He likes that and nods. I think of something else to add.

'You are a great creator of honeymoons.'

It is on this note that I finally go to bed. My planned early nights often end up like this. My head hits the pillow and I don't hear another sound.

It would be good if someone could love Aaron now. Love builds his ego, which needs building. It is still an ego hovering between positive and negative. He certainly can't take any negative observations from me. That not only makes him feel small, it makes him defensive and obtuse. But I don't have the right to say anything while I'm critical. Aaron is so sensitive to energy; I can't fool him into thinking that it's love that makes me speak. He feels the barbs attached to my probing and prodding. I don't know how to really love as I make my observations about him. And so my words are empty and useless anyway.

We sit on the rocking chairs out on the verandah. The weather's getting milder now. We still have a need to talk, as if our closure will take forever. Our souls have wanted to be together and can't understand why we can't resolve our differences.

Aaron tells me his strategy for taking care of himself. 'I'm used to seeing you in a certain way, and I'm deleting those impulses. I'm gradually losing my feelings for you.' He's quiet again, waiting for the words to sink in; waiting, perhaps, for me to start feeling sorry about my decisions. I keep looking at him as he feels out the words he will say next. 'I feel more clear each time, more comfortable and at ease. I'm once more coming into my own integral space.'

I look at him and see the beauty I have often admired coming back into his face. I can imagine how he will look with another girlfriend and what she will see in him. Sex hormones make him wildly attractive and seductive. I am beginning to see more clearly what I'm giving away here.

I once thought that Aaron was compelled to live up to an image of himself as a loving character, the way some Christians do, to follow an injunction. I thought he needed to be a loving person in the eyes of his heavenly Father, who would reward him for being good. But I was doing him a great injustice. He smiled wanly when I told him my thoughts.

'How you don't know me, Carla! I'm just not what you think, but I feel your rejection of me.'

I felt chastened. A blush crept over my face. I just had to voice my thoughts and found that they were way off. Aaron is the peacemaker. His heart is the pure heart of a child who gives all of himself and then doesn't know when it's time to retract.

TAKE ME AWAY FROM YOU

It's time to go.
We have to catch the ferry.
Simon Gladdish, *Images of Istanbul*

 The morning after my latest rebuff Aaron leaves the house at seven o'clock without saying goodbye. Clinton, Margot and I assume he's gone to Darkan, but he turns up at around midday, looking pleased with himself. He doesn't explain his absence, no one questions him, and I have to go out. That evening, when we're having dinner on the verandah, I have the chance to tell him that I was sad to notice he'd gone without a word. And it's then he tells me he went to visit a woman he's been chatting to off and on.

'I've taken my dick elsewhere, Carla,' he says. 'You're a free woman now.'

I look up at the sky, still ablaze with the setting sun of early summer, and feel a deep relief. It's over now. The tensions between us will ease naturally.

'I know what I want and I went to get it,' Aaron says. 'I went somewhere where I'm wanted.'

I'm glad that he can do what he does and find it right. It's so strange, though, to think of Aaron being with another woman. I'm surprised that I'm not in shock. Maybe I am. Maybe there'll be a reaction later.

'She's a good soul,' he says, but I haven't asked for any information.

'I don't need to know who she is.'

Later in the evening, reality sets in for me. Grief hits deeply.

Aaron sees what's going on in me and his compassionate heart wants to save me from the worst. He won't touch me but stands in front of me.

'I still love you, Carla.'

Aaron suddenly collapses in a chair and tells me about the severe pains in his stomach. He squeezes a big fold in his abdomen, trying to comfort it. 'I think I've got an ulcer,' he groans. For days, he's had very little appetite for meals, instead gorging himself on biscuits, peanuts and chocolate-coated almonds.

It's the evening we usually go out to Peter and Pearl's for an Adyashanti video, meditation and discussion. Does he want me to stay and keep him company? No, he doesn't. I go out by myself.

Aaron isn't there when I get home. I assume he's gone away to his girlfriend's for the night and lock up. It's some time past midnight when I hear him come back.

On the verandah that has become our sacred space, he makes the announcement that I have both feared and longed for.

'I'm free of you now, Carla. Last night, I turned myself inside out.'

I look at him, not knowing how to understand him.

'I purged myself of my attachment to you. I went to my girlfriend's and lay in her arms. Then I came home again, and on the way back I vomited. I stopped the car and vomited an incredible amount of stuff. It just kept on coming and coming, like a river.'

My heart is beating rather strongly in my chest. *Aaron's done a telephone job on me at last.* I can feel the difference in him — a certain hardness, coolness, distance; a dryness where once was a flow of sexual interest. *Aaron has reached the point of no return.*

'Even if I wanted to, I couldn't love you any more,' he says. The words cut deep, but I feel their justice. 'You forced me to stop loving you.'

It happened, in spite of his long struggle to keep on loving regardless. Even so, he has no desire to be cruel.

'I will always love you, don't get me wrong, Carla. I love you because of our history and because you are beautiful, but I can't love you any more the way I used to.'

We sit in blessed silence for a while. Aaron, this beautiful, searching, loving soul, is taking the journey of his life the way his God wants him to.

'You've done your healing work on me, Carla.' He looks at me with such appreciation.

It's truly remarkable that he sees what I've done as 'healing work'. All the same, he can't know how difficult this healing work he is referring to has been for me. I am blindly trusting an inner directive to stand apart, to refuse and deny him — to do it and suffer the lonely consequences for myself. I've wanted him so badly at times, and wouldn't have him the way he was. I have to lose Aaron to gain this new version that is now emerging — for his own sake as well as mine. Losing Aaron has been a hell of a process for me too. Loss of a great love is teaching me great lessons.

Aaron wants to make sure I understand his appreciation of what our relationship has meant to him.

'You are the epitome of innocent woman, Carla,' he says, dripping sweet honey over my soul as he sits next to me at the kitchen table, his hands resting on relaxed legs. 'You allowed me to be my own innocent man. I know now that you always loved me, even when you rejected me. You never became bitter and you kept our friendship intact. I thank you for that. You restored my faith in women and in myself. I know I am lovable now. I look around me and notice people that want my friendship, and I welcome their attention. I have no more doubts about my ability to love and be loved. You're in me forever, Carla. I have made the feeling of you my own. I can't have you any more, but I carry you with me. It's been such a good time, Carla.'

My eyes shine with brimming tears.

'I know what I want now, and what I want is being wanted. I'll never again hang on to a person who doesn't want me. I'm free now, to let those into my life who want me. Lots of friendships are coming my way, Carla. My new girlfriend isn't shy about telling me that she wants me, so I am there with her now. I've started a new story with her. What we had, Carla, will never be erased or replaced. We loved each other and both found where we didn't want to go with each other. That's alright with me now. I've complained that you never entered my life like I wanted. I'm not sore about that any more, Carla.'

And so I let him go.

This afternoon he is going to see a movie with his new girlfriend. I don't know who she is and don't need to know. I'm content that he will share some of his new story with me as he once more enters the joy of being wanted for who he is. Even if we both wanted to be together again, it would be an impossibility. The severance had to be real to be effective. We've both learnt the deep lesson of love surviving separation. That warm heart of Aaron's — that is in me, making a more compassionate, affectionate woman out of me. That has been my transformation. I don't have it in me any more to be critical of anyone's shortcomings. That criticalness has evaporated, by some grace of God.

I miss Aaron as I try to fill the house by myself this Sunday afternoon and listen to music. The music evokes deep, erotic memories, and sharp, deep loss stings my belly. At the same time, there is this expansion in my heart and the truth is this: in spite of the grief it is full of exquisite joy.

And suddenly a new and passionate love starts to take me over. What or who can explain the radiant love that now enters my feelings? It comes after a humbling realisation that to a degree, I live 'being true to myself' as a concept and that it has exacted a price. My ego pretended it knew something, when really it knew nothing at all. This becomes plain to me when I remember Aaron's words that I never left the door open for some organic, unplanned changes to happen that might have made it possible for us to stay together in spite of our differences, had we both decided on unconditional acceptance of each other. That truth now comes home to me and I feel betrayed by my ego.

True love, after all, is never judgmental. It never rejects. I was lucky that while I rejected Aaron for his shortcomings, I was still shown his example of love. Aaron drew me back to love by being who he is. That is his greatest gift to me. I love and appreciate him more now than I ever did. Now that it is too late for us.

I sit beside him on the couch while we watch television together. It's seductive, this togetherness. He senses something from me and holds out his hand. I take it gratefully, feeling his warmth and his strength. I lean up against him and want to ask him something, because it hasn't been clear in my mind. He's never actually told me that he's made love to this new friend of his.

'Aaron?'

'Hmm?' He turns his head to me, fully attentive.

'Have you committed yourself sexually then?'

He stirs immediately. 'Commit? I only commit to myself,' he says. And doesn't give any more explanation. Instead, he gets up, my hand still in his, and leads me to my bed.

Everything is wondrously new again as we make love. Every sense is sharply alive; all the knowing we have of each other, the comfort, the pleasure, the joy, the depth, ends in an extraordinary surrender. We lie next to each other and wonder what has happened.

'My new friend said that she doesn't want to share her man,' he says, almost casually. 'So I said, fine, let's be friends then.'

I feel relieved, so relieved. The devil! He made me believe they'd had sex together.

He confides something else about his new friend. 'She has a physical health problem. It's herpes. She doesn't want me to become infected.'

As far as I'm concerned, that is Providence protecting what we still have, allowing us to be together this way.

My heart has once more opened to Aaron like a flower. It absolutely radiates with appreciation of him. The extreme irony of this situation also squeezes my heart with exquisite pain.

An unexpected, unlooked-for but delicious honeymoon ensues. I allow myself to be freely affectionate. Aaron loves it. 'Joan is my friend, and I enjoy her company very much, but you are my lover,' he says.

He's loving, and loving this sex, inviting me to his bed, coming to me in mine, but he's not in love. It's just me in love again. So blindly this time. Which is why I am so totally unprepared for what happens next.

STAY WITH YOURSELF

And I was naked on the top of the mountain.
The view was spectacular, and the voice was within me.
Barbara Barton, *Light from the Universal Mind*

It's Thursday morning, very early. Last night I felt so much like making love with Aaron, but he left to visit his friend, Joan, and came back very late. This morning, I leave him asleep and go off to my now regular meet-up with some women friends for breakfast in Applecross.

When I come home again, Aaron gets up from his office chair to give me the most intimate of hugs. Every centre in our bodies is connected to the other in this long embrace. Aaron sinks his head onto my shoulder, raises it to kiss me, then sinks it down again. I'm ecstatic: we'll make such love tonight. No words are spoken as he returns to his computer station. Without knowing it, I have just completely and utterly misread him.

I'm resting on my bed, as I often do after lunch, when he comes in and leans over me. His face seems serious as he looks long into my eyes. What's he looking for? But he says nothing. It's the look of lovers who need no words to communicate, I think. I'm such an ass.

He's off to visit his parents, who need him to move some furniture for them. 'I might be back late,' he says.

I've waited all day; I can wait a bit longer.

As I wait, I prepare. I do my Pilates exercises and dance to music, saying with mock impatience: 'Hurry up, Aaron! Can't you feel how much I want you!'

He comes home, finally, and takes me into his arms, seemingly delighted. 'Do you like this man, Carla?'

I take this as an invitation and smile happily into his face.

'Yes! And do you want this woman?'

Aaron moves out of our embrace and holds my hands. 'I screwed Joan last night,' he says. 'I can't make love to you because I don't want to risk infecting you.'

A shockwave goes through my system. He's made love to this ... this woman with herpes. *Herpes is forever.* He says he doesn't want to make love to me because he wants to protect me. Instantly I know that herpes or not, it wouldn't have made any difference. I feel cruelly stripped down to bare bones, to empty space where my heart once was.

'It's not about protecting me from herpes, Aaron. Please be honest. We don't do triangles, do we? Not you, not Joan, and not me. The truth is that you've switched.'

I clearly remember Joan's words to Aaron during his first visit to her house, reported back to me: *I don't want to share my man.*

I take a step back from him, still looking into his eyes, which are red-rimmed in a very pale face just now.

'She really wanted me, she really likes me, and I responded to that,' he says, quietly, evenly, only explaining himself because he cares for me. 'I threw caution to the wind, and it was good. It was only good. I have no regrets.' He also has no shame, no guilt. He feels clean.

The words act like knives, cutting things to ribbons inside me. I let go of his limp hands.

'It wasn't a game, Carla.' Meaning that it was a conscious and serious step for him. And then he says, 'It wasn't about sex. It was about warmth and expressing a friendship. I enjoyed her and I made a bubble with her. I own my sexuality with her.'

That is so important to Aaron, to own his sexuality. No one can tell him what to do with it. No one has the power to make him feel guilty about what he does with it.

Listening to Aaron's words gives me a few moments to come to myself somewhat, but there's nothing much for me to say. A hollow voice comes out of my hollow chest. 'Well, goodnight then, Aaron,' and I sleepwalk out of the lounge room towards my bed.

'Come and talk to me if you need me!' he calls after me. Aaron the veteran carer. He knows what will happen to me now, though he has no idea how bad his timing is.

Among the tangle of sheets I begin the long wrestling with my feelings. This grievous pain of loss is the pain Aaron must have felt when I stepped back from him, I realise. Now it's my turn to feel its searing heat, its sickening emptiness, the inclination to vomit. I notice the way my mind wants to compensate. I imagine getting up, packing a bag, disappearing for a couple of days to the beach for endless walks by the shore. Feelings of rage and revenge, of lashing out, come and go. I let the thoughts run their course and then get up to talk to Aaron.

I find him lying on his bed fully clothed. No part of him was going to get undressed during this night when our separation will be sealed.

I sit on the corner of his bed closest to the door and tell him, with a voice as steady as my body will allow, what my thoughts have come to.

'I want to thank you, Aaron, for what you did. You've done me a great service because I didn't really know how to separate from you. Your action has made things definite between us. I know you have been honourable in all this.'

It's dark in his room, but we don't need to see each other's eyes as we speak. Aaron edges over to me and leans on his elbow. He speaks softly.

'I never wanted to hurt you, Carla. I trusted last night that what was said between us about separating was the truth. I wrestled for months with our separation, and came to terms with it. I accepted your love-making and enjoyed you. I always made it clear that I wasn't reattaching myself to you.'

And so did I, I remember. 'I want you to be free!' was my cry as we tumbled once more into a sexual embrace. It was just that, so very recently, we seemed to have fallen in love with each other in spite of ourselves. The electric touch that set me on fire when I first met him, now almost thirty-two years ago, had been reawakened. Just a casual brush past him sent delight through my whole body. But it was obviously a one-sided thing.

'I know how you feel,' he says into the darkness, speaking kindly, trying not to push against the hurt. 'I've been there many times. I want to help you through this, because you haven't had many relationships and you're inexperienced. I'm a veteran.'

'Why didn't you say something earlier in the day?' I ask.

'Because of anxiety.'

'Anxiety about what?'

'I was afraid that you'd blow up and create a scene.'

Ah! That perennial fear of being rejected in any way, especially the loud and emotional way. I understand this about him.

'I don't feel I've violated you or betrayed you by starting a sexual relationship with Joan. You and I had an understanding, Carla.'

I feel ragged and soft at the same time as he leans across and kisses me gently on the mouth before I leave to go to my bed and sleep.

All the next day, the pain rankles. Aaron's attention is on his computer — he's finalising important drawings for Clinton. My head won't function, so I lie down on my bed and try to relax, maybe go to sleep. It's not until the staff have gone home that there's time to talk.

We make our way to the verandah, where some doves soon join us, hoping for some free seed. Young as they are, they're forming couples already, chasing away intruders from their pecking place.

Earlier, I happened to pass through the lounge room when a call came through for Aaron from Joan and I overheard some of the conversation.

'When Joan rang to see how you were, did she also ask about me?' I ask him now.

He thinks back to the call. 'No, she didn't.'

'She's keen to know you're alright because she's protecting her property, her new possession. She couldn't care less about what's happening to me.' Bitterness flashes from my eyes in spite of myself.

'Jealous, are we?'

'Yes. No! I'm angry that you can't see this side of her!'

He smiles indulgently, pitying me, and this infuriates me more. I'm falling to pieces now; starting to lose control of what's coming up in me. I'm due to attend a cooking demo tonight, of all times, at Clinton's place. I decide to go, to give myself a break from Aaron's presence, although once there my attention wanders. I can't eat the delicious food and my eyes threaten to close a few times. I end up buying an expensive German cooking gadget that can do so many things at once.

On the way there, in the private space of my car, the tears had started to crowd behind my eyes. On the way back, they come up again more urgently. I tried to encourage them, but still they're kept behind a dam. And then I arrive home again.

'Been crying?' Aaron asks.

'I wish I could!'

'Lie down on your bed,' he orders. He holds his hand over my tummy, but as the tears start to fall, wrenched from the depths, I roll away from him into a foetal position.

The sobs come unchecked now, from that place of sudden, irrevocable loss. Aaron lies quietly behind me, leaving a delicate space between us as he lightly strokes my fingers that are wrapped around my waist. His concern is a comfort to me; also that he doesn't speak. Eventually he gets up and returns with warm rice milk for me.

'Go to sleep now. Don't do anything unnecessary and just go to sleep.'

I do, and sleep until I wake up to the cloudy skies of early Saturday morning.

* * *

Aaron hears me stir and comes to me immediately. 'Move over so I can sit down,' he orders. I lie sideways to face him. He looks me over and suddenly glows as he reminisces. 'Such magnificent hips! I love the way you melt when you're loved!' But his kindly meant words are no consolation.

'I can't take in what you're saying. I feel like flotsam on the surface of the water.'

'You're dying,' is his instant comment. 'You're burning off the old you, so a new person can come out of the ashes.'

A short silence as I ponder this, then he says, 'A cup of tea on the verandah?'

As we sit in the rocking chairs with our tea, Aaron has questions. He wants to clear up what is, to him, a mystery. 'Why did you love me more than you ever did before? What caused that?'

I think his question over for a bit before I know the answer.

'I tried on unconditional love for size, and it suited me! When Isaac came and gave his talk, that boosted the whole process. He was a catalyst for my living with my heart wide open.' And with my eyes closed and blind, I think, but that's another matter.

Wait, there is more to this.

'The other thing is that I seem to be the kind of person who deliberately creates distance in order to appreciate better what I love — loving what you can't have kind of thing. Close up, I notice all the faults. Further away, I recapture the bigger picture, and the passion. When Joan became a threat, my passion grew. That's also what happened.'

Now I want clarification from Aaron about the behaviour I misinterpreted so badly yesterday. 'What were you doing?' I ask.

'I didn't know how to talk to you. I decided to wait until you approached me for sex before I told you about Joan.'

'Oh.'

The pain of that moment comes flooding back. I remember to breathe, all the way down to the bottom of my abdomen, and find myself again.

Aaron wants to share his memories of being abandoned by previous partners. From his body language, I get an inkling of the anguish he has experienced time and time again. 'I couldn't believe that the woman I loved turned into a woman I couldn't love any more because of her hatred and manipulations. One relationship after another ended the same way; that's why, when I met you, I'd been alone for six years. I swore I'd never be with an ego again.

'When I was left alone after a break-up, my mind would go crazy, endlessly going over everything. I looked in all the corners of my mind for the person who had loved me and I could never find her. It sent me crazy to think all those thoughts and not have any resolution. It wouldn't let up, not after a week, months, even a year. I'd think I was alright, and then some little reminder would send me right back there again. A tiny trigger and all was pain again.

'After a series of these experiences of getting nowhere with my mind, I remembered what I'd learnt in therapy. Thoughts aren't real, they don't contain any reality and they're not the truth, that's why they don't have any energy. I tortured myself with memories and with trying to justify my hurt feelings. It was all worse than useless.'

And then Aaron reveals some thoughts that speak to the innermost part of my heart, and for which I know I will be forever grateful.

'My mind had convinced me that I'd lost my love. But I *can't* lose my love. My love is *my* love. I have the ability to love and the choice to love. I allowed myself to realise that I was that love myself. I'm the one that loves, that's what matters. I'm about creating warmth, and receiving and enjoying it from others who want to give it back to me. You are the love that you give, not the love you receive. The love that others give you passes through you, but you are the source of love.'

Aaron at his best. This is the man I want and can never have again.

We take other precious opportunities to talk. 'A relationship is never between two people,' Aaron says. Two people love each other, and they think they are going to stay in love forever. But there are other people that live in them, and their voices talk to them. They tell them what isn't lovable about the other person, and it all starts going downhill from there because the voices are believed and become more important than the love the two people feel for each other.'

Aaron goes on to explain how he thinks the 'voices' come into being.

'A baby comes in from the realm of love, but has to depend on the faces he sees around him in order to create his own self-image. The only information he has about life and himself is what is reflected back to him by the people near him. Every feeling gets registered in there, and not all of them are positive ones. Those are the voices, the people, that live in him as he grows up. When a person becomes wise, he will hear those voices but not give them too much attention. Love is more important. It was more important for me to love you than to judge you for what I didn't like about you.'

For all his deep wisdom, Aaron hasn't been able to still the voice inside himself that constantly belittles him, constantly doubts his self worth, constantly makes him recoil in horror from criticism. That one voice has infiltrated his system at its core, where it's difficult to face because it seems part of his real being. To challenge it would be to break open the most deeply protected thing in him — a tender heart that has been piteously broken many times. This heart has become wise, wise enough to choose love, and yet it lacks the courage to go to the place that feels like total unlove, to discover what's underneath the burden. The voice is too real for him. Somehow he can't betray this voice, which keeps him humble, in his own terms.

'Why is it that you still won't trace some of your voices?' I ask.

'Because it takes pain to make us go down to the core, the kind of pain that's so bad that it's worse not to look than to keep it hidden.'

'You can become aware of a voice,' Aaron says, 'but it's like talking about a weedy plant that floats on top of a pond. You can know a lot about that weed, but until you go down there into the murky depths and pull out its roots ...'

Oh my, yes! Not only that, but down there Aaron is likely to find a demon; the creature that controls him to such a degree that his eyes and ears and his whole body are weakening under its influence. This demon is mortally afraid of the light, and long ago found a safe home in Aaron. When I challenge Aaron about his reactions to the slightest criticism, his eyes grow dark and his face twitches. A shadow comes over it, warning me: *Don't go there, Carla!* Even in our most unthreatening conversations, the merest mention of this characteristic puts him on the defensive. He deflects it by reminding me of my own patterns.

Aaron is basking in his new friendship now, though, and is confident to tell me what he thinks. 'You are beautiful, Carla, but beauty is not enough for me. Joan is like another Aaron.' I notice the animation and joy as he speaks. 'With her, I can be the man I want to be. I need a person like her in my life, to reflect myself back to me. She is a survivor, like me. I'm an opportunist. I gather things from the side of the road. In her own way, she's like me.'

An unfortunate choice of word: *opportunist*.

'Yes, that's something I'm sure she has in common with you,' I say. 'She's an opportunist. In a different way to you, but still an opportunist.'

Aaron either ignores the implication or doesn't notice it. He continues to tell me his thoughts, clasping a fist inside his hand as he talks. He does this when he feels sure of himself.

'Joan may have the same feelings later on as you're going through now, but that's not my concern. The fear of the future won't stop me from the rightness of loving in the moment. She wants to know me, and I want to get to know her. We're good for each other.'

The fear of the future doesn't seem to contain the reality of herpes as yet, for Aaron. Joan is a new broom. It's so nice, of course, to be with a person who shows you only one face: that of loving appreciation.

'Relationship is about learning from one another,' he goes on. 'It's about providing a mirror for the other. It's about seeing in the other what isn't seen yet in the self. You see that, you fall in love with that, you want that for yourself. Sex is a way of touching the other deeply and sharing those energies you admire in each other. It's about waking up what you love in yourself. I have your innocence now. I have grown in truthfulness because of you. Look at my finger and toe, how they're healing. I'm clean with my energies, so I heal fast.'

A new day and, for me, a new insight. God and his angels have done this to me for my benefit. I didn't know how to break off my attachment to Aaron and so went back on my word and on what I knew clearly, time and time again. So the severance had to be done the rough way, a way to ensure it would end. Aaron had sex with another woman while he was my lover. The pain of that was deep enough to shake me out of my mesmerised state. And he may now have herpes. That knowledge is a safety valve that will make us respect our own boundaries.

We have our last discussions.

'I respected your decisions, Carla. I never stood in your way, but you forced me to stand apart from you. I have myself now.'

It's been a great achievement, this surrender.

'I fell in love with the new light that I saw in you, Aaron. It's my turn now to do the same, to choose to accept and respect your decisions, and choose to love instead of getting angry.'

I realise that my whole soul has longed for this growth for him and for myself. Aaron's not really my soul-mate, as I thought; he seems to be my *twin* soul. One soul that came into this world as a man and a woman: as one part heals, so does the other.

'Can I ask you a point-blank question?' Aaron looks serious as he waits for my permission. 'Would you want us to go back to the way things were?'

I hesitate for a few moments, feeling out the truth. Such a welter of conflicting feelings rush in, but the question is actually immaterial. We both moved on because that's the right thing for us to do, and we can't go against that. We both feel a different future pulling us. There were some egos involved in the process, but who cares? As I've said to Aaron a few times, God, or Life, knows how to use anything at all for our growth.

Aaron is still certain that my belief in the vision I had of the end of our relationship eventually created that end. It is a product of my mind's doing, he says.

Even though mind, or ego, has had a part, I know better. 'I've loved you enough to let you go, so you could become more of yourself.'

He listens, but can't hear. And it doesn't matter.

For days, my heart lurches from the extreme pain of wanting the past to the quiet dignity of accepting the present. I can't eat. I go for early morning walks, drinking in the deep friendship that nature provides in the little park nearby. Sometimes I feel as lonely as a forgotten island. And then I remember that we are all alone, and will die alone. And then it's equally true that I am never alone. I'm at the centre of myself, and myself is the Universe. This, I realise, is abundance. I can have it all now that I need and want no more than what is here.

Isaac Shapiro's words come back to me: *Carla, stay with yourself.*

I will take the opportunity of the pain of this separation to be completely with myself again and learn to never, ever, leave myself. I have myself at my deepest core, where unreasonable happiness wells up eternally. This is how another man will find me — already happy, but ready to share myself in another round of self-discovery.

I, too, feel a future pulling at me. I will be adored once more by someone who can share my vision and whom I can support in our mutual quest for freedom. For freedom never ends. Growth never ends. Joy never ends, and neither does love.

AARON

The beloved of my soul,
Beloved of my heart,
Beloved by my body,
Beloved by Life itself.

Even if Life brought us bodily together for a time that was not to be
forever,
It was a very good time that should not be underestimated or
forgotten.

And you were fun,
You were tender,
You were so present and intimate.
You were passionate
And oh, so appreciative,
Not short of using honey words and words of deep truth to express
what you felt.

I am thankful to have had your precious and unique self in my life.
You have drawn out the best in me.

You have done more than that and educated me in the way of being
   just myself
Just as you were being yourself.

I can never forget you and what you have been to me.
I will miss you terribly and be left with images filled with light and
   gratitude.

I thank you for the many jobs you did for me; the many ways you
   made my life easier.
For teaching me computer skills, for fixing my car door, the garage door,
   the handle in the bathroom, to mention only a very few things.

Thanks for being my companion and showing such different aspects
   of life,
Especially your house and your collection of recyclable things
And your interest in all things stellar, extra-terrestrial and celestial.
And your phenomenal memory re the earth and how it is made and
   wars and how they were fought, and who fought who and why. It
   has been such a wondrous show of how many facts the mind can
   hold all at once and what the emotions can be so engaged in.

Thank you for the purity of your soul — it shines brightly and sweetly.
Thank you for not getting very angry for me, or not for long.
For your patience and persistence, and for letting me go when the
   time was right.

I'm not good at sharing myself when it's time to distance myself
   from you.

I hope my heart's words can speak to you.

All my love forever,
Your Carla

ACKNOWLEDGEMENTS

Thank you to Margot Wiburd, DeVere Mining Technologies' valued copywriter and secretary, who waded through my original writings and completed this book's very first edit. Since all had been based on journal notes, this was an especially difficult task.

I want to thank the staff from every department at HarperCollins for their friendly dealings with me. It makes such a difference when there is cordiality as well as professionalism.

I was fortunate to have Nicola O'Shea work with me again for the official edit. Her phenomenal skills to appropriately cut and slash found a good outlet in this manuscript! Nicola handed over to Anne Reilly, who stayed with me during the processes of further numerous smaller changes, gaining permissions for the quotes I used, and helping me gain a usable perspective regarding some restrictive legal proprieties which curtailed parts of this story.

Of course I owe a great deal of thanks to Aaron, who never wavered in his generous agreement to have his life exposed along with mine. He has courage! We have both moved on since this story was written, but will never move away from the friendship we share.

My first book, *God's Callgirl*, elicited thousands of emails from readers. I take this opportunity to thank you, readers, for your deep appreciation, and hope that this sequel will touch you in a similar way.

For those who want to contact me, there is a way via my website, www.carlavanraay.com

May our spirits touch across the pages of this book.

NOTES ON QUOTATIONS

p. vi, Nirmala (Daniel Erway), *Gifts With No Giver, A Love Affair With Truth*, Endless Satsang Press, Sedona, 1999, p. 16. Nirmala is an Advaita spiritual teacher.

p. 1, *Love Poems from God: Twelve Sacred Voices from the East and West*, Daniel Ladinsky (trans.), Penguin Compass, New York, 2002. All Daniel Ladinsky's poems are copyright and are used with his permission. Chuang Tzu (*c.* 370–301 BCE) is thought to be the author of the classic Taoist text, *Chuang Tzu*.

p. 7, *Love Poems from God (op. cit.)*. St Teresa of Avila (1515–82) was a prominent Spanish mystic and nun.

p. 13, Barbara Barton, *Light From The Universal Mind*, Universal Press, Sydney 1999, p. 75.

p. 15, Leo Buscaglia, *Love, What Life Is All About* …, A Fawcett Crest Book, New York, 1972, p. 111.

p. 22, *Love Poems from God (op. cit.)*. St John of the Cross (1542–91) was a Spanish mystic and Carmelite friar.

p. 26, *Love Poems from God (op. cit.)*. St Catherine of Siena (1347–80) was an Italian mystic who devoted her life to God.

p. 32, Ram Tzu (Wayne Liquorman), *No Way*, Advaita Press, Redondo Beach, 1990, p. 56. Ram Tzu, of California, is a speaker on Advaita spiritual matters.

p. 40, *ibid.*, p. 60.

p. 46, *Love Poems from God (op. cit.)*. Meister Eckhart (1260–1328) was a German-born Dominican monk, scholar and mystic.

p. 52, *Love Poems from God (op. cit.)*. Tukaram (*c.* late 16th century–1650) was an Indian saint and poet.

p. 71, DH Lawrence, *Birds, Beasts and Flowers: Poems*, Martin Secker, London, 1923. Lawrence (1885–1930) was a controversial English writer.

p. 77, *Love Poems from God (op. cit.)*. St Thomas Aquinas (*c.* 1225–74) was an Italian Catholic priest and theologian.

p. 83, Nirmala, *op. cit.*, p. 28.

p. 92, *ibid.*, p. 9.

p. 105, *ibid.*, p. 25.

p. 110, Adyashanti, *Emptiness Dancing*, Sounds True, Inc., Boulder, 2004. Adyashanti, of Northern California, is a teacher of non-dual spirituality.

p. 118, Marianne Williamson, *A Return to Love*, HarperCollins, New York, 2003. This resonant phrase has been quoted by many people, including Nelson Mandela.

p. 126, Robert Rabbin, *Echoes of Silence: Awakening the Meditative Spirit*, Inner Directions Publishing, 2000, p. 12. Robert is an author and teacher of public speaking with a lifelong interest in mysticism and spirituality: www.realtimespeaking

p. 132, *ibid.*, p. 73.

p. 143, Nirmala, *op. cit.*, p. 35.

p. 150, Galway Kinnell, 'Oatmeal', *Risking Everything: 110 Poems of Love and Revelation*, ed. Roger Housden, Harmony Books, New York, 2003, p. 93.

p. 167, Robert Rabbin, *op. cit.*, p. 41.

p. 178, *The Subject Tonight Is Love*, Daniel Ladinsky (trans.), Penguin Compass, New York, 2003, p. 24. Hafiz of Shiraz (Khwaja Shams ud-Din Hafiz-i Shirazi, 1326–90), one of the great Sufi poets, was born in Persia (modern Iran).

p. 185, *ibid.*, p. 47.

p. 190, William Shakespeare, *Twelfth Night*, act 1, scene 1, lines 1–3, Duke Orsino.

p. 201, Robert Rabbin, *op. cit.*, p. 55.

p. 207, Byron Katie, of The Work Foundation, is a wonderful Californian healer and practitioner of spiritual inquiry whom the author met and studied with in Amsterdam.

p. 241, Nirmala, *op. cit.,* p. 51.

p. 257, Simon Gladdish, *Images of Istanbul*, Gladpress, Swansea, 1997, p. 50.

p. 262, Nirmala, *op. cit.,* p. 48.

p. 268, René Descartes (1596–1650) was a French scientist, philosopher and writer.

p. 276, *Love Poems from God (op. cit.)*. Kabir was a 15th-century Indian saint and straight-talking mystical poet.

p. 284, *Speaking of Life: A Rare Collection of Wisdom, Humour and Inspiration*, Peter Stafford (ed.), Omniread, Fremantle, 1998, p. 187. Ralph Waldo Emerson (1803–82) was a North American philosopher, writer and public speaker.

p. 290, *The Selected Poems of Rainer Maria Rilke*, Robert Bly (trans.), HarperPerennial, London 1981. Rainer Maria Rilke (1875–1926) was born in Prague (then Bohemia, now part of the Czech Republic) and is regarded as one of the greatest German-language poets of the 20th century.

p. 297, Nirmala, *op. cit.*, p. 25.

p. 307, *ibid.*, p. 80.

p. 315, *ibid.*, p. 86.

p. 326, Barbara Barton, *op. cit.*, p. 27.

p. 338, Nirmala, *op. cit.*, p. 32.

p. 348, DH Lawrence, *op. cit.*

p. 357, Neale Donald Walsch, *Conversations with God: An Uncommon Dialogue (Book 2)*, Hampton Roads Publishing Company Inc., Charlottesville, 1997, p. 235.

p. 364, Simon Gladdish, *op. cit.*, p. 11.

p. 370, Barbara Barton, *op. cit.*, p. 42.